ADVANCES IN VETERINARY SCIENCE AND COMPARATIVE MEDICINE

VOLUME 29

ADVISORY BOARD

W. I. B. Beveridge
J. H. Gillespie
W. R. Hinshaw

C. E. Hopla
Norman D. Levine
C. A. Mitchell

W. R. Pritchard

CONTRIBUTORS TO THIS VOLUME

Shehu U. Abdullahi
Chris W. Clinton
Robert A. Crandell
Donald P. Griffith
Dwight C. Hirsh

Joel R. Leininger
Carl A. Osborne
David J. Polzin
J. M. Rutter
Saul Tzipori

ADVANCES IN VETERINARY SCIENCE AND COMPARATIVE MEDICINE

Edited by

CHARLES E. CORNELIUS
California Primate Research Center
University of California
Davis, California

CHARLES F. SIMPSON
Department of Preventive Medicine
College of Veterinary Medicine
University of Florida
Gainesville, Florida

Volume 29

1985

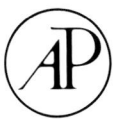

ACADEMIC PRESS, INC.
Harcourt Brace Jovanovich, Publishers

Orlando   San Diego   New York
Austin   London   Montreal   Sydney   Tokyo   Toronto

COPYRIGHT © 1985 BY ACADEMIC PRESS, INC.
ALL RIGHTS RESERVED.
NO PART OF THIS PUBLICATION MAY BE REPRODUCED OR
TRANSMITTED IN ANY FORM OR BY ANY MEANS, ELECTRONIC
OR MECHANICAL, INCLUDING PHOTOCOPY, RECORDING, OR
ANY INFORMATION STORAGE AND RETRIEVAL SYSTEM, WITHOUT
PERMISSION IN WRITING FROM THE PUBLISHER.

ACADEMIC PRESS, INC.
Orlando, Florida 32887

United Kingdom Edition published by
ACADEMIC PRESS INC. (LONDON) LTD.
24–28 Oval Road, London NW1 7DX

LIBRARY OF CONGRESS CATALOG CARD NUMBER: 53–7098

ISBN 0-12-039229-1

PRINTED IN THE UNITED STATES OF AMERICA

85 86 87 88   9 8 7 6 5 4 3 2 1

CONTENTS

CONTRIBUTORS vii
PREFACE ix

Struvite Urolithiasis in Animals and Man: Formation, Detection, and Dissolution

CARL A. OSBORNE, DAVID J. POLZIN, SHEHU U. ABDULLAHI, JOEL R. LEININGER, CHRIS W. CLINTON, AND DONALD P. GRIFFITH

I.	Introduction	2
II.	Terminology	2
III.	Chemical and Physical Characteristics of Uroliths	6
IV.	Etiopathogenesis	18
V.	Struvite Urolithiasis	27
	References	95

The Relative Importance of Enteric Pathogens Affecting Neonates of Domestic Animals

SAUL TZIPORI

I.	Introduction	104
II.	Rotaviruses	105
III.	Enterotoxigenic *E. coli* (ETEC)	125
IV.	*Cryptosporidium*	158
V.	*Clostridium perfringens* Type C	168
VI.	Calf Diarrhea	172
VII.	Piglet Enteritis	179
VIII.	Diarrhea in Foals	186
IX.	Concluding Remarks	192
	References	193

Fimbriae: Relation of Intestinal Bacteria and Virulence in Animals

DWIGHT C. HIRSH

I.	Introduction	207
II.	The Bacterial Cell Surface	210

III.	The Epithelial Cell Surface	226
IV.	Fimbriae in the Clinical Setting (A Summary Statement)	228
	References	231

Atrophic Rhinitis in Swine
J. M. RUTTER

I.	Introduction	240
II.	Occurrence and Importance	242
III.	Clinical and Pathological Features	244
IV.	Etiology	246
V.	Pathogenesis	249
VI.	Epidemiology	259
VII.	Diagnosis	262
VIII.	Control	266
IX.	Immunity and Vaccination	268
X.	Conclusions	274
	References	275

Selected Animal Herpesviruses: New Concepts and Technologies
ROBERT A. CRANDELL

I.	Introduction	281
II.	Equine Rhinopneumonitis	283
III.	Pseudorabies (Aujeszky's Disease, Mad Itch)	295
	References	319

INDEX ... 329

CONTRIBUTORS

Numbers in parentheses indicate the pages on which the authors' contributions begin.

SHEHU U. ABDULLAHI, Department of Veterinary Surgery and Medicine, Faculty of Veterinary Medicine, Ahmadu Bello University, Zaria, Nigeria (1)

CHRIS W. CLINTON, Urolithiasis Laboratory, Department of Urology, Baylor College of Medicine, Houston, Texas 77030 (1)

ROBERT A. CRANDELL, Texas Veterinary Medical Diagnostic Laboratory, College Station, Texas 77841 (281)

DONALD P. GRIFFITH, Department of Urology, Baylor College of Medicine, Houston, Texas 77030 (1)

DWIGHT C. HIRSH, School of Veterinary Medicine, University of California, Davis, California 95616 (207)

JOEL R. LEININGER, Department of Veterinary Pathobiology, College of Veterinary Medicine, University of Minnesota, St. Paul, Minnesota 55108 (1)

CARL A. OSBORNE, Department of Small Animal Clinical Sciences, College of Veterinary Medicine, University of Minnesota, St. Paul, Minnesota 55108 (1)

DAVID J. POLZIN, Department of Small Animal Clinical Sciences, College of Veterinary Medicine, University of Minnesota, St. Paul, Minnesota 55108 (1)

J. M. RUTTER, Agricultural and Food Research Council, Institute for Research on Animal Diseases, Compton, Newbury, Berkshire RG16 0NN, England (239)

SAUL TZIPORI,[1] Attwood Institute for Veterinary Research, Department of Agriculture, Westmeadows 3047, Victoria, Australia (103)

---

[1]Present address: Microbiology Department, Royal Childrens Hospital, Parkville, Victoria 3052, Australia.

PREFACE

This volume of *Advances in Veterinary Science and Comparative Medicine* contains articles evaluating the latest information known about certain important diseases or abnormal conditions of animals.

The article on urolithiasis in cats and dogs is a summary of all the published and unpublished information known about the etiology, diagnosis, and medical dissolution of struvite uroliths in dogs and cats.

The article on enteric pathogens affecting neonates of domestic animals is a current and comprehensive account of data that has been published on this topic since 1980.

The relationship of fimbriae to the virulence of intestinal bacteria is discussed in the third article. The chemical and morphologic characteristics of fimbriae also are identified.

The article on atrophic rhinitis in swine details the important facts known about this complex disease, which is worldwide in distribution.

Two herpesvirus diseases, pseudorabies and rhinopneumonitis, are worldwide in occurrence. New concepts and technologies that relate to the epizootiology, diagnosis, prevention, and control of these two viral diseases are discussed in the final article.

C. E. CORNELIUS
C. F. SIMPSON

Struvite Urolithiasis in Animals and Man: Formation, Detection, and Dissolution

CARL A. OSBORNE,* DAVID J. POLZIN,*
SHEHU U. ABDULLAHI,† JOEL R. LEININGER,‡
CHRIS W. CLINTON,§ AND DONALD P. GRIFFITH**

*Department of Small Animal Clinical Sciences, College of Veterinary Medicine, University of Minnesota, St. Paul, Minnesota, †Department of Veterinary Surgery and Medicine, Faculty of Veterinary Medicine, Ahmadu Bello University, Zaria, Nigeria, ‡Department of Veterinary Pathobiology, College of Veterinary Medicine, University of Minnesota, St. Paul, Minnesota, §Urolithiasis Laboratory, Department of Urology, Baylor College of Medicine, Houston, Texas, and **Department of Urology, Baylor College of Medicine, Houston, Texas*

I.	Introduction	2
II.	Terminology	2
	A. Uroliths and Crystalluria	2
	B. Urolithiasis	3
	C. Names of Uroliths	3
III.	Chemical and Physical Characteristics of Uroliths	6
	A. Overview	6
	B. Mineral Composition	7
	C. Matrix Composition	10
	D. Nuclei and Laminations	15
IV.	Etiopathogenesis	18
	A. Overview	18
	B. Initiation and Growth	19
	C. Summary of Urolith Formation	27
V.	Struvite Urolithiasis	27
	A. Mineral Composition of Struvite Uroliths	27
	B. Matrix Composition of Struvite Uroliths	30
	C. Composition of Matrix Concretions	33
	D. Bacterial Urinary Tract Infections	34
	E. Ureaplasma Urinary Tract Infections	41
	F. Diet	42
	G. Alkaline Urine	45

H.	Genetics	45
I.	Feline Urethral Plugs versus Feline Struvite Uroliths	46
J.	Biological Behavior of Uroliths	52
K.	Diagnosis	57
L.	Medical Management of Struvite Urolithiasis	67
M.	Medical versus Surgical Management	93
	References	95

I. Introduction

For centuries, removal of uroliths from man and animals has been the province of the surgeon. The lifespan of stones formed within the urinary tract has been likened to that of stones in nature formed from quartz, granite, and other minerals and found in fields, along mountains, and under oceans. Most thought that, like stones in nature, uroliths required long periods of time to form and, therefore, would require long periods to dissolve. Surgical removal was deemed the only feasible treatment.

After observing spontaneous dissolution of a struvite nephrolith in a dog in the early 1970s, serious consideration was given to the notion that uroliths might be effectively dissolved by medical rather than by surgical maneuvers. Since that time, development of highly effective and economically feasible noninvasive protocols designed to dissolve struvite uroliths in dogs and cats has become a reality.

The objective of this discussion is to provide an overview of current progress related to the etiology, diagnosis, and medical dissolution of struvite uroliths in dogs and cats. This information may have application to medical dissolution of struvite in man, cattle, sheep, and other species of animals. It is apparent that surgical removal of uroliths may some day become of historical interest.

II. Terminology

A. Uroliths and Crystalluria

In the past, confusion has occurred as a result of various terms used to describe precipitates that form in urine. Depending on the size and consistency of the precipitates, they have been referred to as crystals, sand, sabulous plugs, gravel, pebbles, stones, rocks, uroliths, and/or calculi.

The word crystal is derived from the Greek word "krystallosus," which means "ice," and is used to refer to the solid phase of substances having a specific internal structure and enclosed by symmetrically arranged planar surfaces. The term sabulous is derived from the Latin word "sabulosus" meaning "sand." The Latin word "calculus" means pebble. The Greek word "lithos" means "stone." "_____ uria" is a suffix derived from a Greek word (ouron) meaning "urine." The preferred terminology for abnormal microscopic precipitates in urine is crystalluria, while macroscopic concretions are called uroliths.

B. Urolithiasis

The urinary system is designed to dispose of body wastes in liquid form. However, some waste products are sparingly soluble and occasionally precipitate out of solution.

Urolithiasis may be conceptually defined as the formation of uroliths as a result of multiple congenital and/or acquired pathophysiologic processes that result in increased concentrations of less soluble crystalloids in urine. If the crystals become trapped in the urinary system, they may grow to such size that they cause or contribute to clinical signs. Urolithiasis should not be conceived of as a single disease, but rather as a sequela of one or more underlying abnormalities.

C. Names of Uroliths

Uroliths may be named according to mineral composition (Table I), location (nephroliths, Fig. 1; renoliths, ureteroliths, Fig. 2; cystoliths, Fig. 3; vesical calculi, urethroliths, Fig. 4), or shape (smooth, Fig. 5; faceted, pyramidal, Figs. 3 and 6; laminated, Fig. 7; mulberry, jackstone, Fig. 8; staghorn or branched, Fig. 9; urethral plugs, Figs. 10 and 11).

A mineral is a naturally occurring, inorganically formed substance which has a characteristic chemical composition, and usually has an ordered atomic arrangement which may influence its external geometric form. Minerals commonly found in uroliths often have a chemical name and a crystal (or mineral) name (Table I) (Mitchell, 1979). Magnesium ammonium phosphate hexahydrate is commonly called struvite. The name struvite was coined in 1845 by Ulex, a Swedish geologist, in honor of H. C. G. von Struve (1772–1851), a Russian

TABLE I

GLOSSARY OF SOME CRYSTALLINE SUBSTANCES THAT MAY BE DETECTED IN UROLITHS

Chemical name	Crystal name	Formula
Oxalates		
Calcium oxalate monohydrate	Whewellite	$CaC_2O_4 \cdot H_2O$
Calcium oxalate dihydrate	Weddellite	$CaC_2O_4 \cdot 2H_2O$
Phosphates		
β-Tricalcium phosphate (calcium orthophosphate)	Whitlockite	$\beta Ca_3(PO_4)_2$
Carbonate-apatite	Same	$Ca_{10}(PO_4CO_3OH)_6(OH)_2$
Calcium hydrogen phosphate dihydrate	Brushite	$CaHPO_4 \cdot 2H_2O$
Calcium phosphate	Hydroxyapatite or calcium apatite	$Ca_{10}(PO_4)_6(OH)_2$
Magnesium ammonium phosphate hexahydrate	Struvite	$MgNH_4PO_4 \cdot 6H_2O$
Magnesium hydrogen phosphate trihydrate	Newberyite	$MgHPO_4 \cdot 3H_2O$
Uric acid and urates		
Anhydrous uric acid	Same	$C_5H_4N_4O_3$
Uric acid dihydrate	Same	$C_5H_4N_4O_3 \cdot 2H_2O$
Ammonium acid urate	Same	$C_5H_3N_4O_3NH_4$
Sodium acid urate monohydrate	Same	$C_5H_3N_4O_3Na \cdot H_2O$
Cystine	Same	$(SCH_2CHNH_2COOH)_2$
Silicon dioxide	Same	SiO_2
Xanthine	Same	$C_5H_4N_4O_2$

diplomate and naturalist. Prior to that time, magnesium ammonium phosphate was sometimes referred to as "guanite" because the mineral was detected in bat guano (Polache et al., 1951). Magnesium hydrogen phosphate trihydrate is sometimes called newberyite in honor of James Cosmo Newbery (1843–1895), an Australian geologist. Apatite is derived from the Greek word "apate" meaning "deceit," and was used to name calcium phosphate-containing minerals because they were often mistakenly identified as other minerals. Calcium hydrogen phosphate dihydrate was named brushite after George James Brush (1831–1912), an American mineralogist. β-Tricalcium phosphate (calcium orthophosphate) was called whitlockite in honor of Herbert P. Whitlock, a twentieth century mineralogist. Calcium oxalate dihydrate is commonly called weddellite because it was observed in ocean floor samples obtained from the Weddell sea in Antartica. Calcium oxalate monohydrate was named whewellite in honor of an English mineralogist named William Whewell (1794–1866).

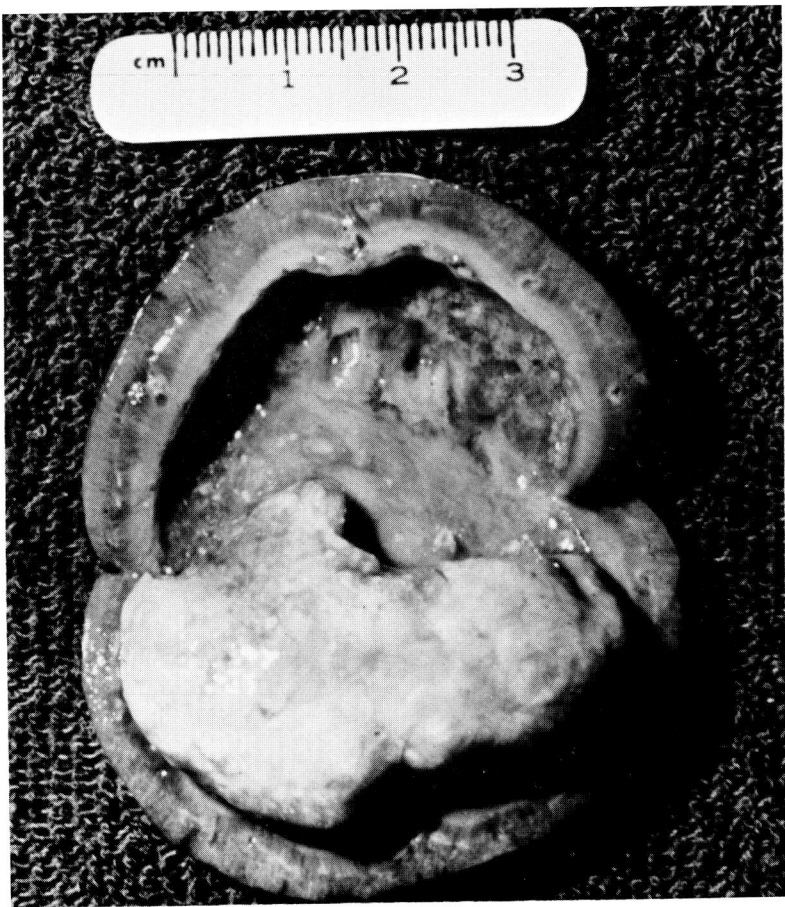

FIG. 1. Infection-induced struvite nephrolith located in the left kidney of a 5-year-old female miniature schnauzer. The urolith has obstructed urine outflow through the ureter and caused severe hydronephrosis. Severe pyelonephritis caused by urease-producing staphylococci affects remaining portions of the renal parenchyma.

Characteristic shapes of crystals and uroliths are influenced primarily by the internal structure of crystals and the environment in which they form (Hinman, 1979). Crystals of calcium oxalate monohydrate tend to fuse, producing smoothly rounded or mammillated uroliths. Crystals of calcium oxalate dihydrate typically appear as sharp spiculated structures. Amorphous silica commonly produces stones that resemble small six-pronged metal pieces used in the children's game of jacks (thus the name jackstone) (Fig. 8). Local factors that influence the size and shape of uroliths include (1) number of

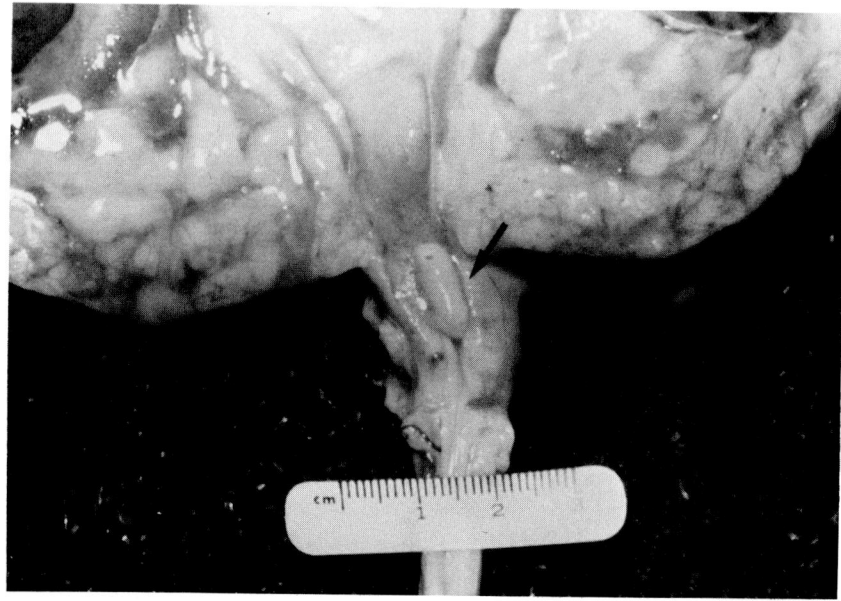

FIG. 2. Ureterolith (arrow) lodged in the proximal lumen of the left ureter of a 4-year-old female malamute. Most of the renal parenchyma has been destroyed by obstruction to urine outflow and a secondary urinary tract infection with urease-producing *Proteus mirabilis*.

uroliths present, (2) mobility or fixation of uroliths, (3) flow characteristics of urine, and (4) anatomical configuration of the structure in which uroliths grow.

III. Chemical and Physical Characteristics of Uroliths

A. Overview

Uroliths are polycrystalline concretions composed primarily of organic or inorganic crystalloids and smaller quantities of organic matrix. They may also contain a number of minor constituents. A variety of different types of uroliths may occur in dogs, cats, and man. Uroliths are not disorganized precipitates of crystalline material, but typically are composed of organized crystal aggregates with a complex internal structure. Such organization implies a definite cause, and argues against their formation by random precipitation. Cross sections of uroliths frequently reveal nuclei and laminations, and less frequently

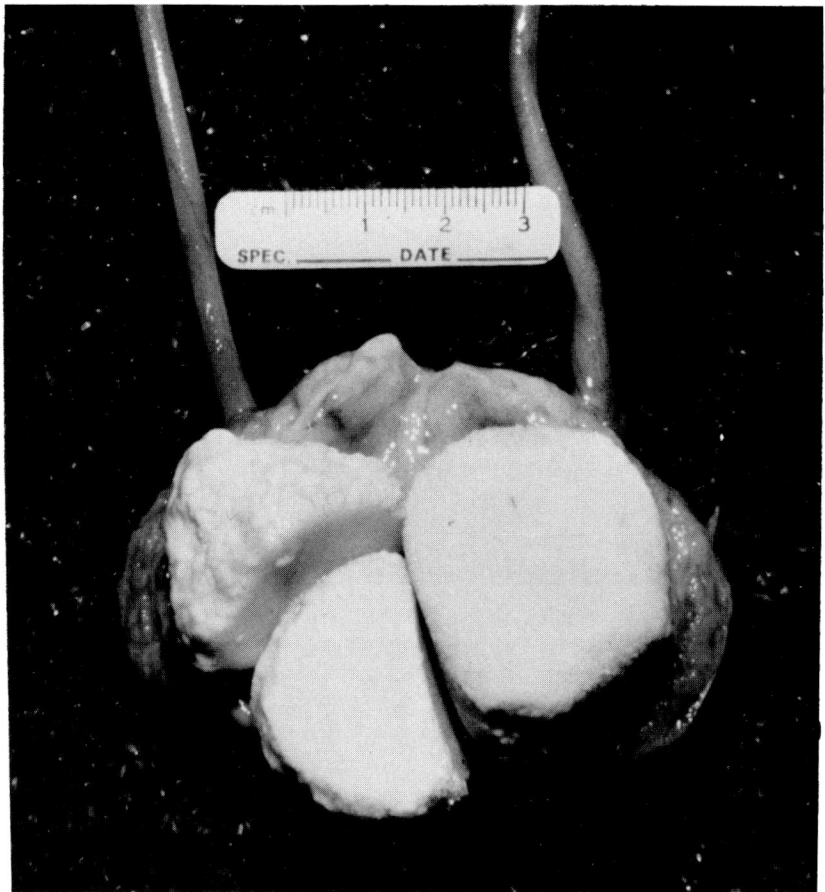

Fig. 3. Pyramidal-shaped urocystoliths associated with a concomitant staphylococcal urinary tract infection in an adult female beagle dog.

reveal radical striations (Fig. 7). The fact that urine that bathes calculi varies in composition (and probably in degree of saturation with calculogenic crystalloids) from day to day, and perhaps from hour to hour, is of conceptual importance in trying to understand the physical characteristics of uroliths.

B. Mineral Composition

Much of the current information pertaining to the physical and chemical characteristics of uroliths is related to their mineral composi-

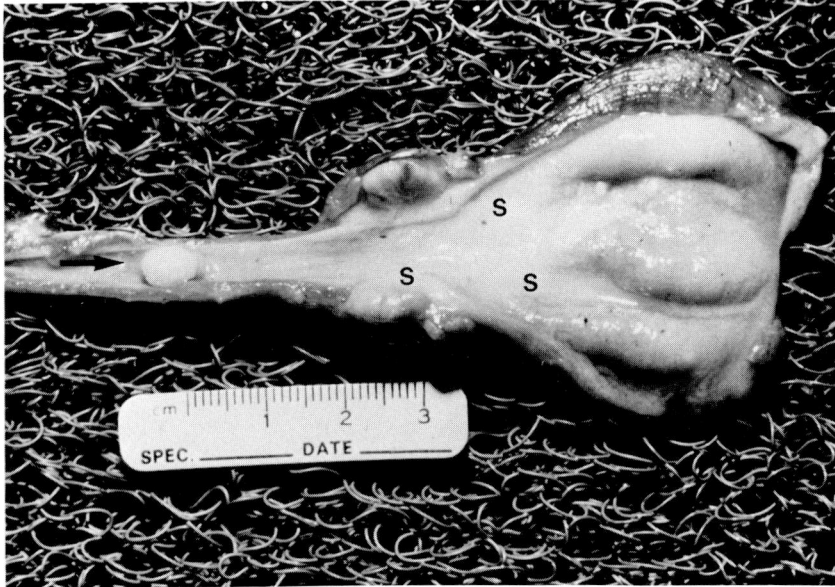

FIG. 4. Struvite urethrolith (large arrow) and large quantities of "sand" (s) induced in the lower urinary tract of an adult male miniature schnauzer by experimental induction of a staphylococcal urinary tract infection.

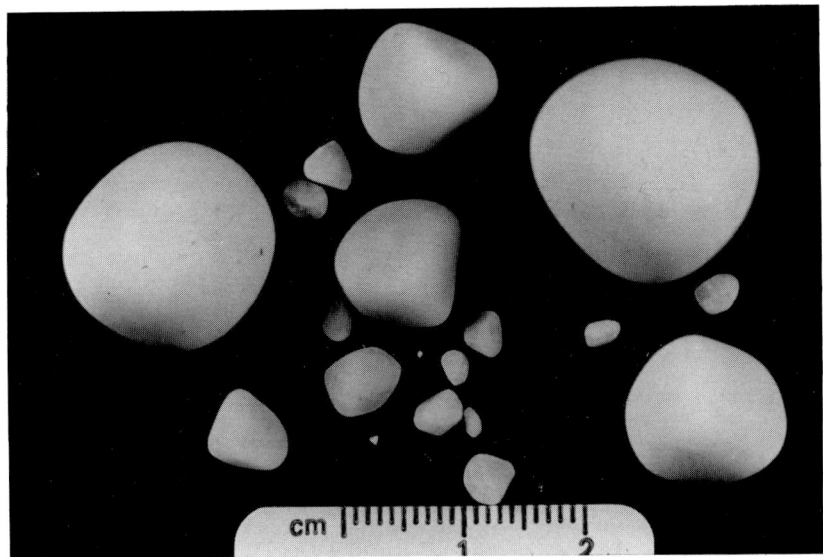

FIG. 5. Multiple smooth uroliths composed of 100% magnesium ammonium phosphate and removed from the urinary bladder of a 12-year-old female dachshund.

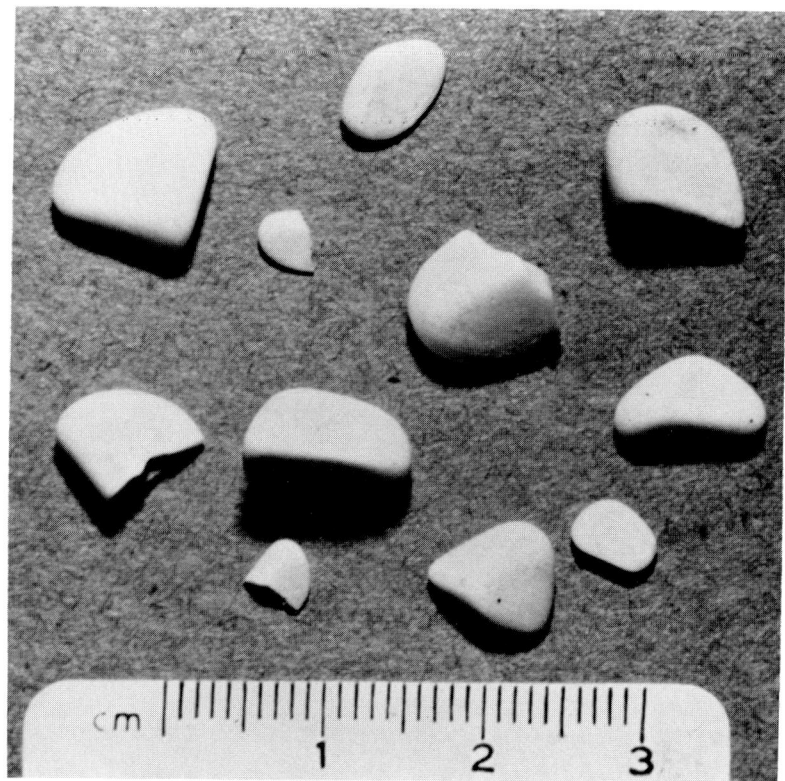

Fig. 6. Multiple struvite uroliths voided from the bladder through the urethra of a 2-year-old female miniature schnauzer with a staphylococcal urinary tract infection.

tion. In fact, it has been suggested that the structure and appearance of calculi are primarily dependent on their mineral composition.

The most common mineral type of calculi encountered in dogs and cats is magnesium ammonium phosphate. Ammonium acid urate, uric acid, calcium phosphate, and calcium oxalate (monohydrate and dihydrate) occur much less frequently. In contrast, calcium-containing uroliths (calcium oxalate and calcium phosphate) are most prevalent in humans living in developed countries of the world (Tables II, III, and IV). Trace elements, including iron, copper, zinc, tin, lead, and aluminum, have been identified in human uroliths (Meyer and Angino, 1977). They may also occur in feline uroliths. These elements appear to be incorporated into calculi by adsorption during growth; they do not appear to play an important role in initation or growth of calculi.

Knowledge of the actual frequency with which various types of min-

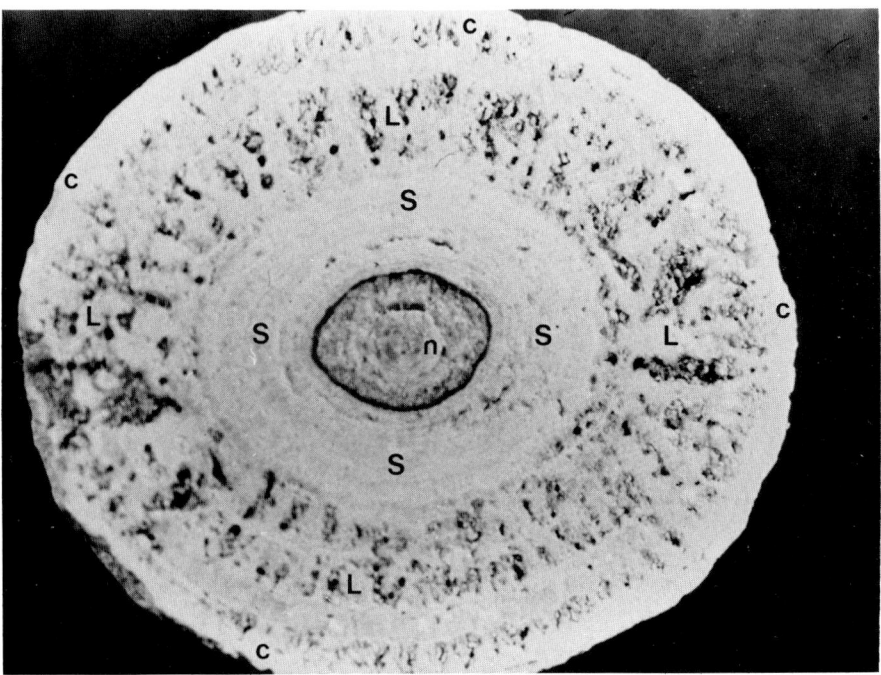

Fig. 7. Laminated urolith removed from the urinary bladder of a 2-year-old spayed Bichon Frise dog. The nidus (n) was composed of 10% calcium apatite, 15% ammonium acid urate, and 75% struvite. The stone (s) was composed of 15% calcium apatite and 85% struvite. The shell (L) was composed of 75% calcium apatite and 25% struvite. The surface crystals (c) were composed of 75% calcium apatite and 25% struvite.

erals and metabolites occur in uroliths of dogs and cats has been severely hampered by widespread use of relatively insensitive qualitative methods of urolith analysis. However, it appears that, even though a particular mineral usually predominates, the mineral composition of many uroliths may be mixed (Tables III and IV). On occasion, the center of a urolith may be composed of one type of crystalloid (for example, silica), whereas outer layers are composed of a different crystalloid (especially struvite) (Fig. 12). The detection, treatment, and/or prevention of the causes underlying urolithiasis are dependent on knowledge of the composition and structure of all portions of uroliths.

C. Matrix Composition

1. Uroliths

The nondialyzable portion of calculi that remains after crystalline components have been dissolved with mild solvents is organic matrix.

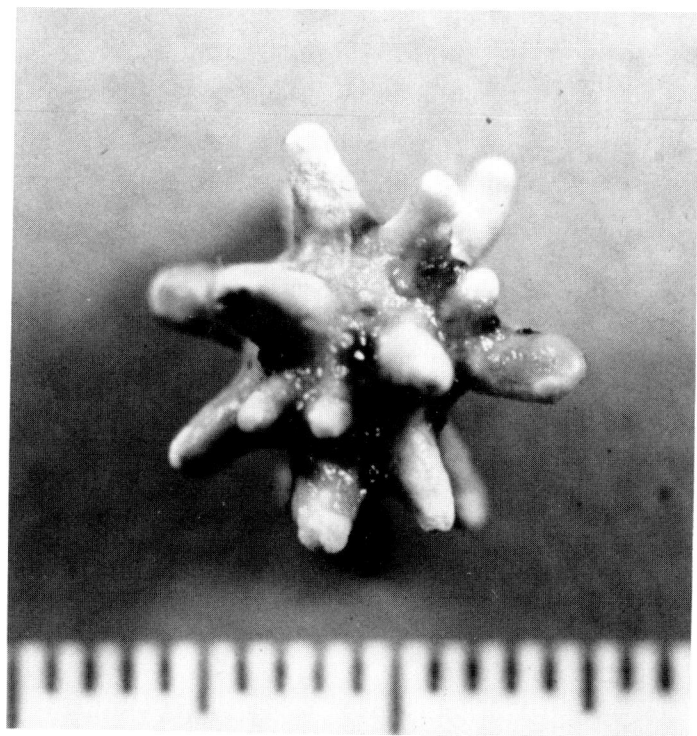

Fig. 8. Jackstone removed from the urinary bladder of a 7-year-old male Yorkshire terrier. The urolith was composed of 100% amorphous silica. Attempts to induce dissolution with a calculolytic diet were unsuccessful. (Scale is marked in millimeters.)

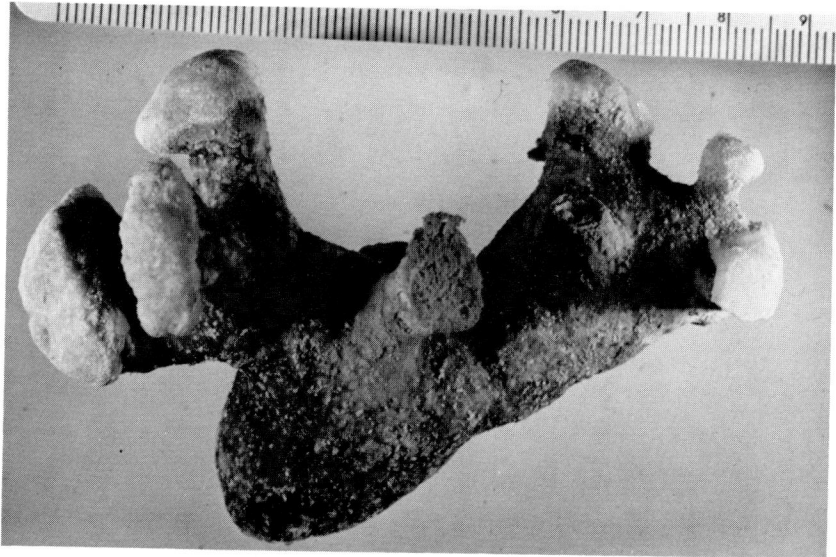

Fig. 9. Staghorn struvite urolith removed from the kidney of an adult human.

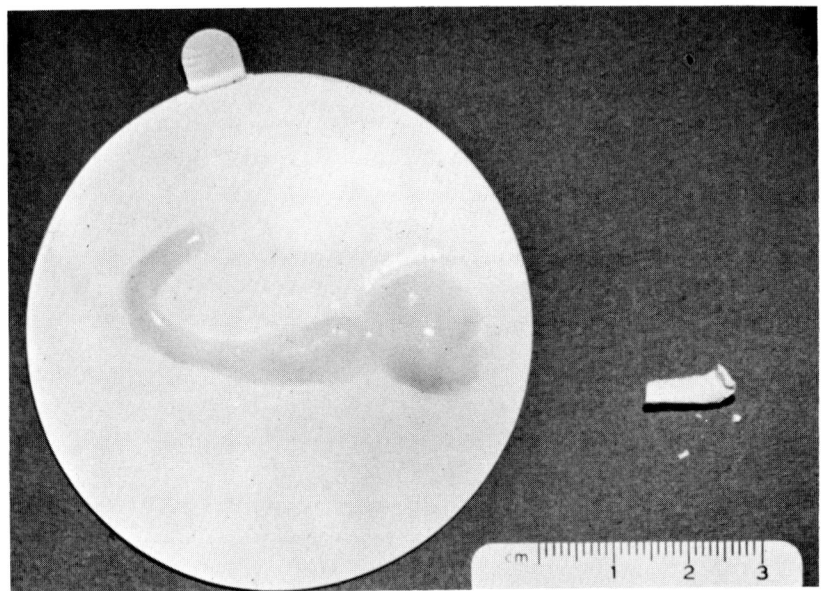

Fig. 10. Urethral plug composed of a large quantity of matrix and struvite removed from the urethra of a 6-year-old male dachshund. The portion of the urolith to the right has been allowed to dry.

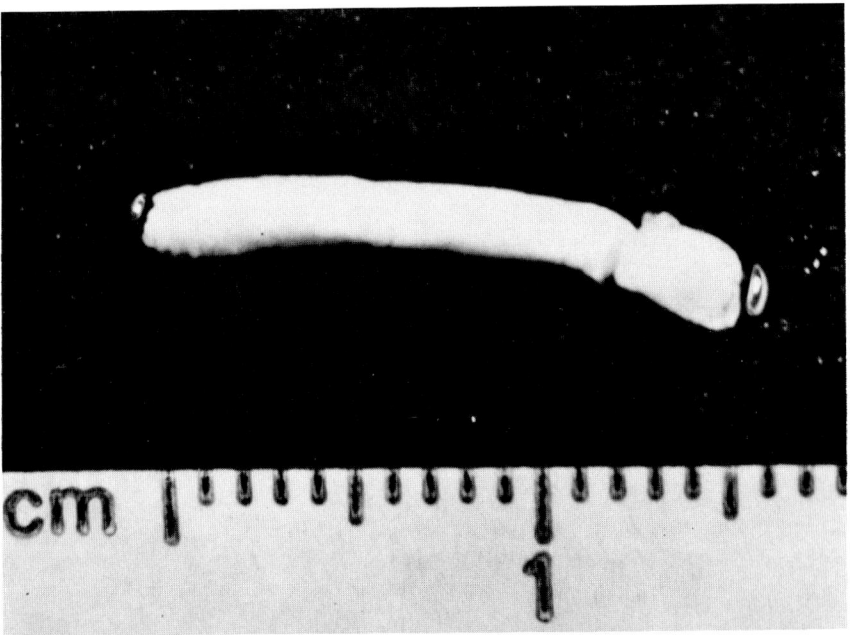

Fig. 11. Urethral plug removed from a 3-year-old castrated male domestic shorthair cat. The mineral composition of the plug consisted of 100% magnesium ammonium phosphate. (From *J. Am. Anim. Hosp. Assoc.* 1984, **20**, 17–32.)

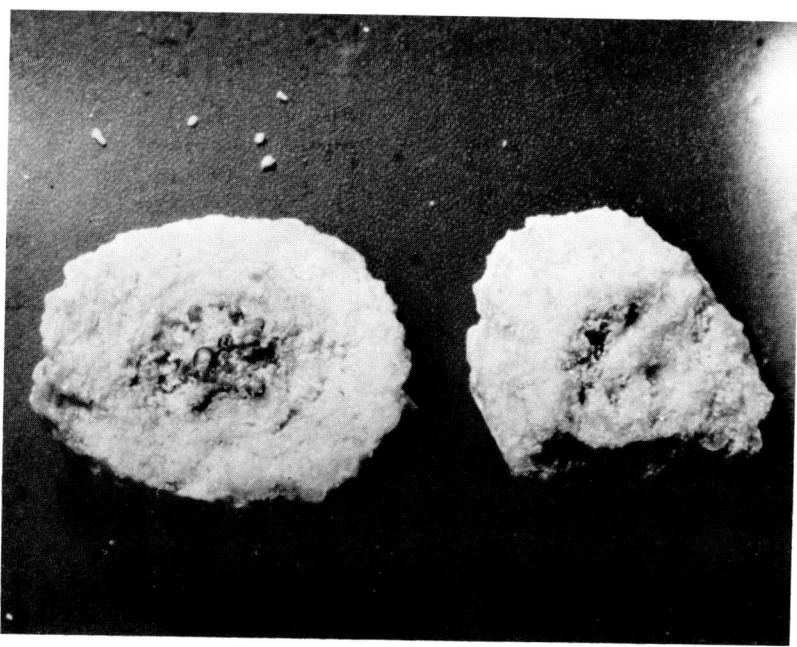

FIG. 12. Urocystolith removed from a 13-year-old male poodle. Note the jackstone composed of silica in the center of the urolith. The shell was composed of 75% struvite and 25% calcium apatite (Courtesy of Dr. D. G. Low, University of California, Davis, California.)

Calculi consistently contain variable quantities of organic matrix substances in addition to crystalloids (Boyce and Garvey, 1956; Cornelius and Bishop, 1961; Malek and Boyce, 1977; Pak, 1976; Spector *et al.*, 1976). Organic matrix substances identified in human uroliths and experimentally produced in animals include matrix substance A, Tamm-Horsfall mucoprotein, uromucoid, serum albumin, and α- and γ-globulins (Wickham, 1976). Of these, matrix substance A, Tamm-Horsfall mucoprotein, and uromucoid appear to be quantitatively more significant than α- and γ-globulins (Sutor *et al.*, 1978).

The macromolecular complexes of diverse mucoprotein compounds comprising matrix substances have been hypothesized by some to represent the skeleton of calculi. Although the physical characteristics of uroliths suggest an organized relationship between the matrix skeleton and crystalline building blocks, the role of each of these components in formation, retention, and growth of calculi is poorly understood. *In vitro* studies utilizing human urine revealed that Tamm-Horsfall protein is related to the formation of calcium oxalate crystals (Rose and Sulaiman, 1982). On the other hand, heparin (a sulfated

TABLE II

Prevalence of Common Minerals Detected in Canine, Feline, and Human Uroliths[a]

Mineral type	Percentage		
	Canine	Feline	Human
Calcium oxalate (mono- and dihydrate)	6	±2	33
Calcium oxalate and calcium apatite	?	2	34
Calcium apatite (pure)	3	<1	4
Brushite (pure or mixed)	<1	0	2
Struvite (major component) and calcium apatite (minor component)	74	88	15
Uric acid	<1	<1	8
Urates (sodium and ammonium)	4	±2	Rare
Cystine	1	0	3
Silica	<1	0	0
Calcium carbonate	0	0	0
Matrix	<1	±1	0
Mixed[b]	9	4	0
Artifacts	0	0	1
Total	100	100	100

[a]Data from Osborne et al. (1984d,f) and Prien (1974).
[b]Uroliths did not contain at least 70% of one mineral type and/or contained an identifiable nucleus and shell.

glycosaminoglycan) was found to prevent calcium oxalate adhesion to chemically injured rat bladder urothelium (Gill et al., 1982).

In summary, organic matrix may affect urolith formation by one or more of several mechanisms: (1) a site for heterogeneous nucleation (refer to Section IV); (2) a template for organizing and modifying growth of crystals; (3) a binding agent that cements calculi particles together and promotes retention of crystals; and/or (4) protective colloids that prevent further growth of calculi (Smith et al., 1978). Organic matrix could also be a passive substance having no effect on stone formation or growth.

2. Matrix Concretions

By definition, a urolith contains some minerals. However, concretions composed primarily (greater than 65%) of matrix may occur. They commonly occur in male cats (Fig. 11) (Osborne et al., 1984a) and male sheep (Kimberling and Arnold, 1983), but rarely occur in dogs (Fig. 10) and man (Griffith and Klein, 1983; Robertson and Peacock, 1982; Wickham, 1967). They are commonly called matrix stones. They

TABLE III

MINERAL COMPOSITION OF 494 FELINE UROLITHS ANALYZED
BY QUANTITATIVE METHODS[a]

Predominant mineral type	Number of uroliths	Percentage
Magnesium ammonium phosphate·6H$_2$O	420	85.0
100%	329	66.6
70–99%[b]	91	18.4
Calcium oxalate		
Calcium oxalate monohydrate	15	3.0
100%	4	0.8
70–99%[b]	8	1.6
Calcium oxalate dihydrate		
70–99%[b]	3	0.6
Calcium phosphate	10	2.0
Calcium phosphate		
100%	4	0.8
70–99%[b]	5	1.0
Calcium hydrogen phosphate·2H$_2$O		
100%	1	0.2
Uric acid and urates	9	1.8
Ammonium acid urate		
100%	1	0.2
Uric acid		
100%	2	0.4
70–99%[b]	1	0.2
Cystine	0	0
Silica	0	0
Mixed[c]	19	3.8
Compound[d]	7	1.4
Matrix	14	2.8
Total	494	100

[a]Analysis performed by optical crystallography and X-ray diffraction.

[b]Uroliths composed of 70–99% of mineral type listed; no nucleus and shell detected.

[c]Uroliths did not contain at least 70% of mineral type listed; no nucleus and shell detected.

[d]Uroliths containing an identifiable nucleus and one or more surrounding layers of different mineral type.

may form a cast of that portion of the excretory pathway in which they are formed, implying a rapid rate of formation (Figs. 10 and 11).

D. NUCLEI AND LAMINATIONS

Examination of cross sections of calculi often reveals a nucleus and adjacent peripheral laminations. Nuclei of calculi are focal points (or

TABLE IV

Mineral Composition of 770 Canine Uroliths Analyzed by Quantitative Methods[a]

Predominant mineral type	Number of uroliths	Percentage
Magnesium ammonium phosphate·$6H_2O$	524	68.0
100%	293	38.0
70–99%[b]	231	30.0
Magnesium hydrogen phosphate·$3H_2O$	1	0.1
Calcium oxalate	53	6.9
Calcium oxalate monohydrate		
100%	13	1.7
70–99%[b]	31	4.0
Calcium oxalate dihydrate		
100%	3	0.4
70–99%[b]	6	0.6
Calcium phosphate		
Calcium phosphate	24	3.1
100%	13	1.7
70–99%[b]	6	0.8
Calcium hydrogen phosphate·$2H_2O$		
100%	4	0.5
70–99%[b]	1	0.1
Uric acid and urates	38	4.9
Ammonium acid urate		
100%	21	2.7
70–99%[b]	13	1.7
Sodium acid urate		
100%	2	0.3
70–99%[b]	1	0.1
Uric acid	1	0.1
Cystine	19	2.5
Silica	23	2.9
100%	18	2.3
70–99%[b]	5	0.6
Mixed[c]	38	4.9
Compound[d]	45	5.8
Matrix	5	0.6
Total	770	100

[a]Analysis performed by optical crystallography and X-ray diffraction.

[b]Uroliths composed of 70–99% of mineral type listed; no nucleus and shell detected.

[c]Uroliths did not contain at least 70% of mineral type listed; no nucleus and shell detected.

[d]Uroliths containing an identifiable nucleus and one or more surrounding layers of different mineral type.

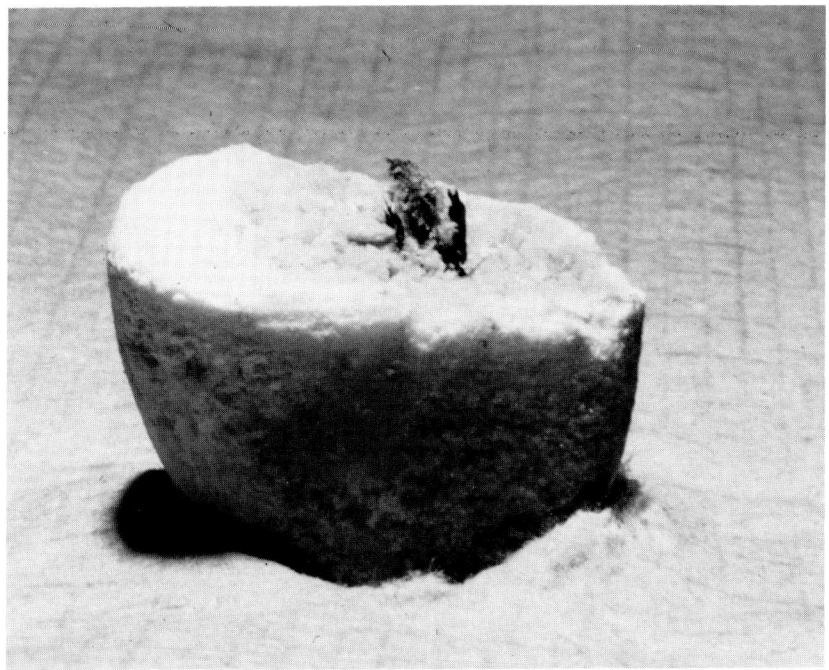

Fig. 13. Suture material in the center of a struvite urolith removed from the urinary bladder of an adult male mixed-breed dog.

cores) that differ in appearance from more peripheral portions of the stone. They are usually, but not invariably, located in the center of uroliths. Nuclei may be of crystalline composition (Figs. 7 and 12), or may be composed of foreign material (Figs. 13 and 14), tissue debris, blood clots, bacteria, etc. The mineral composition of a crystalline nucleus may be identical or different from the remainder of the calculus (Figs. 12 and 15).

Nuclei surrounded by well-defined layers (or lamellae) of solid material suggest that they represent an early phase of stone evolution. Crystalline nuclei that are large enough to be detected visually, however, are far too large to represent an initial crystalline nidus for crystal nucleation in the physiocochemical sense. Centrally located nuclei infer that the urolith was freely accessible to urine from all sides, and that growth proceeded at a similar rate on all sides.

Microradiographic studies of uroliths removed from dogs indicate that nuclei are not essential for calculi formation (Clark, 1976). In addition, when more than one mineral component was present, they

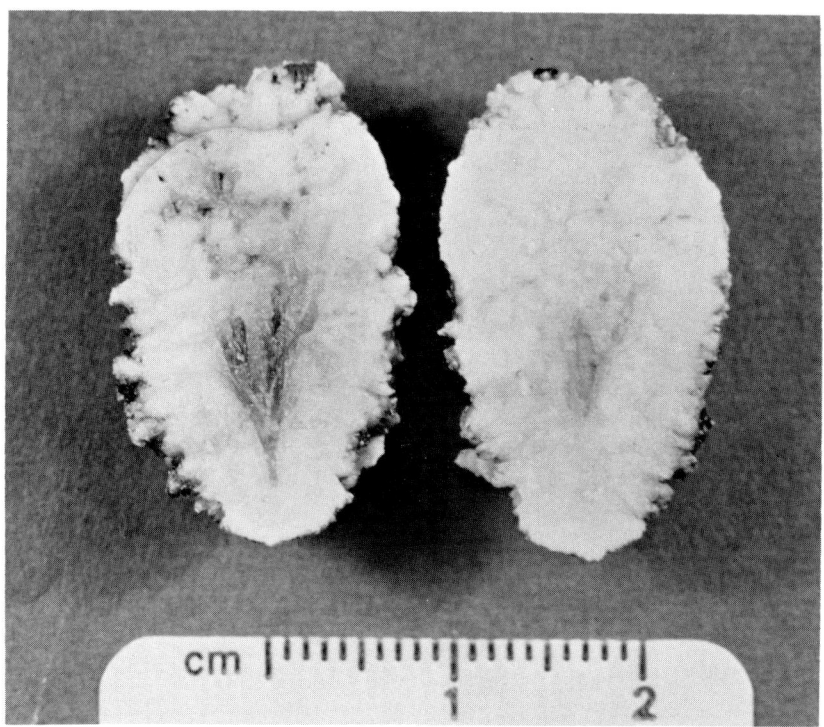

FIG. 14. Cross section of a struvite urolith removed from the urinary bladder of a 3-year-old castrated male domestic shorthair cat. The cat had previously had a perineal urethrostomy. The structure in the center of the urolith is a fox tail. Evaluation of a Gram-stained section of the matrix of the urolith revealed countless Gram-positive bacteria, presumably staphylococci.

were deposited in distinct areas within calculi. Complete intermixing of crystals throughout the same urolith was not detected. Similar studies of cat uroliths have not been reported.

Laminated calculi are common, and may represent alternating bands of different mineral types, periods during which stone growth occurs without interruption, and alternating periods of precipitation of minerals and gel. Although a difference in the appearance of two consecutive layers should prompt one to suspect a difference in composition, this is not always the case.

IV. Etiopathogenesis

A. OVERVIEW

Conceptual understanding of the etiopathogenesis of urolithiasis is an essential prerequisite to medical therapy and prevention of calculi.

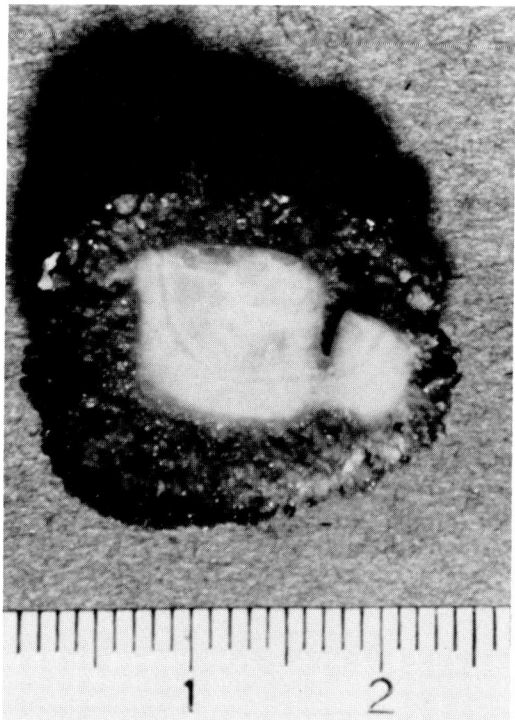

FIG. 15. Cross section of a urolith formed in the urinary bladder of an adult female beagle dog as a result of experimental infection with urease-producing *Proteus* spp. The nucleus of the urolith consists of struvite, and was transplanted into the bladder prior to the induction of infection. The shell also consists of struvite formed after the induction of infection. The darker color of the shell was caused by hematuria. (Scale is marked in millimeters.)

Despite extensive clinical and experimental research, the exact mode(s) of calculogenesis remains speculative. The fact that urolith formation is erratic and unpredicatable indicates that several interrelated complex physiologic and pathologic factors are involved.

B. INITIATION AND GROWTH

Urolith formation is associated with two complementary but separate phases—initiation and growth. It appears that initiating events are not the same for all types of calculi. In addition, factors that initiate urolith formation may be different from those that allow growth.

1. Initiation

The initial step in the development of a urolith is the formation of a crystal nidus (or crystal embryo). This phase of initiation of urolith formation (called nucleation) is dependent on supersaturation of urine with calculogenic crystalloids. The degree of supersaturation may be influenced by the magnitude of renal excretion of the crystalloid, the urine pH, and crystallization inhibitors in the urine. Further growth of the crystal nidus is dependent on its ability to remain in the urinary system; the degree and duration of supersaturation of urine with crystalloids identical to or different from that of the nidus; and physical characteristics of the crystal nidus.

Several theories have been proposed to explain the initiation of calculogenesis. Each theory emphasizes a single factor. On the basis of current knowledge, the most popular hypotheses are the precipitation–crystallization theory, the matrix–nucleation theory, and the crystallization–inhibition theory.

a. Precipitation–Crystallization Theory. This hypothesis incriminates excessive supersaturation of urine with stone-forming crystalloids as the primary event in calculogenesis (Coe and Favus, 1981). In this hypothesis, nucleation (initiation of urolith formation) is considered to be a physicochemical process of precipitation of crystalloids from a supersaturated solution. Calculus formation is thought to occur independently of preformed matrix or inhibitors of crystallization.

According to this hypothesis, production of urine excessively saturated with one or more urolith-forming crystalloids leads to spontaneous nucleation of the crystalloid. If nucleated crystalloids become trapped in the urinary system during continued supersaturation, urolith growth will occur. Mucoprotein matrix is thought to be nonspecifically incorporated into the urolith as calculus growth proceeds.

Oversatuation of urine with urolith-forming crystalloids may be associated with the following: (1) increased renal excretion of crystalloids as a result of increased glomerular filtration, increased tubular secretion, or decreased tubular reabsorption (examples include hypercalciuria, hyperuricosuria, hyperoxaluria, cystinuria, and xanthinuria); (2) negative body water balance associated with increased tubular reabsorption of water and subsequent urine concentration (examples include excessive water loss via other routes, lack of water consumption, and living in a hot, dry climate); and (3) urine pH-favoring crystallization [examples include formation of alkaline urine by urease-producing bacteria, formation of alkaline urine as a result of renal tubular acidosis, formation of alkaline (or less acid) urine as a result of diet composition and/or feeding patterns, and administration of alkalinizing drugs].

The precipitation–crystallization hypothesis provides a plausible explanation for the formation of cystine, urate, and magnesium ammonium phosphate uroliths. It is also applicable to those patients with oxalate calculi in which hypercalciuria, hyperoxaluria, hyperuricosuria, or a combination of these can be detected (Coe, 1978; Wickham, 1976).

b. Matrix–Nucleation Theory. This hypothesis states that matrix substances are "promoters" of nucleation, and incriminates preformed organic matrix as the primary determinant in calculogenesis (Finlayson, 1974; Hallson and Rose, 1979; Malek and Boyce, 1977; Wickham, 1976). Organic matrix substances are thought to be mucoproteins with crystal-binding properties. The matrix–nucleation theory is based on the assumption that preformed organic matrix forms an initial nucleus that subsequently permits stone growth by precipitation of crystalloids. The theory is somewhat analogous to bone formation in its requirement for organic matrix (Pak, 1976).

The role of organic matrix in calculogenesis has not been identified with certainty; however, the similarity of the overall composition of matrix from human uroliths of various mineral composition has been used to support this hypothesis (Malek and Boyce, 1977). The observation that the specific amino acid composition differed for human stones of different mineral content also supports this hypothesis (Spector *et al.*, 1976). It has been hypothesized that the overall negative charges of some forms of urolith matrix may provide binding sites for cations such as calcium and magnesium (Chow *et al.*, 1973; Chow *et al.*, 1983).

Immunologic techniques have provided most of the current information about matrix components (Malek and Boyce, 1977). Matrix substance A is a potent antigenic component of human uroliths and comprises a large portion of the matrix of most calciferous (that is, nonmatrix) stones. Matrix substance A has been consistently identified in human uroliths of all types, can be detected in renal tissue of stone formers, and is present in varying quantities in the urine of stone formers (Boyce and King, 1963; Boyce *et al.*, 1962; Keutel and King, 1964). Matrix substance A cannot be detected in normal human kidneys or in the urine of non-stone formers (Moore and Gowland, 1975).

The exact composition of matrix substance A is unknown, although it does not contain hydroxyproline (Pak, 1976). It is reported to have a molecular weight of 30,000 to 40,000 (Wickham, 1976). Recent studies using contemporary immunologic methods indicate that matrix substance A may not be a single antigenic entity, but rather may comprise a group of substances called stone specific antigens (Moore and Gowland, 1975).

Other matrix components, identified in human uroliths include serum albumin, α- and γ-globulins, uromucoid, and Tamm-Horsfall mucoprotein (Pyrah, 1979; Wickham, 1976). There is no substantial evidence to suggest that stone matrix is a product of an immune response. *In vitro* studies of human urine have provided results that indicate that uromucoid may promote calcium oxalate and calcium phosphate crystal formation (Hallson and Rose, 1979).

A unique, but as yet unidentified, protein has been detected by immunologic methods in urine and urethral plugs of a small number of male cats with naturally occurring urethral obstruction (Rich and Norcross, 1969). It was hypothesized that viruses may directly or indirectly cause production of this protein, and that the protein may serve as a matrix to aid conglomeration of struvite crystals (an example of the matrix–nucleation hypothesis).

Matrix has been incriminated in the etiopathogenesis of "feline urolithiasis" by another group of investigators (Duch *et al.*, 1978). Differences in the characteristics of urine polyelectrolytes (thought to be components of matrix) in control cats, cats with experimentally induced urolithiasis, and cats with naturally occurring urethral obstruction were interpreted to support the matrix–nucleation theory. Unfortunately, the specific characteristics of the naturally occurring disease were not specified in this study.

c. *Crystallization–Inhibition Theory.* This hypothesis incriminates reduction or absence of organic and inorganic inhibitors of crystallization as the primary determinant of calcium oxalate and calcium phosphate calculogenesis. This theory is based on the fact that several crystalloids, especially calcium, are maintained in solution at concentrations significantly higher than occur in water (that is, urine is a metastable supersaturated solution). Because normal urine can hold larger amounts of some crystalloids in solution than can simple aqueous solutions, reduction or absence of specific crystal inhibitors is a logical hypothesis of calcium calculogenesis. The following have been reported to inhibit calcium crystallization: organic acids (especially citrates); magnesium; inorganic pyrophosphates; urea; mucopolysaccharides; glycosaminoglycans; RNA-like material; and as yet unidentified substances (Finlayson, 1974; Fleisch, 1978; Fleisch and Russel, 1977; Pyrah, 1979; Robertson and Peacock, 1982; Sutor *et al.*, 1978). The role, if any, of crystallization inhibitors in urolithiasis is of clinical importance, since it is feasible that therapy could be designed to increase the amount and/or potency of some natural inhibitors in stone-forming patients. Unfortunately, specific inhibitors of struvite, urate, cystine, and silica crystallization have not been identified.

Citrates and other organic acids may form soluble chelates with calcium. Urinary citrate inhibits the precipitation of calcium oxalate and calcium phosphate and growth of both crystal types. A low excretion and a low concentration of urine citrate have been reported in patients with uroliths containing calcium (Schwille et al., 1979).

Magnesium has been hypothesized to act as a crystallization inhibitor of calcium salts by nonspecific attachment to crystal surfaces, and this interferes with migration of solutes to crystal growth sites (Pak, 1978). Experimental studies in rats revealed that increasing the magnesium content of the diet reduces the incidence and severity of calcium salt deposition in renal tubules (Bunce et al., 1980; Harwood, 1982). High magnesium diets promote experimental formation of struvite uroliths in cats (Finco and Barsanti, 1984; Kallfelz et al., 1980; Lewis et al., 1978; Rich et al., 1974). Therefore, the role of magnesium in calculogenesis may vary, depending on the mineral composition of the urolith. In patients with uroliths containing calcium, high urine levels of magnesium may help to inhibit initiation and/or growth of uroliths. In contrast, high urine levels of magnesium may augment initiation and/or growth of struvite (magnesium ammonium phosphate) uroliths.

Inorganic pyrophosphates, which are products of intermediary metabolism, inhibit crystallization of calcium salts. Results of studies of humans with recurrent calcium urolithiasis indicate that they excrete only about half as much pyrophosphate in urine as do normal control persons, and have less inhibitory activity toward calcium phosphate crystallization in their urine (Fleisch and Russell, 1977). Inhibitory activity remaining after treatment of urine with pyrophosphatase was not significantly different from that of control patients, suggesting that diminished excretion of pyrophosphate is of major importance. Pyrophosphates apparently do not influence the precipitation of magnesium ammonium phosphate or uric acid (Fleisch and Russel, 1977).

d. *Summary.* To date, several lines of evidence have been reported to support the precipitation–crystallization hypothesis, the matrix–nucleation hypothesis, and the crystallization–inhibition hypothesis. This evidence has not been completely accepted, however. The balance of evidence suggests that the most likely cause of nucleation and formation of a crystal embryo is precipitation from a supersaturated solution. An organic matrix is not required for precipitation, and inhibitors may be more important in growth than in initiation of urolith formation.

Irrespective of the theory proposed for nucleation and nidus formation, an essential requirement is supersaturation of urine with a urolith-forming crystalloid. A crystal nidus cannot be formed if urine is undersaturated with the crystalloid in question. The matrix–nucleation and crystallization–inhibition theories imply that only a low degree of supersaturation is required to initiate urolith formation. The precipitation–crystallization theory is based on the supposition that a greater degree of supersaturation is required to initiate urolith formation. Thus, the greater the degree of urine supersaturation, the greater the predisposition to urolith formation.

These hypotheses are not mutually exclusive; calculogenesis may be dependent on more than one initiating factor. In one study of humans with recurrent idiopathic calcium oxalate urolithiasis, evidence was presented that implicated both supersaturation with calcium oxalate and reduction in the concentration of crystal inhibitors as underlying events (Robertson et al., 1976). It was suggested that normal individuals did not form large crystals in their urine because of low levels of supersaturation and high concentrations of crystallization inhibitors.

2. Growth

Once a crystal nidus has formed, it may grow into a urolith of the same composition. As was the situation with the initiation of urolithiasis, however, the exact events leading to stone growth have not been identified. Calculi do not appear to grow haphazardly because they are composed of an orderly arrangement of crystals (Clark, 1976). It has been suggested that a crystalline nidus may grow by (1) crystal growth; (2) epitaxial growth; and/or (3) crystal aggregation (Finlayson, 1977; Fleisch, 1978; Pak, 1978; Robertson et al., 1971).

a. Crystal Growth. Once a nidus is formed, it may develop into a stone of the same composition by a process of crystal growth, provided the urine is supersaturated. Formation of a new crystal nidus requires a greater degree of urine supersaturation than does its subsequent growth (Coe, 1978). For example, addition of calcium oxalate seed crystals to a supersaturated solution of calcium oxalate will change a metastable solution to an oversaturated one with rapid crystal growth and formation of pure calcium oxalate stones. The critical factor for crystal growth appears to be persistent production of supersaturated urine, rather than reduced excretion of inhibitors of crystallization.

b. Epitaxial Growth. Growth by epitaxy indicates organized growth of one type of crystal upon the surface of another type. The physical characteristics of the initiating crystals and growth crystals must permit proper alignment with respect to each other; thus, growth by epitaxy implies a regular alignment of crystals.

Epitaxial growth may provide a plausible explanation for the finding that uroliths frequently are of mixed composition. It may represent a heterogeneous form of nucleation. Thus, calcium phosphate may serve as a nidus leading to epitaxial growth by calcium oxalate. Likewise, a nidus of monosodium urate or uric acid may lead to epitaxial growth with calcium oxalate, and brushite (calcium hydrogen phosphate dihydrate) may serve as a nidus for further growth of calcium phosphate or calcium oxalate (Coe, 1977).

  c. *Crystal Aggregation.* This hypothesis of growth of uroliths is based on the supposition that further aggregation of nucleated crystals may be normally inhibited by substances present in urine (Fleish and Russel, 1977; Hansen *et al.*, 1976; Pak, 1978; Robertson *et al.*, 1971). In stone formers, crystals may bind to one another, leading to formation of large clusters.

  It has been suggested that the crystal aggregation phenomenon distinguishes simple crystalluria, which occurs in most normal animals, from stone formation (Figs. 16 and 17). In the presence of crystal aggregation inhibitors, crystals that form do not grow and are readily passed through the urinary tract. If crystal aggregation inhibitors are deficient, or have impaired function, growth by aggregation will occur. This hypothesis is supported by the observation that only individual

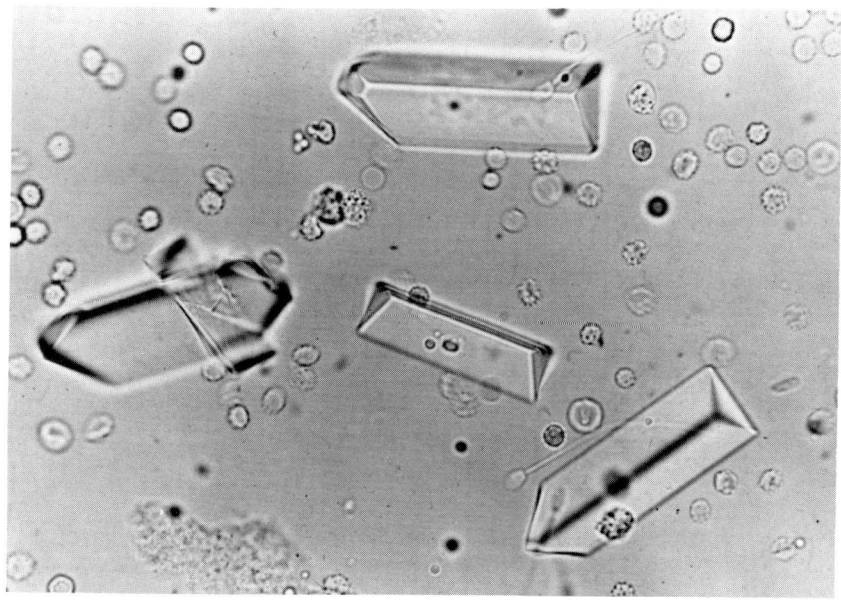

FIG. 16. Isolated struvite crystals in the urine of a normal adult male dog. Unstained ×66.

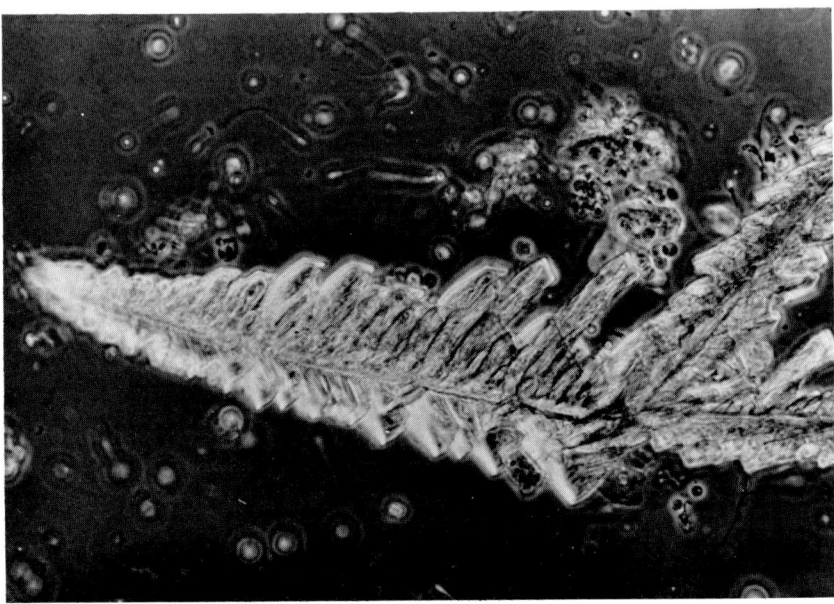

FIG. 17. Aggregate of struvite crystals formed in the urine of an adult male dog. Notice the orderly alignment of individual struvite crystals. Unstained phase microscopy; ×42.

calcium oxalate crystals are found in normal humans, whereas stone formers often excrete large aggregates of this salt (Robertson and Peacock, 1982). Substances thought to have crystal-aggregation inhibiting properties for calcium salts include glycosaminoglycans, citrates, pyrophosphates, and diphosphonates (Fleisch, 1978).

  d. *Growth versus Time.* Although the time required for naturally occurring uroliths to form has not been determined, radiographically detectable struvite uroliths have been experimentally induced in dogs within 2 weeks (Klausner *et al.,* 1980a). Dissolution of naturally occurring struvite uroliths in dogs and cats has been induced in a period as short as 2 weeks (C. A. Osborne, 1984, unpublished data). These observations suggest that urolith kinetics should be conceived in terms of days to weeks rather than months to years.

  The highly structured and organized arrangement of classical uroliths as compared to the disorganized arrangement of urethral plugs may also be related to time. The implication is that the unstructured, apparently disorganized, urethral plugs form more rapidly than do the highly structured uroliths.

C. Summary of Urolith Formation

1. Classical Uroliths

The initial step in formation of a urolith is formation of a crystal nidus (or crystal embryo). This phase of initiation of urolith formation, called nucleation, is dependent on supersaturation of urine with calculogenic crystalloids. A greater degree of supersaturation is required for homogeneous nucleation than for heterogeneous nucleation. The degree of urine supersaturation may be influenced by the magnitude of renal excretion of the crystalloid, urine pH, and/or the presence of crystallization inhibitors in urine. Noncrystalline proteinaceous matrix substances may also play a role in nucleation in some instances.

Further growth of the crystal nidus is dependent on the following: (1) its ability to remain in the lumen of the excretory pathway of the urinary system; (2) the degree and duration of supersaturation of urine with crystalloids identical or different from that in the nidus; and (3) physical characteristics of the crystal nidus. If they are compatible with other crystalloids, epitaxial growth with different crystalloids may occur.

2. Matrix Concretions

In contrast to classical uroliths, the initiation and growth of matrix concretions are poorly understood. Available data suggest that matrix materials produced from tissue surrounding the excretory pathway of the urinary system are of greater importance in the formation of feline urethral plugs than are proteinaceous substances excreted into urine from plasma. It is probable that crystals present in urine at the time matrix concretions form and grow may become trapped within their matrix in a fashion analogous to the formation of a gelatin salad that contains fruit or vegetables. The contribution of locally produced matrix to urethral plugs found in sheep has apparently not been evaluated. Likewise, little information is available regarding matrix concretions that form in dogs, humans, and other species of animals.

V. Struvite Urolithiasis

A. Mineral Composition of Struvite Uroliths

The mineral composition of struvite uroliths may be pure magnesium ammonium phosphate hexahydrate, or they may contain varying

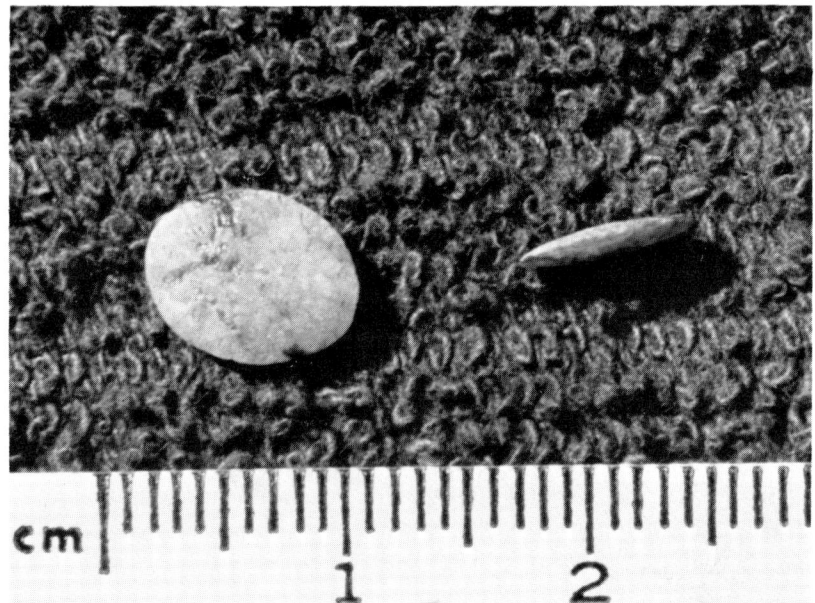

FIG. 18. Disk-shaped 100% struvite uroliths removed from the urinary bladder of a 3-year-old male domestic shorthair cat.

quantities of calcium apatite, carbonate-apatite, and/or ammonium acid urate. Pure struvite uroliths occur predominantly in cats (Fig. 18 and Table III), frequently in dogs (Table IV), and uncommonly in man (Table II). Struvite uroliths removed from dogs may be pure magnesium ammonium phosphate (Fig. 5), but frequently contain small quantities of calcium apatite, carbonate-apatite, and ammonium acid urate (Figs. 7 and 12). The quantity of calcium apatite in human struvite uroliths is often greater than that observed in dogs and cats (Tables V and VI).

Struvite uroliths have been called MAP (magnesium ammonium phosphate) calculi, phosphate calculi, "infection stones," "urease stones," and triple phosphate stones. Triple phosphate is a misnomer that originated because qualitative chemical analyses of uroliths revealed calcium, magnesium, ammonium, and phosphate (three cations and one anion). The name is incorrect, since struvite does not contain calcium (Table I). However, human and canine uroliths are frequently impure, containing minor quantities of calcium phosphate (calcium apatite) and carbonate-apatite. As will be discussed, carbonate-apatite is thought to occur in patients with urinary tract infections caused by

TABLE V

COMMON CHARACTERISTICS OF CANINE, FELINE, AND HUMAN STRUVITE UROLITHS

Chemical name
  Magnesium ammonium phosphate hexahydrate
Crystal name
  Struvite
Formula
  $MgNH_4PO_4 \cdot 6H_2O$
Variations in composition
  Struvite only
  Struvite mixed with lesser quantities of calcium apatite and/or ammonium acid urate
  Nucleus of a different mineral surrounded by variable layers composed primarily of struvite. Small quantities of calcium apatite and/or ammonium acid urate may also be present
Physical characteristics
  Color: Struvite uroliths are usually white, cream, or light brown in color. The surface of uroliths is commonly red because of concomitant hematuria, and may be green (caused by bile pigments)
  Shape: Variable
  Density: Variable; soft if they contain a large quantity of matrix; dense and harder to cut if little matrix is present. A combination of hard and soft internal density may occur within the same urolith. Radiodense compared with nonskeletal tissue on survey radiographs. Degree of radiodensity is related to the quantity of matrix (inversely proportional) and other minerals, especially calcium apatite (more proportional).
  Number: Single or multiple
  Size: Subvisual to a size limited by the capacity of the structure (kidney and urinary bladder) in which they form
Predisposing factors
  Urinary tract infections with urease-producing microbes in patients whose urine contains a large quantity of urea
  Alkaline urine pH
  Unidentified factors
Characteristics of affected patients
  May occur at any age, but more commonly detected in middle-aged adults

urease-producing microbes. Generation of carbonate anions (CO_3^{2-}) apparently is associated with displacement of some phosphate anions in calcium apatite molecules (Table I).

Following exposure to air, struvite may lose water and ammonia and change into magnesium hydrogen phosphate trihydrate (newberyite) (Table I). Although newberyite is not reported to be a primary constituent of human uroliths (Sutor, 1972), we have experimentally induced it in cats by feeding them 1% dietary magnesium in the form of magnesium oxide (Fig. 19) (C. A. Osborne, 1984, unpublished data).

TABLE VI

DIFFERENCES IN THE CHARACTERISTICS OF CANINE, FELINE,
AND HUMAN STRUVITE UROLITHS

Variations in composition
  Calcium apatite occurs more frequently and in greater quantity in human struvite
    uroliths than in canine and feline struvite uroliths
  Calcium apatite occurs more frequently and in greater quantity in canine struvite
    uroliths than feline struvite uroliths

Physical characteristics
  Shape: Branched or staghorn uroliths can only form in man (not dogs or cats), due
    to the branched nature of their renal pelves. Sterile struvite uroliths
    obtained from the urinary bladders of cats commonly have a wafer or disk
    shape; they are typically thicker at their center than at the periphery.
    Sterile feline struvite uroliths may also have a rough, jagged, quartz-like
    appearance
  Nuclei and laminations: Common in infection-induced uroliths of all species.
    Uncommon in sterile struvite uroliths of cats.
  Location: May be located in the kidney, ureter, urinary bladder, and/or urethra of
    all species. Most occur in the renal pelves of humans; most occur in the
    urinary bladders of dogs and cats. Urethral uroliths are more common
    in male dogs and cats than in male humans

Urinary tract infections
  Proteus spp. appear to be the most prevalent calculogenic microbes of humans
  Staphylococci are the most prevalent calculogenic microbes of dogs
  Staphylococci may cause struvite uroliths in cats, but most feline struvite uroliths
    form in sterile urine
  Ureaplasmas have been isolated from urine and stones of humans with struvite
    uroliths, and from urine of dogs with struvite uroliths

Characteristics of affected patients
  No obvious race predisposition in man or breed predisposition in cats.
  May occur in any breed of dog, but especially common in miniature schnauzers,
    dachshunds, poodles, Scottish terriers, beagles, pekingese, and Welsh corgis.
  In humans and dogs, infection-induced struvite uroliths are more common in
    females than males. No apparent sex predisposition in cats

---

B. MATRIX COMPOSITION OF STRUVITE UROLITHS

Most experimental and clinical studies of struvite uroliths have been designed to study their mineral composition. There is a paucity of information concerning the origin, specific composition, and quantity of matrix in sterile and infection-induced struvite stones. In man, calcium oxalate and calcium phosphate uroliths typically contain greater than 95% organic or inorganic crystalloids, and less than 5% organic matrix (weight versus weight ratio) (Boyce and Garvey, 1956). Howev-

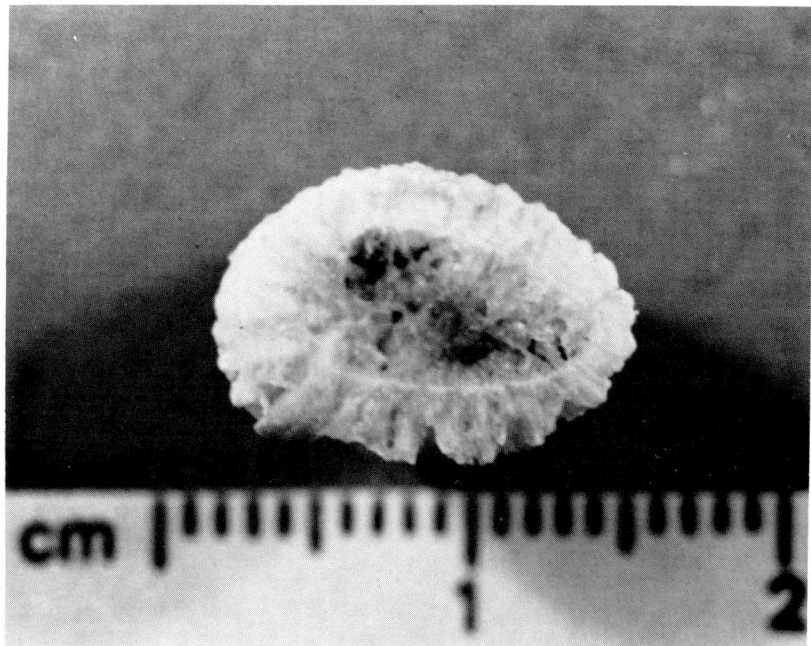

FIG. 19. Urolith removed from the urinary bladder of an adult female domestic shorthair cat. The nucleus formed naturally and was composed of 100% magnesium ammonium phosphate. The shell was induced by adding 1% magnesium to the diet and is composed of 100% magnesium hydrogen phosphate trihydrate.

er, there is a general consensus of opinion that larger quantities of matrix may occur in struvite uroliths that form in patients with urinary tract infections caused by urease-producing microbes (Fig. 20) (Grant et al., 1973; Osborne et al., 1984a). It is probable that a substantial portion of this matrix results from inflammatory changes induced in the urothelium and adjacent tissues by toxic products of ureolysis (Griffith and Klein, 1983; Krawiec et al., 1984a,b). This observation

$$NH_2\text{-}\overset{O}{\overset{\|}{C}}\text{-}NH_2 + H_2O \xrightarrow{urease} 2NH_3 + CO_2$$

$$CO_2 + H_2O \leftrightarrow H_2CO_3 \leftrightarrow H^+ + HCO_3^- \leftrightarrow CO_3^{2-}$$

$$NH_3 + H_2O \leftrightarrow NH_4^+ + OH^-$$

FIG. 20. Schematic illustration of factors leading to the formation of struvite, calcium apatite, and carbonate-apatite as a consequence of degradation of urea by microbial urease.

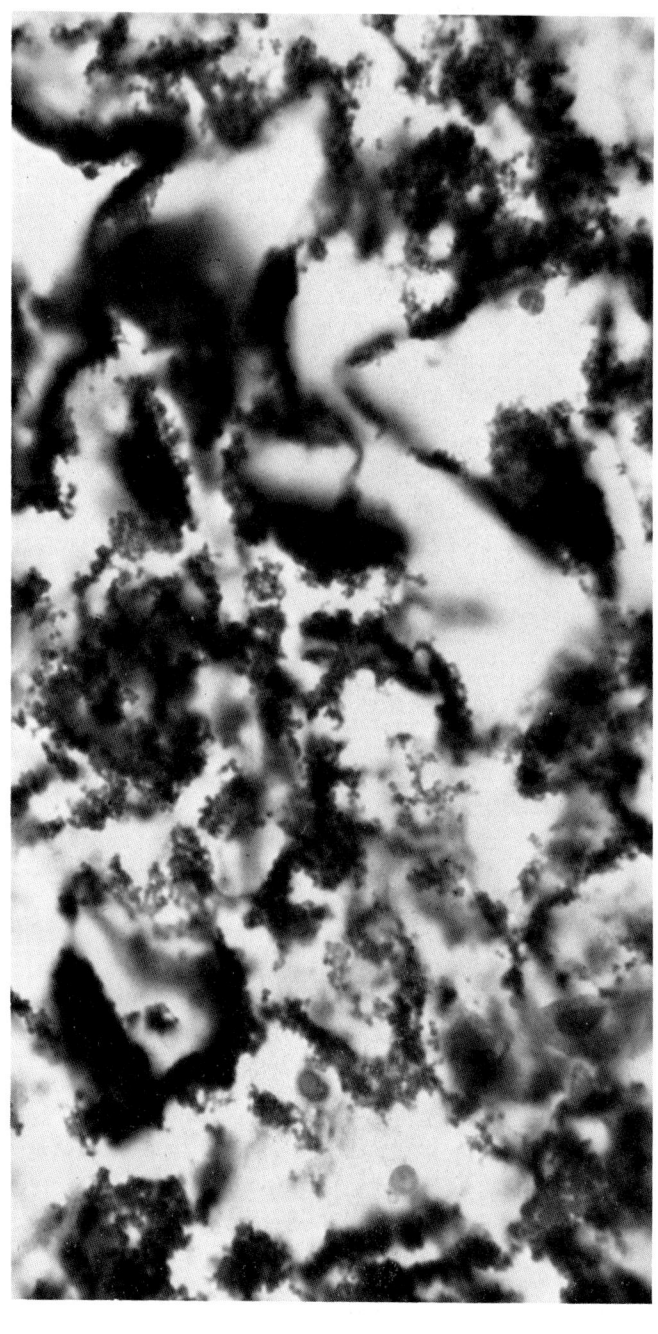

FIG. 21. Photomicrograph of a section of struvite urocystolith removed from a 3-year-old female miniature schnauzer. Microscopic evaluation revealed countless Gram-positive cocci (presumably staphylococci) in an acellular pale eosinophilic matrix. H & E stain; ×100. [From *Proc. 27th Gaines Vet. Symp.* (1977), pp. 25–37.]

provides a plausible explanation of the variability of density among different infection-induced struvite uroliths and in different regions of the same infection-induced struvite urolith.

Light microscopic examination of demineralized, naturally occurring, canine struvite uroliths suggests that the matrix is not deposited in a haphazard fashion (Cornelius et al., 1961). Light microscopic examination of struvite uroliths that have formed in humans, dogs, or cats with urease-positive urinary tract infections typically reveals bacteria dispersed throughout the stone (Clark, 1974a; Stamey, 1980) (Fig. 21). Preliminary studies of the matrix of human struvite–apatite uroliths revealed that it contained a substantial quantity of acidic amino acids (Spector et al., 1976). It is conceivable that negatively charged amino acids could attract and/or retain cations such as magnesium and ammonium.

C. Composition of Matrix Concretions

1. Man and Dogs

In man and dogs, matrix concretions usually occur secondary to infection, especially with urease-producing bacteria. In man, matrix concretions are characteristically composed of gels containing mucopolysaccharides, inflammatory and desquamated cells, proteinaceous debris, and scattered crystalline material (usually struvite and carbonate-apatite) (Griffith and Klein, 1983; Wickham, 1976). The organic matrix that commonly occurs in association with these concretions is poorly understood. Preliminary investigations indicate that the matrix contains large quantities of glycosaminoglycans. It has been hypothesized that the alkalinity and ammonia generated from bacterially induced ureolysis cause chemical injury to the urothelium, which in turn stimulates production of glycosaminoglycans by mucosal or submucosal cells. It has been suggested that matrix concretions form in patients that produce urine that contains very low concentrations of calculogenic minerals (Robertson and Peacock, 1982). It is not known whether or not such matrix is capable of promoting mineral deposition if the concentration of calculogenic minerals in urine increases.

2. Cats

Matrix concretions (urethral plugs) that form in the urethras of male cats are also poorly understood. They frequently, but not invariably, contain struvite (Table VII). The origin and composition of matrix in

TABLE VII

CHARACTERISTICS OF FELINE STRUVITE URETHRAL PLUGS

Chemical name
Magnesium ammonium phosphate hexahydrate

Formula
$MgNH_4PO_4 \cdot 6H_2O$
Variations in composition
Struvite only
Struvite mixed with relatively small quantities of calcium apatite

Physical characteristics
Color: Struvite urethral plugs are typically white, cream, or light brown in color
Shape: Often have a cylindrical shape; sometimes they form a shapeless gelatinous mass
Nuclei and laminations: None grossly visible
Density: Soft and easily compressible
Number: Apparently single
Size: Diameter conforms to diameter of urethra. Length varies from a few millimeters to several centimeters

Predisposing factors
Reduced diameter of the penile urethra
Locally produced matrix?
Factors affecting struvite crystalluria?

Characteristics of affected feline patients
Mean age = 3.8 years (range <1 to >12 years)
No obvious breed disposition
Consistently (if not invariably) in males

urethral plugs which commonly occur in cats with lower urinary tract disease, have not been determined (Osborne et al., 1984b). However, matrix typically occurs in the absence of detectable bacterial urinary tract infections (consult Section V,I,1 for additional information).

D. BACTERIAL URINARY TRACT INFECTIONS

1. Overview

Several factors, which may be interrelated, appear to play a role in promoting supersaturaton of urine with struvite, including urinary tract infections with urease-producing microbes, alkaline urine, genetic predisposition, and diet. Of these factors, urinary tract infections appear to be more important in man (Griffith et al., 1978), most dogs

(Osborne et al., 1981), mink (Nielsen, 1956), and some rats (Kinter et al., 1982). Other mechanisms are probably involved in cats (Osborne et al., 1984a, b,c) and sheep (Bartos and Palmore, 1981; Emerick, 1969; Kimberling and Arnold, 1983; White and Porter, 1969), since the majority of struvite uroliths in these species are apparently not associated with urease-positive bacterial urinary tract infections.

2. Stoichiometry

There is a general consensus of opinion that urine must be supersaturated with magnesium ammonium phosphate hexahydrate for struvite uroliths to form. However, acid urine from humans and, presumably, dogs and cats is normally undersaturated with respect to magnesium ammonium phosphate (Elliot et al., 1958, 1959). Normally, urine ammonium (NH_4^+) concentration rises only when acid catabolites are excreted in high concentration by the kidneys. This rise in urine concentration of ammonium ions represents a normal compensatory response by the renal tubular cells to secrete ammonia (NH_3) into the tubular lumina in order to reduce acidity by the subsequent formation of ammonium (NH_4^+). Whereas ammonia is lipid soluble and can penetrate tubular cell walls, ammonium is lipid insoluble and cannot penetrate cell walls (so-called ion trapping). Likewise, excretion of alkaline urine under physiologic conditions is associated with a reduction in renal production of ammonia, and, thus, reduced quantities of ammonium ions in urine.

When urinary tract infections with urease-producing microbes occur in man or animals forming urine with a sufficient quantity of urea, the unique combination of concomitant elevation in the concentrations of ammonium and carbonate (CO_3^{2-}) ions in an alkaline environment may develop. These conditions favor formation of uroliths containing struvite ($MgNH_4PO_4 \cdot 6H_2O$), calcium apatite [$Ca_{10}(PO_4)_6(OH)_2$], and carbonate-apatite [$Ca_{10}(PO_4)_6CO_3$]. The following mechanisms are involved (Fishbein, 1981; Griffith, 1978a; Griffith and Klein, 1983) (1) urease (a metallo-enzyme containing nickel) produced by bacteria or ureaplasma hydrolyzes urea to form two molecules of ammonia and a molecule of carbon dioxide (Fig. 20); (2) the ammonia molecules react spontaneously with water to form ammonium and hydroxyl ions (pK of NH_3 = 9.03), which alkalinize urine by reducing its hydrogen ion concentration. The solubility of struvite and calcium apatite decreases in alkaline urine. In addition to alkalinizing urine, the newly generated ammonium ion is available for the formation of magnesium ammonium phosphate crystals; (3) the newly generated molecule of carbon dioxide combines with water to form carbonic acid, which in turn dissociates to form bicarbonate (pK = 6.33) and hydrogen ions. In an extremely alkaline environment, bicarbonate may lose its proton to become carbonate (pK = 10.1). Anions of carbonate may displace anions of phosphate in calcium apatite crystals to form carbonate-apatite crystals; (4) in the progressively alkaline environment induced by microbial hydrolysis of urea, dissociation of monobasic hydrogen phosphate ($H_2PO_4^-$) results in an increased concentration of dibasic hydrogen phosphate (HPO_4^{2-}) and anionic phosphate (PO_4^{3-}). Given a constant concentration of total phosphate, a change in pH from 6.80 to 7.40 increases the PO_4^{3-} concentration by a factor of approximately 6 (Burns and Finlayson, 1982). Anionic phosphate is then available in increased quantities to combine with magnesium and ammonium to form struvite, or with calcium to form calcium apatite; (5) ammonium ions may combine with urates to form ammonium acid urate (He et al., 1984; Garcia de la Pena and Cifuentes Delatte, 1981).

Studies of canine struvite uroliths associated with urinary tract infections revealed that staphylococci were capable of producing phosphatase in addition to urease (Clark, 1974a). This observation prompts the hypothesis that bacterial phosphatase might increase the concentration of urine inorganic phosphate by its action on organic phosphates.

Both urea (60 MW) and urease (±483,000 MW) are required for ammonia production, alkalinization, supersaturation, and subsequent precipitation of struvite, calcium apatite, and carbonate-apatite crystals. The majority of urea in urine originates from dietary protein (Abdullahi et al., 1984), while the urease in vertebrates must be derived from microbes (some bacteria, some yeasts, or ureaplasmas) (Delluva et al., 1968; Griffith and Klein, 1983; Kornberg et al., 1954a,b; Levensen et al., 1959). The high concentration of urea normally present in urine of individuals who consume dietary protein in excess of daily requirements for protein anabolism makes urine an environment well suited to support the pathogenic effects of urease-producing microbes. Because of the importance of urease in the etiopathogenesis of struvite urolithiasis in man and many animals, the name "urease stones" has been proposed (Griffith, 1978a). Following a parallel line of reasoning, the name "urea stones" would also be appropriate.

Continued production of ammonia, and perhaps other toxic reactants as a consequence of urease-induced ureolysis, appears to induce an inflammatory response in the urothelium and adjacent structures (Griffith, 1978b; Krawiec et al., 1984a,b). In fact, urease production contributes to the virulence of uropathogens that produce this enzyme (Brande and Siemienski, 1960; MacLaren, 1968; 1969; Parsons et al.,

1984; Rosenstein and Hamilton-Miller, 1984). The associated increase in urine concentration of proteinaceous inflammatory products may contribute to calculogenesis by acting as a form of matrix.

Another mechanism that has been hypothesized to predispose patients with urinary tract infections to urolithiasis has been bacterially mediated reduction in the urine concentration of citrate (Conway *et al.*, 1949; Robertson and Peacock, 1982; Scott *et al.*, 1943). Citrate is often called a crystallization inhibitor, since it can combine with cations such as calcium and magnesium to increase their solubility (Schwille *et al.*, 1979). It has also been suggested that bacteria may produce calculogenic matrix substances (Stegmeyer and Stegmeyer, 1983).

3. Experimental and Clinical Observations

Clinical studies of dogs (Brodey, 1955; Brown *et al.*, 1977a; Clark, 1974a; Finco *et al.*, 1979; Goulden, 1968; Klausner *et al.*, 1980a; Osborne and Klausner, 1978; Weaver and Pillinger, 1975) and man (Griffith, 1978a, 1982; Stamey, 1980) and experimental studies in dogs (Klausner *et al.* 1980b), rats (Brande and Siemienski, 1960; Vermuelen and Goetz, 1954), mink (Nielsen, 1956), and rabbits (Davolos, 1943; Keyser, 1945; Suby and Suby, 1947) have repeatedly demonstrated a close relationship between the formation of struvite uroliths and urinary tract infections caused by urease-producing bacteria. Bacterial urinary tract infections have been such a common finding in man and dogs with struvite uroliths that they are sometimes called infection stones (Griffith, 1978a; Osborne *et al.*, 1981).

Several *in vitro* observations indicate that bacterial urease-induced supersaturation of urine with magnesium ammonium phosphate is the primary (but not necessarily the only) cause of infection-induced struvite uroliths (Griffith and Musher, 1975; Griffith *et al.*, 1976; Griffith, 1978a): (1) growth of urease-producing *Proteus* spp. in urea-free urine, or in urine containing a urease inhibitor, did not cause alkalinization, supersaturation, or crystallization of struvite and apatite; (2) growth of weak urease-producing bacteria (*Klebsiella* spp. and *Pseudomonas* spp.) and nonurease-producing bacteria (*Escherichia* spp.) was not associated with alkalinization, supersaturation, and subsequent precipitation of struvite and apatite crystals.

Staphylococcus and *Proteus* spp. are consistent and potent urease producers, and have been commonly isolated from animals and man with infection-induced struvite uroliths (Chute and Suby, 1940; Griffith, 1978a, 1982; Osborne *et al.*, 1981). For reasons that are unexplained, staphylococci have been more commonly associated with struvite uroliths in dogs than *Proteus* spp. (Table VIII) (Brown *et al.*,

TABLE VIII

Prevalence of Naturally Occurring Uroliths in 168 Dogs with Bacterial Urinary Tract Infections[a]

Isolates	Number of dogs with UTI[b]	Number of dogs with struvite uroliths	Number of dogs with nonstruvite uroliths	Mean urine pH[c]
Escherichia coli	50	0	3	6.3
Staphylococcus aureus	48	39	1	7.8
Proteus mirabilis	35	10	0	7.9
Klebsiella pneumoniae	10	0	0	7.1
Staphylococcus epidermidis	3	1	0	6.5
Streptococci species	4	1	0	5.8
Pasteurella aeruginosa	1	0	1	6.0
Mixed infection	17	3	1	7.1
Total	168	54	6	

[a] All dogs had ≥ 10^5 bacteria per milliliter of urine.
[b] UTI, Urinary tract infection.
[c] Mean urine pH of dogs at the time of detection of urinary tract infection and uroliths.

1977a; Clark, 1974a; Finco *et al.*, 1970; Osborne and Klausner, 1978; Weaver and Pillinger, 1975), while *Proteus* spp. are most commonly associated with struvite uroliths in humans (Feit and Fair, 1979; Griffith and Klein, 1983; Krojden *et al.*, 1984; Lewi *et al.*, 1984; Stamey, 1980). In pilot studies of dogs performed in our laboratories at the University of Minnesota, we have had better success in experimentally inducing struvite uroliths with clinical isolates of staphylococci than with *Proteus* spp. (C. A. Osborne, 1984, unpublished data). Likewise, results of experimental studies in rats indicated that different strains of staphylococci had different calculogenic potentials (Vermuelen and Goetz, 1954). It is of interest that staphylococci were a predominantly reported isolate from human patients with urolithiasis 4 decades ago (Scott, 1975). It appears that some strains of *Proteus mirabilis* have special affinity for the urinary tract of human patients (Senior, 1979). Large numbers of urease-producing *Staphylococcus aureus* were isolated from urine and a calcium oxalate–calcium phosphate renolith removed from a 50-year-old man (Droller and Freiha, 1977). Struvite was not detected.

It is conceivable that differences in calculogenic activity of different uropathogenic microbes are related to differences in properties of urease produced by various microbes. It has been reported that urease produced by different microbes varies in activity, inducibility, optimum pH required for urease activity, and susceptibility to urease inhibitors (Rosenstein et al., 1981, 1984). Specific strains of *Proteus* spp. have been shown to produce characteristic isoenzymes (Senior et al., 1980). In one study of urease produced by *Proteus* spp. isolated from human patients, *P. morganii* was more resistant to the effects of acetohydroxamic acid and other urease inhibitors than *P. mirabilis, P. rettgeri*, and *P. vulgaris*.

Although other organisms such as *Klebsiella* spp. and *Pseudomonas* spp. have the potential to produce varying quantities of urease (Griffith, 1978a), they have not been as commonly associated with the initiation of struvite urolith formation in man or dogs (Table VIII). Likewise, *Escherichia coli* and other nonurease-producing microbes have not been linked to naturally occurring struvite uroliths, presumably because they infrequently produce urease (Griffith, 1978a; Leshler and Jones, 1978). However, it has been reported that urease activity may be transferred by bacterial plasmids (Grant et al., 1981).

Clinical and experimental studies indicate that infections with urease-producing bacteria, primarily staphylococci, often precede development of struvite uroliths in dogs. Evaluation of a litter of five miniature schnauzers that were the offspring of parents with recurrent struvite urolithiasis revealed that struvite uroliths developed in four by the time they were approximately 1 year old (Klausner et al., 1980a). Males and females were affected. A significant number of urease-producing staphylococci were isolated from the urine of three of four dogs prior to radiographic detection of uroliths, and from the urine of one dog 1 month following detection of uroliths. Periodic evaluation of serum electrolyte, urea nitrogen, creatinine concentration, and serum enzyme activity over a 26-month period revealed no abnormalities. Anatomic abnormalities that might predispose to urinary tract infection were not identified by radiography or necropsy studies. In one dog, bladder uroliths recurred following surgical removal of multiple cystoliths. In another, urethral and ureteral obstruction associated with acute generalized pyelonephritis induced a lethal uremic crisis. Gross and microscopic lesions detected by necropsy in all dogs with uroliths were typical of bacterial infection. In another study, inoculation of urease-producing staphylococci into the urinary bladders of normal beagles and miniature schnauzers related to parents with struvite urolithiasis resulted in formation of almost pure struvite uroliths in 8 of 13 dogs with staphylococcal urinary tract infections (Fig. 4) (Klausner et al., 1980b). Bladder uroliths were detected by abdominal survey radiography 2 to 8 weeks following infection of their urinary tracts. Abnormalities in systemic cell-mediated immunity were not detected in dogs before or after establishment of urinary tract infections. However, the design of the study precluded critical evaluation of local microbial defense mechanisms of the urinary tract of miniature schnauzers related to struvite urolith-forming parents.

Urease-producing bacteria have frequently been cultured from the interior of struvite uroliths removed from humans (Rocha and Santos, 1969; Thomas and Stamey, 1973) and dogs (Clark, 1974a; Klausner et al., 1977; Klausner et al., 1980b; Weaver and Pillmer, 1975), and occasionally from struvite uroliths removed from cats (Osborne et al., 1984a,b). Light microscopic examination of Gram-stained sections of uroliths removed from dogs and cats with urease-positive urinary tract infections frequently reveals Gram-positive cocci, presumably staphylococci (Figs. 13 and 21). In contrast, urease-producing bacteria have been uncommonly cultured from the interior of nonstruvite uroliths.

Bacteria that become trapped within struvite uroliths may remain viable for long periods. For example, we repeatedly (weekly for 3 months) isolated viable urease-producing staphylococci from the inner portions of struvite uroliths surgically removed from the urinary bladder of a female miniature schnauzer and incubated them at room temperature in a sterile container. Several studies have revealed that calculogenic bacteria harbored within uroliths are protected from the destructive effects of antimicrobial agents in urine (Fowler, 1984; Nemoy and Stamey, 1971; Rocha and Santos, 1969; Takeuchi et al., 1984).

After formation of struvite uroliths in dogs, as a result of staphylococcal urinary tract infections, the bacterial flora of urine may change. The change in bacterial flora may be associated with damage to local host defense mechanisms by uroliths, iatrogenic infection induced by urinary catheters, or administration of antimicrobial agents.

A small percentage of dogs with struvite urolithiasis have sterile urine. In some of these cases, however, bacteria have been isolated from the inside of calculi. This observation indicates that bacterial infection of the urinary tract may undergo spontaneous remission after initiating urolith formation in some patients.

In contrast to struvite uroliths, bacterial infection of the urinary tract is not a consistent finding in dogs with nonstruvite uroliths (ammonium urate, calcium oxalate, cystine, silica, etc.). When infection does occur in association with these so-called metabolic uroliths, it appears to be a sequela rather than a predisposing cause of urolith formation. The results of one clinical study in dogs were interpreted to indicate that secondary urinary tract infections were more commonly associated with cystine (25 or 53 cases) and urate (10 of 12 cases) uroliths than oxalate uroliths (none infected) (Brown *et al.,* 1977a).

E. UREAPLASMA URINARY TRACT INFECTIONS

T-mycoplasmas (or "tiny" mycoplasmas) differ from other mycoplasmas by their production of urease, and, therefore, their ability to hydrolyze urea (Shepard and Lunceford, 1967; Ford and MacDonald, 1967). Urea is required for growth of these organisms (Ford and MacDonald, 1967; Shepard and Lunceford, 1967). Urease produced by T-mycoplasmas is not homogeneous; it has at least three distinct isozymic forms (Delisle, 1977; Romano *et al.,* 1979). Because of their distinguishing property of producing urease, T-mycoplasmas have been assigned to a separate genus (*Ureaplasma*) within the Mycoplasmatales family (Shepard *et al.,* 1974). At least eight distinct serotypes of human *Ureaplasma urealyticum* have been identified (Shepard and Lunceford, 1978).

Ureaplasmas have been isolated from the urinary tract of humans (Birch *et al.,* 1981; MacDonald *et al.,* 1982; Petterson *et al.,* 1983; Taylor-Robinson *et al.,* 1977). There apparently has been little effort to isolate them from the urinary tracts of dogs, cats, and other species. Consideration of ureaplasmas as etiologic agents in struvite urolithiasis was catalyzed by the results of an experimental study in rats in which struvite uroliths were rapidly produced in male rat urinary bladders by intrarenal or intravesical injection of urease-producing ureaplasmas isolated from humans (Friedlander and Brude, 1974; Lamm *et al.,* 1977). For unexplained reasons, both viable and killed ureaplasmas appeared to have struvitogenic properties. Results of subsequent studies, however, indicate that viable ureaplasmas are the most calculogenic (Grenabo *et al.,* 1984).

Ureaplasma urealyticum has been isolated from struvite uroliths removed from the renal pelves of human patients (Hedelin *et al.,* 1984; Pettensson *et al.,* 1983). They could not be isolated from renoliths composed of calcium oxalate, calcium phosphate, or uric acid. We have repeatedly isolated large numbers of *Ureaplasma* from an adult female basset hound with uroliths presumed to be composed of struvite, and located in the renal pelves and urinary bladder (C. A. Osborne, 1984, unpublished data). Although the urine from this dog contained urease, urease-producing bacteria could not be isolated from it.

Preliminary efforts at the University of Minnesota to isolate ureaplasmas from urine of cats with struvite uroliths have been unsuccessful. Further studies are desirable, however, because ureaplasmas are fastidious and cell-associated. Factors reported to limit growth of ureaplasmas in broth cultures include pH > 7.5 (Ford and MacDonald, 1967; Shepard and Lunceford, 1965), osmotic activity > 600 mOsm/kg (Kenney and Cartwright, 1977), and high ammonia concentrations (Ford and MacDonald, 1967; Sayed and Kenney, 1978).

F. DIET

1. Infection Stones

The quantity of dietary protein catabolized for energy influences formation and dissolution of infection-induced struvite uroliths. Consumption of dietary protein in quantities that exceed daily protein requirements for anabolism results in the formation of urea from catabolism of amino acids. Hyperammonuria, hypercarbonaturia, and alkaluria mediated by microbial urease are dependent on the quantity of urea (the substrate of urease) in urine.

Abnormal urinary excretion of minerals as a result of an enhanced glomerular filtration rate, reduced tubular reabsorption, and/or enhanced tubular secretion is not required for initiation and growth of infection-induced uroliths. However, metabolic and anatomic abnormalities may indirectly induce struvite uroliths by predisposing to urinary tract infections (Table VII).

2. Sterile Stones

Clinical studies indicate that microbial urease is not involved in the formation of struvite uroliths in most cats and some dogs. Several observations suggest that dietary or metabolic factors may be involved in the genesis of sterile struvite uroliths in these species.

Pilot studies of clinical cases of struvite uroliths in dogs revealed a population of patients (9 of 20) whose urine was frequently alkaline, but did not contain identifiable bacteria, and did not contain detectable quantities of urease. Microscopic examination of demineralized Gram-stained sections of some struvite uroliths removed from dogs with bacteriologically sterile urine revealed no Gram-positive bacteria (Clark, 1974a; C. A. Osborne, 1984, unpublished data). Whereas infection-induced human struvite uroliths frequently contain calcium apatite or carbonate-apatite, a large number of the canine sterile uroliths were 100% struvite (Table IV).

Pilot studies performed in our laboratories revealed that the pH of urine of cats with naturally occurring struvite uroliths was commonly acid (pH 6.5) (C. A. Osborne, 1984, unpublished data). Their urine did not contain detectable bacteria or ureaplasma, and did not contain identifiable quantities of urease. Microscopic examination of demineralized Gram-stained sections of some sterile struvite uroliths did not reveal evidence of Gram-positive microbes. Unlike infection-induced struvite uroliths in man and dogs, the majority of sterile struvite uroliths removed from cats were 100% magnesium ammonium phosphate hexahydrate.

Results of experimental studies of cats also indicate that sterile struvite uroliths may be initiated by altering dietary composition. Four groups of investigators have reported convincing data concerning experimental production of magnesium phosphate and magnesium ammonium phosphate uroliths in cats consuming calculogenic diets (Chow et al., 1976; Jackson, 1972; Kallfelz et al., 1980; Lewis, 1981, 1983; Rich et al., 1974). Uroliths experimentally produced in cats by one group of investigators were similar in gross appearance and mineral composition to one subset of struvite uroliths commonly encountered in male and female cats with naturally occurring urolithiasis (Taton et al., 1984). Consumption, absorption, and excretion of comparatively high quantities of magnesium appeared to be one of the most important factors of the calculogenic diets, although other factors may also play a role. The calculogenic diets contained significantly more magnesium than was found in many commercially prepared cat foods (Kallfelz et al., 1980; Lewis et al., 1978). Uroliths produced during early experimental studies were composed of magnesium phosphate (Kallfelz et al., 1980; Lewis et al., 1978; Rich et al., 1974), while those produced in subsequent studies were found to contain magnesium, ammonium, and phosphate. Results of further studies indicate that the precise mineral composition of uroliths induced by dietary excess of magnesium is influenced by urine pH (Finco et al., 1984). Administration of a sufficient quantity of magnesium oxide alkalinizes urine produced by cats. Uroliths formed in this situation contain magnesium hydrogen phosphate trihydrate (newberyite) (C. A. Osborne, 1984, unpublished data) (Fig. 19). They are nearly devoid of ammonium ions. However, if the composition of the diet is modified so that urine of neutral pH is produced, uroliths composed of magnesium ammonium phosphate may be induced (Finco et al., 1984).

On the basis of currently available data, it appears that the composition of diets may play a primary role in the formation of sterile struvite uroliths in cats with naturally occurring urolithiasis. Further studies are required to confirm this hypothesis.

The relationship of diets to the formation of urethral plugs is not clear. Although dietary ingredients could contribute to the mineral component of urethral plugs, it is not known whether or not they contribute to the matrix component of urethral plugs. It is conceivable that formation of large quantities of crystalline material could stimulate production of matrix substances by tissues lining the urethral lumen. Hypercalciuria has recently been incriminated in the pathogenesis of hematuria in children (Stapleton et al., 1984). However, further studies are necessary before meaningful conclusions can be formulated about the etiopathogenesis of naturally occurring urethral plugs in cats. Progress to date has been hindered by lack of a reproducible model of feline lower urinary tract diseases characterized by urethral plug formation.

Formation of ruminant uroliths containing phosphate may be influenced by dietary factors. It has been difficult to interpret reports of ruminant urolithiasis because modern methods of quantitative urolith analysis have not been consistently utilized. Unfortunately, it has been common practice to refer to nonsiliceous uroliths in ruminants as "phosphate uroliths." However, available data indicate that ruminant phosphate uroliths often contain magnesium phosphate [$Mg_3(PO_4)_2$], calcium phosphate, and occasionally magnesium ammonium phosphate. Diets high in grains rather than roughage appear to be the most calculogenic (Johnston, 1981; Kimberling and Arnold, 1983; Sorensen, 1980; Udall et al., 1958; White and Porter, 1969). It has been suggested that hyperphosphaturia and alkaline urine pH associated with high grain diets predispose to the formation of uroliths with calcium, magnesium, and/or ammonium as cations, and phosphate as the anion. Administration of stilbestrol to stimulate growth of ruminants may contribute to urolith formation by increasing urinary mucoprotein (matrix) concentration (Udall and Jensen, 1958). The relationship of ruminant uroliths containing phosphates to urease-producing microbes is not clear. This association is deserving of further study since urinary tract infections with *Corynebacterium spp.* of bacteria are common in ruminants (Sorensen, 1980); some species of *Corynebacterium* produce urease (Gillespie and Timoney, 1981; Griffith, 1982). Urease-producing *Corynebacterium* spp. have been linked to struvite crystalluria in human patients (Cifuentes Delatte and Soriano, 1984).

In vitro studies consisting of addition of magnesium ($MgSO_4$), ammonium (NH_4 or NH_4Cl), or phosphate ($NH_4H_2PO_4$ or NaH_2PO_4) to sterile human urine ranging in pH from 5.0 to 9.6 revealed that struvite crystals could be induced in an acid or an alkaline environment (Boistelle et al., 1984). High ammonia concentrations were not necessary for formation of struvite crystals provided the concentration of $[Mg] \times [NH_4] \times [PO_4]$ was of sufficient magnitude at a given pH.

The applicability, if any, of these results to struvite urolith formation in dogs and cats in the absence of microbial urease is unknown.

G. ALKALINE URINE

Struvite is less soluble in alkaline than acid urine (Elliot et al., 1979; Burns and Finlayson, 1982). However, under physiologic conditions associated with alkaluria, urine contains low concentrations of ammonia (and, thus, ammonium ions) (Tannen, 1983). Thus, alkaline urine formed in the absence of ureolysis would not be expected to favor the formation of crystals that contain ammonia ions (such as magnesium ammonium phosphate hexahydrate). Clinical studies of naturally occurring urolithiasis in human patients support this generality (Griffith and Klein, 1983). Although oral administration of a sufficient quantity of sodium bicarbonate to alkalinize the urine of cats was reported to increase struvite crystalluria, it did not cause urolithiasis (Rich and Kirk, 1968).

Formation of persistently alkaline urine in the absence of urease-mediated ureolysis may predispose to the formation of uroliths containing hydroxylapatite [$Ca_{10}(PO_4)_6(OH)_2$], but not carbonate-apatite. Pathologic conditions that may result in this sequence of events include distal renal tubular acidosis (Coe and Favus, 1981; Thornhill, 1977), incomplete distal renal tubular acidosis (Backman et al., 1981), and perhaps primary hyperparathyroidism (Coe and Favus, 1981; Klausner et al., 1985). Since alkaline urine favors the dissociation of monobasic phosphate ($H_2PO_4^-$) to dibasic phosphate (HPO_4^{2-}) and phosphate ions (PO_4^{3-}), the formation of calcium phosphate is enhanced. Patients with distal renal tubular acidosis have an impaired ability to acidify urine that is associated with hypercalciuria and excretion of reduced concentrations of urine citrate (Coe and Favus, 1981; Dedmond and Wrong, 1962; Morrissey et al., 1963; Thornhill, 1977).

H. GENETICS

The high incidence of struvite urolithiasis in some breeds of dogs, such as miniature schnauzers, suggests a familial tendency. We hypothesize that susceptible miniature schnauzers inherit some abnormality of local host defenses of the urinary tract that increases their susceptibility to urinary tract infections (Klausner et al., 1980a,b). Hereditary factors thought to be associated with inbreeding have been reported to increase the incidence of struvite uroliths in beagles (Kasper *et al.*, 1978). The incidence of struvite uroliths was 10.7% in an inbred line of beagles as compared to only 2.0% in an outbred line of beagles.

The role of genetics, if any, in the formation of struvite uroliths in humans, cats, and other species is unknown.

I. Feline Urethral Plugs versus Feline Struvite Uroliths

1. Feline Urethral Plugs

a. Gross Appearance. Urethral plugs formed in male cats often resemble toothpaste that is forced through the narrowed, circular opening of a toothpaste tube (Figs. 11 and 22). Typical, soft, paste-like compressible plugs sometimes have a cylindrical shape when they are forced out of the external urethral orifice of male cats. At other times, they form a shapeless gelatinous mass. It is probable that their cylindrical shape, when present, is influenced by the distended urethral lumen and the shape of the external urethral orifice. Although urethral plugs may be readily distorted and compressed by external pressure, classical uroliths are rocklike in consistency.

b. Radiographic Appearance. The radiodensity of urethral plugs as compared to that of soft tissue has not been evaluated in a large population of male cats with confirmed urethral disorders associated with intraluminal plugs. One conceptual error has been a paucity of radiographic evaluation of naturally obstructed male cats. Even when survey and contrast radiographic studies have been performed, interpretation of negative findings has been complicated by the lack of verification that obstructing plugs were present within the urethral lumen. Results of clinical studies indicate that urethral plugs formed *in vivo* may be influenced by a variety of factors: (1) size, (2) location (within or exterior to the bony pelvis), (3) composition (ratio of mineral to matrix), (4) the quantity of tissue that must be penetrated by X rays, and (5) the radiographic technique used to evaluate them. It is well known that uroliths that are composed primarily of matrix (so-called matrix calculi) in humans and dogs are radiolucent because they have radiodensities similar to soft tissue.

c. Microscopic Appearance. Microscopic examination of a limited number of fresh plugs (composed of crystalline material and matrix) removed from the urethras of male cats during the initial episode of dysuria, fixed in formalin, and stained with hematoxylin and eosin or Gram's stain, failed to demonstrate Gram-positive bacteria within

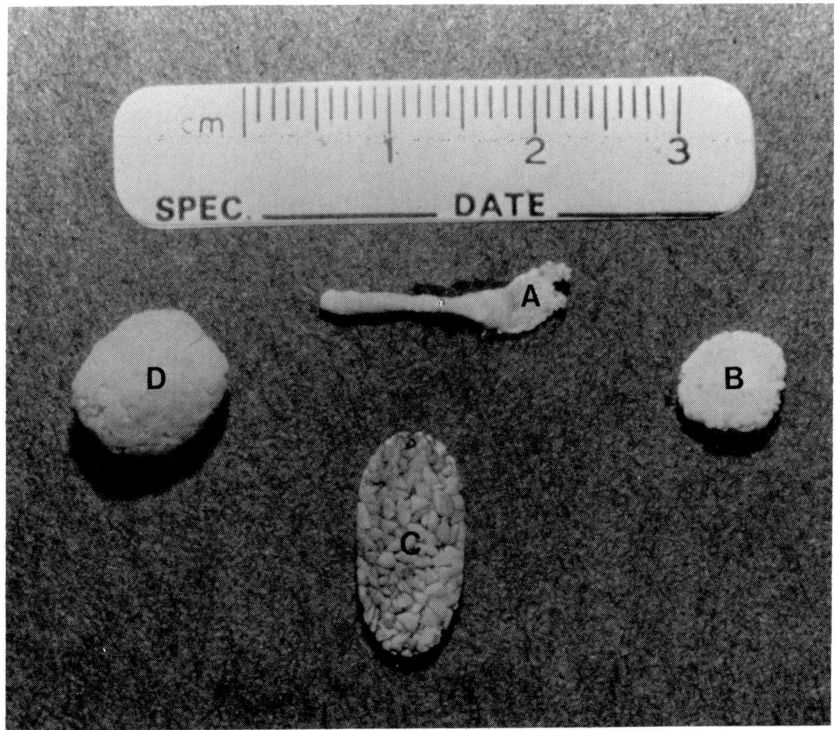

FIG. 22. Photograph of a urethral plug (A), two wafter-like sterile struvite uroliths (B and C), and an infection-induced struvite urolith (D) removed from the urinary tracts of male cats. One end of the urethral plug was crushed with an index finger to illustrate its friable nature. (From *Minn. Vet.*, 1982, **22**, 33–38.)

their matrix (Osborne *et al.*, 1984a). This observation suggests that urease-producing staphylococci were not involved in the initiation of urethral plug formation. Gram-positive bacteria have occasionally been identified in the matrix of classical feline struvite uroliths, and probably were involved in the initiation of their formation and maintenance of their growth (see Section I,2,c).

d. Mineral Composition. Although it has been generally accepted that male feline urethral plugs are composed of varying quantities of minerals and matrix, there have been only a few reports of the evaluation of the mineral composition of a limited number of plugs (Carbone, 1965; Rich and Kirk, 1968; Sutor and Wooley, 1970). Quantitative mineral analysis of 266 male feline urethral plugs submitted to the University of Minnesota by colleagues in private practice in North America revealed that 78% (205) were composed of 100% struvite; 13%

(35) were composed primarily (greater than 70%) of struvite, less than 2% (4) were composed primarily of calcium phosphate, less than 2% (3) were composed of calcium oxalate, and less than 1% (1) were composed of ammonium acid urate. About 4% (10) were composed almost entirely of matrix, and less than 2% were composed of a mixture of minerals. The infrequency with which nonstruvite minerals were recognized in urethral plugs suggests that they are not of great clinical importance. However, they are of great conceptual importance because they suggest that any type of crystal may become trapped in plug matrix. The importance of this observation is that it suggests that matrix may play an important primary role in the formation of some urethral plugs, whereas crystals may play a secondary role in their development.

e. Matrix Composition. When typical male feline urethral plugs are allowed to soak in solutions that are not supersaturated with calculogenic materials (water, physiologic saline solution, formalin, and lactated Ringer's solution), a portion of their crystalline components frequently migrates into the surrounding medium, leaving behind varying quantities of gelatinous substances that are presumed to be matrix. When classical uroliths are allowed to soak in such solutions, they occasionally become more friable, but there is no perceptible, visible change in their composition.

The specific composition and origin (urine and/or tissue surrounding the lumen of the urinary tract) of the matrix in urethral plugs have not been identified, nor has it been established whether or not matrix components of different plugs are consistently similar. It appears that most urethral plugs composed of matrix and crystalline material contain a similar type of as yet unidentified matrix.

The fact that urethral plugs are typically nonstructured with a paste-like consistency, and that they often have poor radiodensities indicates that they contain a substantially greater quantity of matrix than do classical uroliths. Future studies should focus on the origin(s) and composition of the matrix of urethral plugs.

f. Males versus Females. Although females develop naturally occurring classical uroliths almost as often as male cats (Osborne *et al.*, 1984d), available evidence indicates that urethral plugs composed of a large quantity of matrix and variable quantities of minerals are extremely uncommon in females (if they occur). The explanation of this difference is unknown. Although it is possible that plugs form in female cats and are voided during micturition, lack of detection of pluglike material in the feline lower urinary tract of females makes this explanation improbable. We are considering an alternative explanation related to sex differences in periurethral glandular tissue (Osborne et al., 1984b).

2. Feline Uroliths

a. Gross Appearance and Location. The gross appearance and consistency of classical uroliths commonly encountered in male and female cats, dogs, and humans are unquestionably different from feline urethral plugs that occur in male cats. Unlike urethral plugs, uroliths are not disorganized precipitates of crystalline material; they are typically composed of organized crystal aggregates with a complex internal structure.

The majority of uroliths observed in cats have occurred in the urinary bladder; however, on occasion small uroliths formed in the bladder have passed through, or obstructed, the urethra (Osborne et al., 1983a). Renoliths are less common than bladder uroliths in cats; ureteroliths have been rarely encountered.

Although uroliths removed from the urinary tracts of cats may assume any of a variety of shapes, many calculi located in the urinary bladders of cats have been shaped like wafers or disks (Figs. 18 and 22). Such uroliths are typically thicker at their center than at the periphery. The gross appearance of some of these uroliths resembles those induced with calculogenic diets (Osborne et al., 1984a).

b. Radiographic Appearance. Spherical uroliths with a diameter greater than 3 mm are usually radiodense when evaluated by survey radiography. However, since smaller uroliths frequently occur in the urinary bladders of cats, double contrast radiography may be required to detect their presence (Johnston et al., 1982). Flattened circular uroliths are also commonly encountered in the urinary systems of cats and are less radiodense than spherical uroliths of similar maximum circumference.

c. Microscopic Appearance. The microscopic appearance of the matrix of uroliths removed from cats is influenced by whether or not they were formed in association with urinary tract infections. Gram-positive bacteria cannot be identified in the inner portions of struvite uroliths formed in bacteriologically sterile urine. In contrast, large numbers of Gram-positive bacteria can be readily identified in the inner portions of struvite uroliths formed in infected urine, especially those associated with urease-producing staphylococci. On occasion, a combination of a Gram-negative struvite nidus surrounded by infected struvite laminations may occur (Figs. 23 and 24).

d. Mineral Composition. Uroliths similar in appearance to those

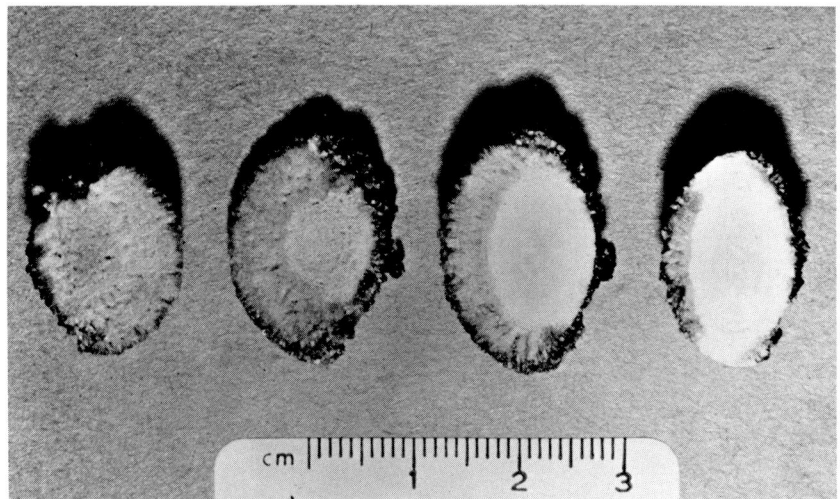

FIG. 23. Serial cross sections of a urolith removed from the urinary bladder of a 7-month-old female domestic shorthair cat. The nucleus and shell of this urolith were composed of 100% magnesium ammonium phosphate (see Fig. 24). (From *J. Am. Anim. Hosp. Assoc.* 1984, **20**, 17–32.)

encountered in dogs and other species have frequently been observed in the urinary systems of male and female cats. Struvite uroliths are the most common form of feline uroliths; ammonium urate, uric acid, calcium phosphate, and calcium oxalate uroliths occur less frequently (Table III) (Osborne *et al.*, 1984c).

In man and dogs, uroliths predominantly composed of struvite commonly contain smaller quantities of calcium apatite and/or carbonate-apatite (Griffith, 1978a; Klausner *et al.*, 1980a; Osborne *et al.*, 1984c). However, the majority of struvite uroliths in cats are pure (100%) magnesium ammonium phosphate (Table III). This observation supports the hypothesis that the initiation of one type of struvite urolith in cats is not linked to infection with urease-producing bacteria.

3. Conclusion

In summary, it appears that at least three different mechanisms may result in feline urinary struvite precipitates that are qualitatively similar, but quantitatively and etiologically dissimilar (Osborne *et al.*, 1984a,c). Formation of amorphous urethral plugs with a large quantity of matrix that is a result of as yet unidentified mechanisms is one form. Formation of sterile struvite uroliths, perhaps as a result of certain

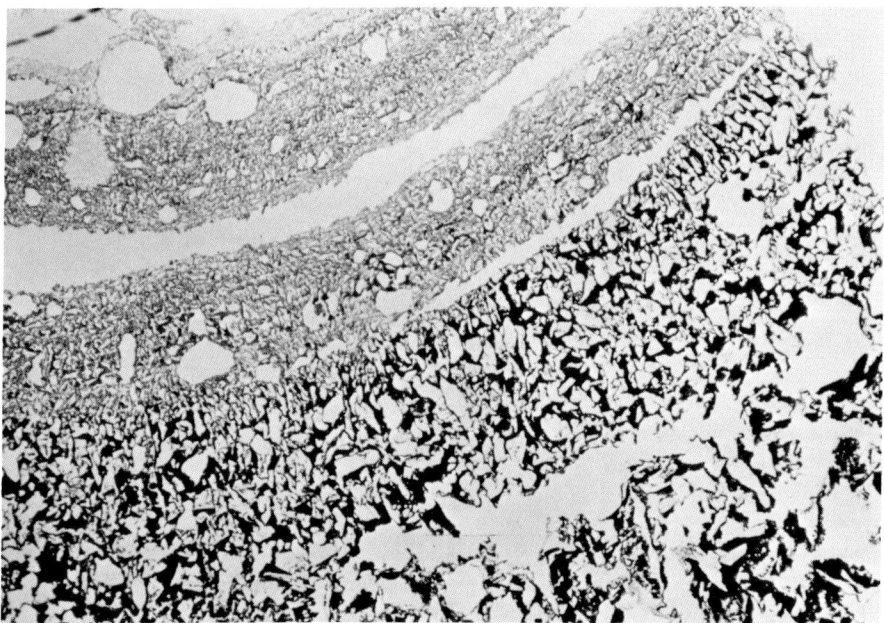

FIG. 24. Photomicrograph of a section of the urolith removed from the cat described in Fig. 23. The center portion of the urolith does not contain bacteria; the shell around the center portion contains a large quantity of Gram-positive material, presumably staphylococci. The sterile struvite urolith in the center appears to have predisposed to urinary tract infections with staphylococci, which caused infection-induced struvite to form an outer shell. Gram's stain; ×17.

dietary ingredients, is another form. Sterile struvite uroliths typically have less matrix than urethral plugs. Formation of "infected" or "urease" struvite uroliths as a sequela to urinary tract infections with urease-producing bacteria is a third form. Infection-induced feline struvite uroliths appear to contain more matrix than sterile uroliths, but typically contain less matrix than urethral plugs. A combination of a sterile struvite nidus that predisposes to urinary tract infections with urease-producing bacteria and subsequent formation of infected struvite laminations around the sterile nidus may also occur.

It is emphasized that not all feline uroliths are composed of struvite. Other mineral forms may also occur. Recognition and corroboration of these differences are of paramount importance to the clarification of the etiopathogenesis of feline lower urinary tract disorders and subsequent formation of effective forms of therapy and prevention.

J. BIOLOGICAL BEHAVIOR OF UROLITHS

1. Overview

Calculi may undergo spontaneous dissolution, remain active (growth occurs), or become inactive (no growth occurs). *Surgical activity* is defined as urolithiasis associated with colic, obstruction to urine outflow, or infection requiring surgical intervention (Smith, 1974). *Metabolic activity* occurs when one or more of the following are present: (1) radiographic evidence of stone growth within the past year, (2) radiographic evidence of a new stone growth within the past year, and (3) documented voiding of uroliths within the past year.

Intermediate activity is a term used to designate those situations in which radiographs are not available, or are inadequate to evaluate the status of urolithiasis during the past year. In a study of 101 consecutive human patients with calculi of intermediate activity, 64 (63%) were found to have inactive urolithiasis, while 37 (37%) had active urolithiasis (Smith, 1974).

The concept of metabolic activity is of prognostic and therapeutic relevance, especially if urolith treatment is likely to be associated with complications. Detection of a urolith is not always justification for medical or surgical management. Calculi may remain asymptomatic within the urinary tract, especially the renal pelvis, for months or years. However, the underlying cause(s) of uroliths and the sequelae of uroliths (partial or total obstruction, urinary tract infection) remain as potential hazards. In those situations in which uroliths are fortuitously detected in asymptomatic patients without significant bacteriuria, the option of monitoring urolith activity by appropriate procedures remains as an accepted option to surgery. If the urolith(s) remains inactive, therapy is not mandatory. If the urolith(s) becomes active, appropriate medical and/or surgical therapy are recommended.

2. Recurrence

Recurrence of struvite uroliths is a common event in all species. Unfortunately, the likelihood of recurrence following therapy is unpredictable. The rate and speed of recurrence of struvite uroliths may be influenced by several variables. Possibilities include (1) persistence of underlying causes of metabolic or infection-induced uroliths (Table IX), (2) failure to remove all uroliths from the urinary tract, including stones and stone fragments inadvertently left behind (pseudorecurrence) and microliths which are subvisual in size, (3) persistence or recurrence of urinary tract infections with calculogenic microbes, (4) surgical use of nonabsorbable suture material that is exposed to the

TABLE IX

CLASSIFICATION OF SOME IDENTIFIABLE CAUSES OF COMPLICATED
URINARY TRACT INFECTIONS

Causes	Potential for surgical correction
I. Interference with normal micturition	
A. Mechanical obstruction to outflow	
1. Calculi and strictures (especially of urethra)	++++
2. Herniated urinary bladder	++++
3. Prostatic cysts, abscesses, or neoplasms	++
4. Obstructing urothelial neoplasms	+
B. Incomplete emptying of excretory pathway	
1. Damaged innervation	
a. Vertebral fractures, luxations, subluxations	++
b. Intervertebral disc disease	++
c. Vertebral osteomyelitis	−
d. Neoplasia	++
e. Vertebral or spinal cord anomalies	±
f. Reflex dyssynergia	−
2. Anatomic defects	
a. Diverticula of urethra, bladder, ureters, renal pelves (especially urachal diverticula)	++++
b. Vesicoureteral reflux	+
II. Anatomic defects	
A. Congenital or inherited	
1. Urethral anomalies	++
2. Ectopic ureters	+++
3. Urachal diverticula	++++
4. Primary vesicoureteral reflux	+
B. Acquired	
1. Disease of the urinary tract, especially lower portions	++++
2. Secondary vesicourteral reflux	+
III. Alteration of urothelium	
A. Trauma	
1. External force	++
2. Palpation	−
3. Urachal diverticula	±
4. Urolithiasis	+
B. Metaplasia	
1. Administration of estrogens	−
2. Estrogen-producing sertoli cell neoplasms	+++
C. Neoplasia	++
D. Urinary excretion of cytotoxic drugs such as cyclophosphamide	−
E. Others	?

(*continued*)

TABLE IX (*Continued*)

	Causes	Potential for surgical correction
IV.	Alterations in the volume, frequency, or composition of urine	
	A. Decreased urine volume	
	1. Negative water balance	
	a. Decreased water consumption	−
	b. Vomiting and/or diarrhea	−
	2. Primary oliguric renal failure	−
	B. Voluntary or involuntary retention	+
	C. Glucosuria	−
	D. Formation of dilute urine[a]	−
	E. Others	?
V.	Impaired immunocompetence	
	A. Diseases	
	1. Congenital immunodeficiency?	−
	2. Acquired	
	a. Hyperadrenocorticism?	±
	b. Uremia	−
	B. Immunosuppressant drugs	−

[a] Formation of dilute urine predisposes the patient to lower urinary tract infections, but may prevent or minimize bacterial infections of the renal medulla.

lumen of the urinary tract, and (5) lack of owner or patient compliance with therapeutic or prophylactic recommendations.

Recurrent uroliths are usually similar in mineral composition to those present during the initial episode, except when a urinary tract infection with urease-producing microbes develops following removal of metabolic stones. In this circumstance, stones originally composed of ammonium acid urate, uric acid, calcium oxalate, calcium phosphate, cystine, or silica may be followed by struvite uroliths.

3. Biological Behavior in Dogs

The natural course of struvite urolithiasis has not been well documented in dogs. This is undoubtedly related to the fact that the two most common choices of management of urolithiasis have been surgical removal or euthanasia.

Clinical and experimental studies performed at the University of Minnesota revealed that struvite uroliths can form within 2 to 8 weeks following infection with urease-producing staphylococci (Klausner *et al.,* 1980a,b). Struvite uroliths associated with urinary tract infections caused by staphylococci or *Proteus* spp. have been detected in puppies as young as 5 weeks of age (Hardy *et al.*, 1972). Retrospective analysis of clinical cases of urolithiasis in immature dogs indicates that struvite uroliths are more common than metabolic uroliths (Hardy *et al.*, 1972).

Although spontaneous dissolution of uroliths appears to be uncommon, it can occur. We have observed five cases (two renoliths and three cystic uroliths) of struvite urolithiasis in dogs in which uroliths underwent spontaneous dissolution (Klausner and Osborne, 1979). Spontaneous dissolution of canine nephroliths has also been reported by others (Kirby *et al.*, 1983). Bilateral renal uroliths were reported to exist for approximately 4 years in a miniature schnauzer before causing death from renal failure (Pollack and Wagner, 1976).

Uroliths located in the urinary bladder commonly pass into the urethra. They commonly lodge behind the os penis in male dogs, but are frequently voided to the exterior by females (Fig. 6). Although renoliths are much less common in dogs than in man (Finco *et al.*, 1970), when formed they may pass into the ureters. The rapid rate at which struvite uroliths form, and the potential that they have to migrate to lower portions of the urinary tract are of clinical importance. If several days have elapsed between the date of diagnostic radiography and the date of surgery scheduled to remove uroliths, the number and location of the stones should be reevaluated by radiography.

Struvite uroliths have a tendency to recur following surgical removal or medical dissolution (Brodey, 1955; Brown *et al.*, 1977b; Clark, 1974b). In a recent retrospective survey of 438 dogs with urolithiasis, 111 patients had 155 known recurrences (Brown *et al.*, 1977b). Recurrence was observed in 17% of dogs with urate uroliths, 47% of dogs with cystine uroliths, and 25% of dogs with oxalate uroliths. Recurrence was most commonly detected within the first year following surgery. Although the highest prevalence of struvite uroliths was observed in females, the highest rate of recurrent struvite uroliths was observed in males. We have evaluated miniature schnauzers with more than seven known recurrences following surgery. However, most instances of multiple recurrences have been associated with poor control of recurrent urinary tract infections with urease-producing microbes. With the advent of effective therapeutic and preventative antimicrobial protocols to control recurrent or persistent urinary tract infections the frequency of recurrent struvite urolithiasis in dogs has declined.

To date, clinical studies of recurrence of canine uroliths have been based on postsurgical evaluations. The rate of recurrence following medical dissolution of canine struvite uroliths has not yet been evaluated in a large population of patients. However, preliminary observations indicate that the rate of recurrence is less frequent than that associated with surgery. In addition, time lapse between recurrent episodes is longer following medical dissolution. The apparent higher rate of recurrence associated with surgical removal of uroliths may be associated with inability to remove all uroliths, especially those located in inaccessible places and/or those that are subvisual in size. The tendency for uroliths to recur following surgery may also be associated with the persistence of an environment that favors initiation and growth of struvite at the time of removal.

4. Biological Behavior in Cats

The natural course of struvite urolithiasis has not been well documented in cats. Feline uroliths have been detected in cats ranging in age from 2 months to more than 16 years (Osborne et al., 1984d). We have observed spontaneous dissolution of naturally occurring bladder uroliths presumed to be struvite in two adult cats. In one, a 5-year-old female domestic shorthair, uroliths spontaneously dissolved 18 days following radiographic detection. Radiographic evidence of uroliths was not detected during seven monthly follow-up examinations. However on the eighth month, multiple urocystoliths were detected. Subsequently, they dissolved spontaneously during the next 3.5 months.

Uroliths that form in the urinary bladder may pass into the urethra of male or female cats (Fig. 4). Likewise, renoliths may pass into the ureters. Feline struvite uroliths have a tendency to recur. In one retrospective study of uroliths in cats, there were 25 known recurrences in 131 patients (Bohonowych et al., 1978). Twenty-one cats had two recurrent episodes, while three cats had three recurrences and one cat had four recurrences.

It is generally accepted that feline urethral plugs are associated with a frequent but unpredictable tendency to recur. However, this generally appears to be an overstatement since most investigators have considered urethral obstruction in male cats and struvite urethral plugs interchangably. Recent clinical studies, however, indicate that urethral obstruction in male cats may be initiated and maintained at one or more sites by one, or a combination of primary, secondary, and/or iatrogenic causes (Osborne et al., 1984a,b,c). Even in instances in which recurrent obstruction is caused by urethral plugs, there have been no studies specifically designed to evaluate comparisons of the nature and composition of first-occurrence plugs and recurrent obstructing material.

5. Biological Behavior in Man

The biologic behavior of struvite renoliths has been studied in human patients. As was the situation in dogs, struvite uroliths in humans may reach a large size within a few weeks (Griffith and Klein, 1983; de la Pena and de la Pena, 1944).

Uroliths in children are uncommon. When they occur, however, many are composed of struvite and carbonate-apatite, and form in association with urease-positive bacterial urinary tract infections (Bartone and Johnston, 1977; Carson and Malek, 1982; Marquardt and Naqel, 1977; Noronha et al., 1979; Sinno et al., 1977). Similar observations have been made in puppies.

Dissolution of struvite uroliths in humans is rare, but has been reported (Elliot, 1954). Failure to remove struvite renoliths by surgical procedures, percutaneous lithotripsy, nephrostomy irrigation, or shockwave lithotripsy is likely to result in progressive destruction of the affected kidneys due to a combination of infection and obstruction to urine outflow (Griffith, 1978a; Stamey, 1980). Persistent renoliths or fragments of renoliths have been commonly associated with persistent urinary tract infections, hematuria, and renal pain, and may lead to renal failure and/or systemic sepsis resulting in death (Rous and Turner, 1977; Singh et al., 1973; Wojewski and Zajaczkowski, 1973).

Surgical removal of struvite renoliths from human patients has been associated with a high rate of recurrence (30%) (Griffith, 1978a,b; Sutherland, 1954). Recurrence is commonly attributed to residual stone fragments which harbor urea-splitting organisms, persistent abnormalities that result in recurrent urinary tract infection, and use of indwelling urinary catheters (Nemoy and Stamey, 1971; Russell et al., 1981; Sutherland, 1981). Because of the high rate of morbidity associated with struvite renoliths in man, they are sometimes called "cancer stones" or "malignant stone disease" (Griffith, 1978a; Griffith et al., 1979).

K. Diagnosis

1. Overview

Uroliths are usually suspected on the basis of typical findings obtained by history and physical examination. Urinalyses, urine culture, and radiography may be required to differentiate uroliths from urinary tract infections, diverticula of the bladder, inflammatory polyps, and neoplasia (Table X).

TABLE X
Problem-Specific Data Base for Urolithiasis

1. Obtain appropriate history and perform physical examination, including rectal examination of urethra
2. Perform complete urinalysis; save aliquot for possible determination of mineral concentrations[a]
3. Perform complete blood count
4. Freeze aliquot of serum collected at time of venipuncture to obtain complete blood count for possible determination of urea nitrogen, creatinine, calcium and/or uric acid concentration
5. Obtain quantitative urine culture and determine urine urease activity; obtain antimicrobial susceptibility if bacterial pathogens are identified. Consider attempts to isolate ureaplasmas if urease-positive urine is bacteriologically sterile
6. Obtain radiographs
    a. Take survey radiographs of entire urinary system
    b. Consider IV urography for patients with renal or ureteral calculi
    c. Consider IV urography or contrast cystography for patients with bladder calculi
    d. Consider contrast urethrography for patients with urethral calculi
    3. Ultrasonography is recommended if equipment is available
7. Remove bladder or kidney biopsy specimens for microscopic examination during nephrotomy or cystotomy
8. Correct anatomic defects during surgical procedure performed to remove uroliths
9. Compare number of uroliths removed during surgery with number of uroliths identified by radiography; postsurgical radiographs should be obtained to evaluate completeness of urolith removal, if necessary
10. Save all uroliths for qualitative or quantitative analysis
11. Initiate therapy to promote dissolution or arrested growth of uroliths, if necessary
12. Initiate therapy to eradicate urinary tract infection
13. Initiate therapy to prevent recurrence of uroliths
14. Formulate follow-up protocol with clients

[a]The patient should be consuming food utilized at time of urolith formation. Alternately, a standardized diet designed to promote reproducible excretion of minerals in the urine of normal animals may be used.

A variety of methods have been used to evaluate the composition of uroliths including gross appearance (Tables V, VI, and VII), crystalluria (Table XI), radiographic appearance (Table XII), qualitative analysis, quantitative analysis, and urolith culture. Of these, quantitative analysis provides the most definitive diagnostic, prognostic, and therapeutic information. With the exception of qualitative chemical analysis, information gained by other methods of evaluation also may be of clinical value.

TABLE XI

CHARACTERISTICS OF SOME COMMON URINE CRYSTALS

Type	Appearance	pH where usually found		
		Acid	Neutral	Alkaline
Cholesterol	Flat colorless plates with corner notch	+	+	−
Calcium oxalate monohydrate	Small spindles, "hemp seeds" or dumbells	+	+	±
Calcium oxalate dihydrate	Small colorless envelopes (octahedral form)	+	+	±
Cystine	Flat colorless hexagonal plates	+	−	−
Magnesium ammonium phosphate	3- to 6-sided colorless prisms	±	+	+
Calcium phosphate	Amorphous, or long thin prisms	±	+	+
Ammonium urate	Yellow-brown spherulites; thornapples	−	±	+
Tyrosine	Fine, colorless or yellow needles arranged in sheaves or rosettes	+	−	−

2. Crystalluria

Crystalluria, by definition, is the appearance of crystals in urine. Routine laboratory procedures for detection of crystalluria are qualitative, not quantitative. Caution must be used in interpreting the significance of crystalluria because crystal formation is influenced by several *in vivo* and *in vitro* variables. *In vivo* variables include (1) the concentration of crystallogenic substances in urine (which in turn is influenced by their rate of excretion and urine concentration of water), (2) urine pH, (3) the solubility of crystallogenic substances in urine, and (4) excretion of medications (such as sulfonamides and ampicillin).

In vitro variables include (1) temperature, (2) evaporation, (3) pH, and (4) the technique of specimen preparation (i.e., centrifugation versus noncentrifugation, volume of urine examined, etc.). Significant *in vitro* changes which occur following urine collection may enhance formation or dissolution of crystals. When knowledge of *in vivo* urine crystal type and quantity is especially important, fresh specimens

TABLE XII

Typical Radiographic Characteristics of Uroliths Commonly Encountered in Dogs and Cats

Mineral type	Degree of radiopacity	Shape
Cystine[a]	+ to ++	Smooth, usually small, round to oval
Oxalate	++++	Usually rough, round to oval
Magnesium ammonium phosphate (struvite)	+ to ++++	Smooth, round or faceted, often wafer-shaped in cats; sometimes assume shape of renal pelvis, ureter, bladder, or urethra, especially in dogs; sometimes laminated
Calcium phosphate (calcium apatite)	++++	Smooth, round or faceted
Ammonium urate and uric acid	0 to ++	Smooth, round or oval; sometimes jackstone, especially in cats
Silica[a]	++ to ++++	Typically jackstone
Mixed	+ to ++++	Varies with composition; may have detectable nucleus and shell
Matrix	0 to +	Usually round, but may be influenced by location

[a]Not yet reported in cats.

should be examined. Ideally, they should be at body temperature. If this is not possible, they should be at room temperature, and not at refrigeration temperature.

Care must be used not to overinterpret or underinterpret the significance of crystalluria. Because crystals only occur in urine that is supersaturated with crystallogenic substances, it represents a risk factor for urolithiasis. However, in most instances, crystalluria that occurs in association with an anatomically and functionally normal urinary tract is harmless. Identification of crystals in such patients does not justify therapy. On the other hand, detection of some types of crystals, or large aggregates of others, may be of diagnostic, prognostic, and/or therapeutic importance. For example, ammonium urate crystalluria may be indicative of portal vascular anomalies or primary hepatic disorders. Calcium oxalate monohydrate and calcium oxalate dihydrate crystalluria may occur in dogs with ethylene glycol toxicity or hypercalcemia; cystine crystalluria is pathognomonic of cystinuria.

Although there is not a direct relationship between crystalluria and urolithiasis, detection of crystals in urine is proof that the urine sample is oversaturated with crystallogenic substances. As previously emphasized, however, oversaturation may occur as a result of *in vitro* events in addition to *in vivo* events. In addition, crystalluria may be influenced by diet (including water). Urine crystal formation, which occurs while patients are consuming hospital diets, may be dissimilar to urine crystal formation which occurs while patients are consuming diets fed at home.

With the advent of medical therapy to induce dissolution of struvite (magnesium ammonium phosphate) uroliths in dogs and cats, the clinical significance of crystalluria has increased. When formulating therapy for medical dissolution of uroliths, knowledge of mineral composition is extremely important. However, since a medical approach to therapy precludes surgical collection of uroliths, one is forced to make a "guesstimate" of their mineral composition on the basis of available clinical data. The only exception to this generality is the availability of one or more uroliths voided through the urethra. In addition to evaluation of pertinent aspects of the history, physical examination, complete urinalysis (including sediment), urine culture, serum chemistries (especially calcium, phosphorus, uric acid, chloride, and bicarbonate), and radiography, it may be of value to attempt to prepare a large pellet of crystals by centrifugation of a large volume (25 to 100 ml) of urine in a conical-tipped centrifuge tube. Evaluation of the pellet of sediment by quantitative methods designed for urolith analysis may provide meaningful clues about urolith composition.

It is emphasized that detection of crystalluria is not synonymous with urolithiasis, nor is it irrefutable evidence of urolithiasis or a stone-forming tendency. In addition, identification of urine crystals should not be relied upon as definitive identification of the mineral composition of uroliths. The latter should be determined by quantitative urolith analysis.

Magnesium ammonium phosphate hexahydrate crystals typically appear as orthorhombic coffin-like prisms in dogs (Table I) (Fig. 16). In cats, they often appear as flattened (or plate-like) prisms. They are variable in size, and may have square or rectangular dimensions (Osborne and Stevens, 1981). Struvite crystals may develop a feathery appearance as they go into solution.

In humans with oxalate urolithiasis, there is a tendency for oxalate crystals to occur in increased numbers and to aggregate together (Cifuentes Delatte, 1983; Werness *et al.*, 1981). There have been no quantitative studies of crystalluria or crystal aggregation in dogs or cats with struvite urolithiasis.

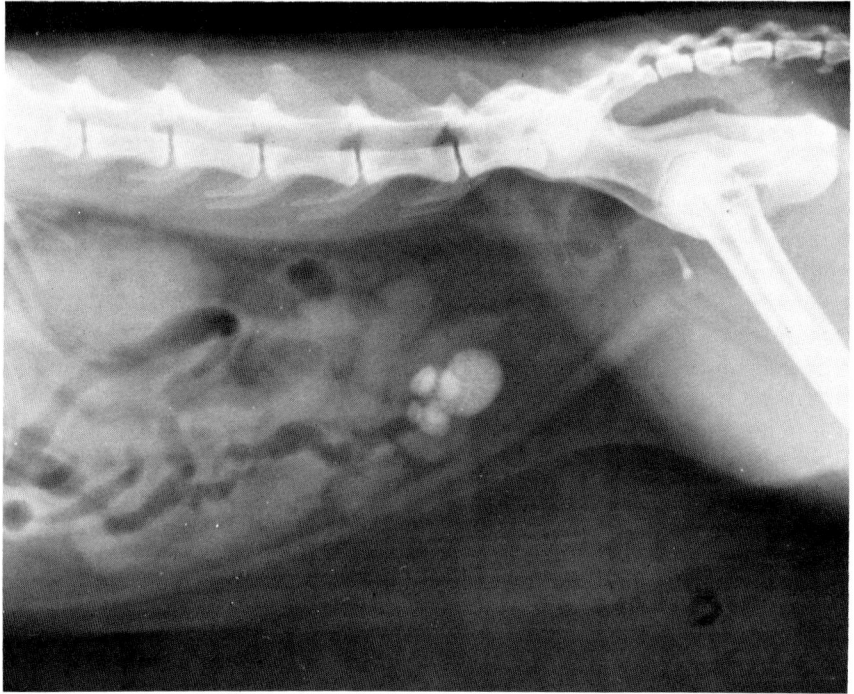

FIG. 25. Laterial view of a survey abdominal radiograph of a 7-year-old male domestic shorthair cat with multiple staphylococcal-induced struvite uroliths in the urinary bladder.

3. Radiographic Characteristics

The primary objective of radiographic evaluation of patients suspected of having uroliths is to determine the site(s), number, density, and shape of calculi. Once urolithiasis has been confirmed, radiographic evaluation is also an important technique to detect predisposing abnormalities.

The radiographic appearance of uroliths is influenced by their size, number, location, and mineral composition. Most uroliths have varying degrees of radiodensity, and therefore can be detected by survey abdominal radiography (Fig. 25) (Table XII). Very small uroliths (less than approximately 3 mm) may not be visualized by survey radiography. Oxalate, phosphate, and silica uroliths are typically, but not invariably, more radiodense than cystine and urate calculi. Urate uroliths may be radiolucent, but usually are radiodense. Because of significant variation, the radiodensity of uroliths is not a reliable index of mineral composition.

Uroliths must be differentiated from: (1) nephrocalcinosis associated with dystrophic or metastatic calcification of the renal parenchyma, (2) radiodense medications or ingesta in the gastrointestinal system, (3) calcified mesenteric lymph nodes, (4) osseous metaplasia of transitional epithelium or mineralization of a neoplasm, (5) radiodensities in the gall bladder (uncommon in dogs and cats), and (6) large thelia in female dogs. Calcifications of the renal parenchyma typically are in the proximity of, but not within, the renal pelvis. Radiodense calculi within the excretory pathway may disappear or become radiolucent following excretion of radiopaque contrast agents. Radiodense objects outside the excretory pathway remain radiodense.

In our experience, radiolucent uroliths are uncommon in dogs. Uric acid uroliths in humans are typically radiolucent. However, in our experience, most (but not all) ammonium acid urate uroliths of dogs are radiodense. This may be related to a variable quantity of phosphates in urate uroliths of dogs. Matrix uroliths may be radiolucent or have some radiodensity. They have not been commonly recognized in dogs, but may occur in cats. Blood clots are radiolucent and may be mistaken for radiolucent uroliths. Radiolucent uroliths may be detected with the aid of positive contrast, or double contrast radiography, or by ultrasonography.

Uroliths which appear radiodense by survey radiography may appear to be radiolucent when evaluated by positive contrast radiography (Fig. 26). This is so because many caluli are more radiodense than body tissue, but less radiodense than the contrast material. A diagnosis of radiolucent stones should be based on their radiodensity as compared to body tissues, and not their radiodensity as compared to positive-contrast material.

It is possible for a urolith to be larger than that depicted by its radiodensity if only a portion of it contains radiodense minerals. This phenomenon is most likely to occur with rapidly growing struvite uroliths.

4. Analysis of Uroliths

The location of the uroliths removed from the urinary tract should be recorded, in addition to their size, shape, color, and consistency. All uroliths should be saved in a container (preferably a sterile one) for future analysis. Do not give uroliths to owners. One or more uroliths may be placed into a container of 10% buffered formalin if microscopic examination is desired.

Because many uroliths contain more than one mineral component, it is important to examine representative portions. The mineral composi-

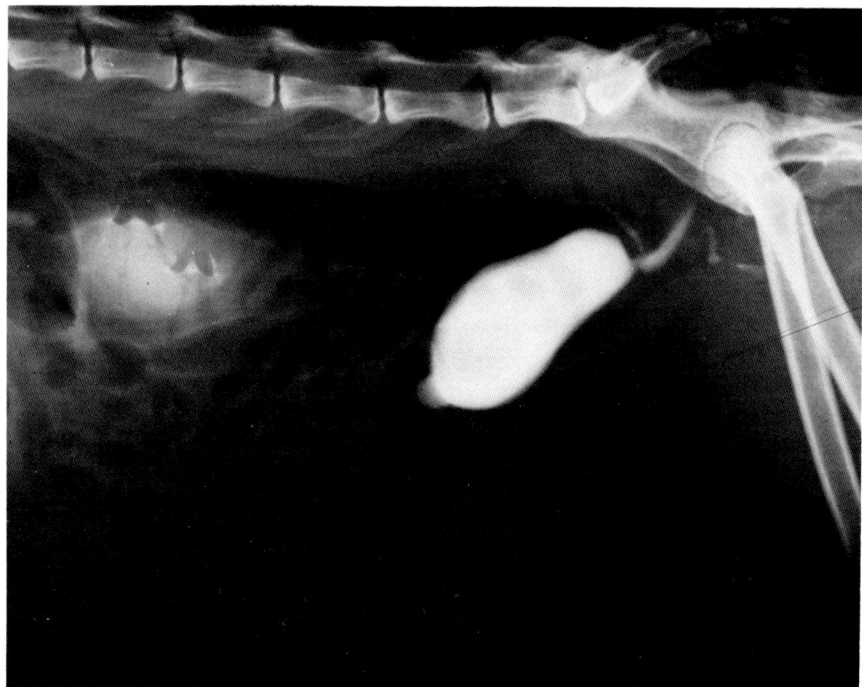

Fig. 26. Lateral view of an intravenous urogram of the cat described in Fig. 25. The uroliths appear less dense than the contrast medium in the bladder lumen. Note the diverticulum located at the vertex of the bladder wall. It is probable that the diverticulum was the predisposing cause of staphylococcal urinary tract infection, which in turn predisposed to struvite urolithiasis.

tion of crystalline nuclei may be identical or different from the remainder of calculi. The nuclei of uroliths should be analyzed separately from outer zones when possible, since the underlying cause of their presence may be suggested by knowledge of the mineral composition of the nuclei (Figs. 7 and 12).

We do not recommend analysis of uroliths by single qualitative chemical analysis. The major disadvantage of this procedure is that only some of the chemical radicals and ions can be detected. In addition, the proportions of the different chemical constituents in the urolith cannot be quantified. One kit commonly used by veterinarians and veterinary laboratories is the Oxford Stone Analysis set.[1] In our

---

[1]Oxford Stone Analysis Set, Oxford Laboratories, 107 North Bayshore Blvd., San Mateo, California 94401.

TABLE XIII

Comparison of Results of Quantitative[a] and Qualitative[b] Methods of Analysis in Detecting Minerals Present in 223 Canine Uroliths

Quantitative analysis		Qualitative analysis	
		Agreement with quantitative analysis	
Mineral type	Number of uroliths[c]	Number	Percentage
Magnesium ammonium phosphate	196	193	98.5
Calcium phosphate[d]	106	3	2.8
Calcium oxalate[e]	11	7	63.6
Ammonium acid urate	18	15	83.3
Sodium acid urate	2	0	0
Uric acid	0	0	0
Cystine	5	4	80

[a] Optical crystallography and X-ray diffraction techniques were used for quantitative analysis.

[b] The Oxford Stone Analysis Kit was used for qualitative analysis.

[c] The total number of stones containing various minerals exceeds 223 because 109 contained only one mineral, 110 contained 2 minerals, and 3 contained 3 minerals.

[d] All uroliths in this group contained calcium apatite; brushite and whitlockite were not detected.

[e] No distinction between calcium oxalate monohydrate and calcium oxalate dihydrate was made in this table since the qualitative method of analysis was not designed to distinguish between these two mineral types.

experience, this chemical kit is unreliable for accurate detection of the composition of uroliths (Table XIII). It is not designed to detect infrequently occurring uroliths, including those composed of silica or xanthine. The kit is also unreliable for consistently detecting calcium in uroliths, and may give false positive results.

In contrast to chemical methods of analysis, physical methods have proven to be far superior for the identification of crystalline substances. They also permit differentiation of various subgroups of minerals (i.e., calcium oxalate monohydrate and calcium oxalate dihydrate, or uric acid and ammonium acid urate), and allow semiquantitative determinations of various mineral components. Physical methods commonly used by laboratories[2] which specialize in

[2] Urolithiasis Laboratory, P.O. Box 25375, Houston, Texas 77055. Veterinary Teaching Hospital, School of Veterinary Medicine, University of California, Davis, California 95616.

quantitative urolith analysis include a combination of polarizing light microscopy, X-ray diffractometry, infrared spectroscopy, and thermogravimetry. Some laboratories are also equipped to perform elemental analysis with an energy-dispersive X-ray microanalyzer (EDX). On occasion, chemical methods of analysis and paper chromatography may be used to supplement information provided by the physical methods mentioned.

We recommend that veterinarians utilize the services provided by laboratories equipped to provide quantitative urolith analysis. At this time, most (but not all) veterinary clinical pathology and veterinary diagnostic laboratories are not equipped to provide quantitative urolith analysis. Caution must be used to avoid irrevocable loss of uroliths by unreliable qualitative chemical studies. If qualitative studies are performed, representative uroliths should be saved for subsequent quantitative analysis. Although the cost of quantitative urolith analysis is about double that of qualitative analysis (approximately $10 versus $20), it is minute as compared to the costs caused by patient mismanagement based on erroneous results.

5. *Urolith Culture*

Bacteria harbored inside uroliths are not always the same as those present in urine. Bacteria detected within uroliths probably represent those present at the time the stone was formed, and may serve as a source of recurrent urinary tract infection. Bacteria may remain viable within the uroliths for long periods. In a pilot study, we were able to culture viable staphylococci from struvite uroliths removed from a miniature schnauzer up to 3 months following surgery. When all the uroliths cannot be removed from the patient, knowledge of the type of associated bacterial pathogens and their antimicrobial susceptibility may be of therapeutic significance.

We use the following procedure to sterilize the outside of uroliths so that the inner aspect may be cultured (Rocha and Santos, 1969). (1) Place uroliths in an alcoholic solution of 3% iodine for 2 hr. (2) Wash uroliths with 1000 ml of sterile physiologic saline solution. (3) Culture the last portion of the saline in contact with the surface of the urolith by inoculating 1 ml into 9 ml of trypticase soy broth. (4) Crush the uroliths with a sterile mortar and pestle and add a small quantity of sterile physiologic saline solution to the crushed crystalline material. (5) Inoculate 1 ml of the saline–calculi suspension into 9 ml of trypticase soy broth. (6) Incubate the broth tubes at 37°C for 48 hr. (7) Make appropriate subcultures utilizing blood agar and MacConkey agar plates.

Detection of bacterial growth in the saline that contacted the surface of the uroliths indicates inadequate sterilization and invalidates the results of culture of the crushed calculi. Baterial growth in saline mixed with crushed calculi, but not in saline in contact with the surface of calculi, indicates that the organisms were within the calculi. Antimicrobial susceptibility tests may be performed on bacteria isolated from the inside of calculi, especially if they are different from those isolated from the urine.

L. MEDICAL MANAGEMENT OF STRUVITE UROLITHIASIS

1. Overview

Therapy of struvite urolithiasis encompasses (1) relief of obstruction to urine outflow when necessary, (2) elimination of existing uroliths, (3) eradication or control of urinary tract infections, and (4) prevention of recurrence of uroliths. Detailed descriptions of nonsurgical and surgical methods of reestablishing urine outflow are beyond the scope of this discussion, but are available elsewhere (Osborne et al., 1985; Smith, 1982). Likewise, details pertaining to surgical removal of uroliths (Osborne et al., 1985; Resnick, 1983; Roth, 1976; Stone, 1984), endoscopic and percutaneous manipulation of uroliths (Castinada-Zuniga, 1982; Drach, 1983), chemolysis via nephrostomy (Dretler and Pfister, 1983; Sheldon and Smith, 1982; Smith and Lee, 1983), disintegration of renal and ureteral uroliths via ultrasound (Alken, 1982; Marberg, 1983), and shock wave lithotripsy (Chaussy and Schmiedt, 1983) have been described.

The objective of the following discussion is to provide the rationale and effectiveness of noninvasive medical protocols designed to induce struvite urolith dissolution. As with all forms of therapy, cautious and careful judgment is in order. The unpredictable and erratic rate at which uroliths form, grow, recur following removal, and undergo dissolution mandates carefully designed and controlled experimental trials before a particular regimen of therapy is judged to be of benefit. The following recommendations should not be used as a standardized approach to treatment, since no two patients have identical therapeutic needs. Within the guidelines outlined herein, individualization of therapy is essential.

2. Indications

Surgery has been a time-honored approach for management of all types of urolithiasis in dogs, cats, and other species of animals. Although surgery has been an effective method that provides immediate elimination of uroliths, it is associated with several limitations. These include (1) persistence of underlying causes and a high rate of recurrence of uroliths despite surgery, (2) patient factors that enhance adverse consequences of general anesthesia or surgery, and (3) inability to remove all uroliths or fragments of uroliths during surgery. In addition, situations occasionally arise in which owners of companion animals will not consent to surgical therapy, but will consider medical therapy. For these and other reasons (i.e., the urolith is asymptomatic), an effective noninvasive medical regimen that will induce urolith dissolution has been a desired but elusive goal. However, results of several experimental and clinical investigations support the feasibility of medical dissolution of uroliths, especially canine and feline struvite uroliths (Abdullahi *et al.*, 1984; Krawiec *et al.*, 1984a,b; Osborne *et al.*, 1982, 1984c,d,e,f,g) and possibly canine ammonium urate uroliths (Osborne *et al.*, 1984f).

Despite the feasibility of dissolution of some types of uroliths, it is emphasized that this form of therapy is associated with potential hazards. Uroliths represent a predisposing cause of urinary tract infections, and are always a predisposition to obstructive uropathy. Both risks and benefits of medical versus surgical therapy must be considered for each patient (consult Section V, M for additional information).

3. Objectives

The objectives of medical management of uroliths are to arrest further urolith growth and/or to promote urolith dissolution by correcting or controlling underlying abnormalities. For therapy to be effective, it must induce undersaturation of urine with calculogenic crystalloids by (1) increasing the solubility of crystalloids in urine, (2) increasing the volume of urine in which crystalloids are dissolved or suspended, and (3) reducing the quantity of calculogenic crystalloids in urine. For example, attempts to increase the solubility of crystalloids in urine often include administration of medications designed to change urine pH, in order to create a less favorable environment for crystallization. Likewise, induction of diuresis is a method commonly used to increase the volume of urine in which crystalloids are dissolved or suspended. Examples of methods to reduce the quantity of calculogenic crystalloids in urine include changes in diet, administration of allopurinol to decrease the formation of uric acid, and administration of cellulose phosphate to minimize intestinal absorption of calcium.

These objectives may be hampered because the underlying causes, and therefore the treatment, of different types of uroliths are dissimilar. They may also be hampered by uroliths that are not homogeneous in composition. This has not been a significant problem in dogs with uroliths composed primarily of magnesium ammonium phosphate and, to a lesser degree, of calcium phosphate, because the solubility characteristics of the two minerals are similar. However, it is logical to expect difficulty in attempting to induce dissolution of a urolith with a nucleus of cystine or silica (Fig. 8) and a shell of struvite, because the solubility characteristics of these two minerals are dissimilar. This phenomenon should be considered if medical therapy seems to become ineffective after initially reducing the size of a urolith.

4. Definition of Urolith Composition

Formulation of therapy to reduce the composition of specific calculogenic crystalloids in urine is dependent on knowledge of the composition of uroliths. For example, administration of D-penicillamine would be of no benefit to patients with calcium oxalate uroliths. Likewise, administration of ascorbic acid, a commonly used acidifier, might potentiate calcium oxalate urolithiasis, since it is a precursor of oxalic acid. In situations in which consideration is being given to medical therapy, but uroliths are not available for analysis, one may be forced to make an educated guess about their composition (Table XIV).

5. Increasing Urine Volume

Diuresis induced by augmenting water consumption is a logical method to decrease the urine concentration of calculogenic substances. It has been a time-honored component of protocols to dissolve and prevent uroliths. However, there have been no controlled studies in dogs or cats with naturally occurring uroliths that document its efficacy. In fact, we have been successful in inducing dissolution of presumed struvite uroliths in cats by dietary alteration that did not augment urine volume (Osborne *et al.*, 1984e).

A potential hazard in inducing diuresis in patients that have urolithiasis associated with urinary tract infections is that it may reduce the concentration of pharmacologic or host-produced antimicrobial agents in the urine (Lees *et al.*, 1981; Osborne *et al.*, 1979). In addition, if compensatory polyuria is stimulated by augmenting thirst with orally administered sodium chloride, hypertension-prone patients may be adversely affected. The therapeutic value of induced diuresis in the treatment of urolithiasis should be reevaluated by appropriately controlled experimental and clinical studies.

TABLE XIV

CHECKLIST OF FACTORS THAT MAY AID IN GUESSTIMATION OF
MINERAL COMPOSITION OF UROLITHS

1. Radiographic density and physical characteristics of uroliths

2. Urine pH
   a. Struvite and calcium apatite uroliths—usually alkaline in dogs. Sterile struvite commonly occurs at a pH of 6.5 in cats.
   b. Ammonium urate uroliths—variable
   c. Cystine uroliths—acid
   d. Calcium oxalate—variable
   e. Silica—variable

3. Identification of crystals in uncontaminated fresh urine sediment, preferably at body temperature

4. Type of bacteria, if any, isolated from urine
   a. Urease-producing bacteria, especially staphylococci and less frequently *Proteus* spp., are typically associated with canine struvite uroliths. Less commonly, urease-producing staphylococci cause feline uroliths. Ureaplasmas may cause struvite uroliths
   b. Urinary tract infections are often absent in patients with calcium oxalate, cystine, ammonium urate, and silica uroliths
   c. Calcium oxalate, cystine, ammonium urate, and silica uroliths may predispose patients to urinary tract infections; if infections are caused by urease-producing bacteria, struvite may precipitate around metabolic uroliths

5. Serum chemistry evaluation
   a. Hypercalcemia may be associated with calcium-containing uroliths
   b. Hyperuricemia may be associated with uric acid or urate uroliths
   c. Hyperchloremia, hypokalemia, and acidemia may be associated with distal renal tubular acidosis and calcium phosphate uroliths

6. Urine chemistry evaluation
   a. Patient should be consuming a standardized diagnostic diet, or the diet consumed when uroliths formed
   b. Although no controlled studies have been performed in dogs or cats, excessive quantities of one or more minerals contained in the urolith are expected

7. Breed of dog and history of occurrence of uroliths in patient's ancestors or littermates

8. Analysis of uroliths fortuitously passed and collected during micturition

6. Canine Struvite Urolithiasis

a. Overview. Current recommendations include (1) eradication or control of urinary tract infections with appropriate antimicrobial agents, (2) use of calculolytic diets, (3) induction of diuresis *if* polyuria does not occur in patients who maintain their uroliths while consuming calculolytic diets, (4) administration of urine acidifiers *if* antimicrobial agents and calculolytic diets do not result in formation of acid urine, and (5) administration of urease inhibitors (acetohydroxamic acid) to patients with persisitent urinary tract infections caused by urease-producing microbes (Table XV).

b. Eradication or Control of Urinary Tract Infections. The importance of urinary tract infections with urease-producing bacteria in the formation of most struvite uroliths in dogs emphasizes the importance of therapy to eliminate or control them. Because of the quantity of urease produced by bacterial pathogens, it may be impossible to acidify urine with urine acidifiers administered at dosages which prevent systemic acidosis (Musher *et al.*, 1974a). Therefore, sterilization of urine appears to be an important prerequisite for creating a state of struvite undersaturation that may prevent further growth of uroliths, or that promotes their dissolution.

Appropriate antimicrobial agents selected on the basis of susceptibility or minimum inhibitory concentration tests should be used at therapeutic dosages. That diuresis reduces the urine concentration of the antimicrobial agent should be considered when formulating antimicrobial dosages (Ling and Hirsh, 1983). Antimicrobial agents should be administered as long as the uroliths can be identified by survey radiography. This recommendation is based on the fact that bacterial pathogens harbored inside uroliths may be protected from antimicrobial agents. Whereas the urine and surface of calculi may be sterilized following appropriate antimicrobial therapy, the original infecting organisms may remain viable below the surface of the urolith. Discontinuation of antimicrobial therapy may result in relapse of bacteriuria and infection.

Although use of antimicrobial agents alone may result in dissolution of struvite uroliths in some patients, experimental studies of rats (Lamm *et al.*, 1977) and dogs (C. A. Osborne, 1984, unpublished data), and clinical studies of humans (Feit and Fair, 1979; Lewis *et al.*, 1983; Stamey, 1980) and dogs (C. A. Osborne, 1984, unpublished data) indicate that this phenomenon represents the exception rather than the rule. In addition to the unpredictable response to this form of therapy, the time required to induce urolith dissolution with antimicrobial agents is usually measured in months rather than in weeks.

TABLE XV

Summary of Recommendations for Medical Dissolution of Canine Struvite Uroliths

A. Adult dogs with urinary tract infections
   1. Perform appropriate diagnostic studies including complete urinalyses, quantitative urine culture, and diagnostic radiography. Determine precise location, size, and number of uroliths. The size and number of uroliths are not a reliable index of probable efficacy of therapy

   2. If available, determine mineral composition of uroliths. If unavailable, guesstimate their composition by evaluation of appropriate clinical data (Table XIV)

   3. Consider surgical correction if uroliths are obstructing urine outflow, and/or if correctable abnormalities predisposing to recurrent urinary tract infections are identified by radiography or other means

   4. Eradicate or control urinary tract infections with appropriate antimicrobial agents. Maintain antimicrobial therapy during, and for 3 to 4 weeks following, urolith dissolution

   5. Initiate therapy with calculoytic diets. No other food or mineral supplements should be fed to the patient. Compliance with dietary recommendations is suggested by reduction in SUN concentration (usually ≤ 10 mg/dl)

   6. Feed patients calculolytic diets for 1 month following the disappearance of uroliths as detected by survey radiography

   7. If possible, avoid diagnostic follow-up studies requiring urinary catheterization

   8. Consider administration of acetohydroxamic acid (25 mg/kg/day divided into two equal doses) to patients with persistent urease-producing microburia, despite use of antimicrobial agents and calculoytic diets

   9. Devise a protocol for periodic follow-up including
      a. Serial urinalyses. Urine pH, specific gravity, and microscopic examination of sediment for crystals are especially important. Remember, crystals formed in urine stored at room or refrigeration temperatures may represent artifacts
      b. Serial radiography at monthly intervals to evaluate stone location(s), number, size, density, and shape
      c. Quantitative urine culture where indicated

B. Adult dogs with sterile urine
   1. Follow the protocol described above, but do not administer antimicrobial agents or acetohydroxamic acid

TABLE XV (Continued)

  2. Periodically culture urine specimens obtained by cystocentesis to detect secondary urinary tract infections. If a urinary tract infection develops, initiate antimicrobial therapy

C. Immature dogs
  1. Use caution in consideration of use of protein-restricted diets for growing pups

  2. Short-term therapy with calculolytic diets may be considered. If initiated, monitor the patient for evidence of nutritional deficiencies (especially protein malnutrition)

  3. Acetohydroxamic acid has not been evaluated in growing pups

  4. Pending further studies, surgery remains the safest means of removing uroliths from immature dogs

---

c. Urease Inhibitors. Clinical studies of man (Burns and Gauthier, 1984; Griffith *et al.*, 1978, 1979, 1981; Griffith and Musher, 1973; Rodeman *et al.*, 1983, Williams *et al.*, 1984), experimental studies of rats (Griffith and Musher, 1973; Lamm *et al.*, 1977), and experimental and clinical studies of dogs (Krawiec *et al.*, 1984a,b; C. A. Osborne, 1984, unpublished data; Senior *et al.*, 1984) have revealed that microbial urease inhibitors administered in pharmacologic doses are capable of inhibiting struvite urolith growth and/or promoting struvite urolith dissolution. Hydroxamic acids are specific inhibitors of urease (Fishbein, 1981; Griffith and Musher, 1975; Kobashi *et al.*, 1971; Rosenstein *et al.*, 1981; Rosenstein and Hamilton-Miller, 1984). They apparently owe at least a portion of their inhibitory activity to their molecular structure which is similar to that of urea (Fig. 27). The terminal —CO—NHOH structure of acetohydroxamic acid may noncompetitively block the active site of urease molecules, because its similarity to the amide groups of urea allows access to the active site (Burr, 1977; Fishbein and Daly, 1970; Fishbein, 1981). Because hydroxamic acids also chelate nickel, they may bind to nickel atoms in urease, thereby interfering with urease activity (Fishbein, 1981; Griffith and Klein, 1983). Of the variety of hydroxamic acids, acetohydroxamic acid (AHA) combines an acceptable level of toxicity with a relatively rapid inhibitory effect against urease (Burr, 1979; Fishbein and Daly, 1970; Griffith and Klein, 1983; Rosenstein *et al.*, 1981, Williams *et al.*, 1984).

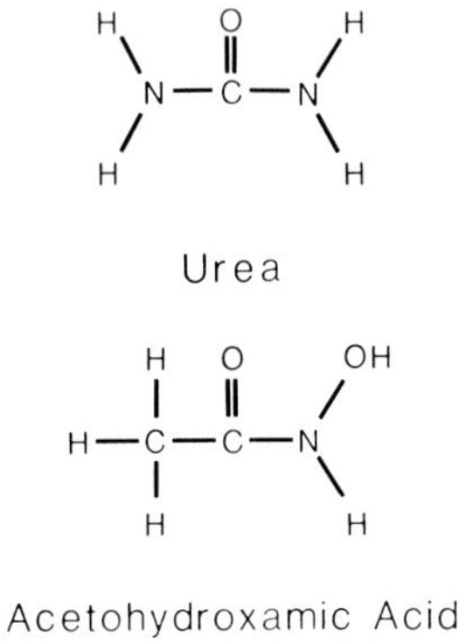

$$\begin{array}{c} H O H \\ \diagdown \| \diagup \\ N - C - N \\ \diagup \diagdown \\ H H \end{array}$$

Urea

$$\begin{array}{c} H O OH \\ | \| \diagup \\ H - C - C - N \\ | \diagdown \\ H H \end{array}$$

Acetohydroxamic Acid

FIG. 27. Schematic illustration of similarity in structural configuration of urea and acetohydroxamic acid.

Acetohydroxamic acid is rapidly and completely absorbed from the gastrointestinal tract of dogs and is excreted and concentrated in urine (Feldman et al., 1978; Rosenstein et al., 1981; Rosenstein and Hamilton-Miller, 1984; Summerskill et al., 1968). When given orally at pharmacologic doses, AHA retards alkalinization of urine caused by urease-producing microbes. Its urease-inhibiting activity is effective between urine pHs of 5 and 9, but is most effective at pH 7. AHA has been reported to have a dose-related bacteriostatic effect against some Gram-positive and Gram-negative bacteria (Griffith, 1978a, 1982; Krawiec et al., 1984a,b). It may also potentiate the antimicrobial effect of antibiotics (especially trimethoprim and sulfamethoxazole) and urine antiseptics (methenamine) (Griffith and Musher, 1973; Griffith et al., 1978; Griffith and Klein, 1983; Musher et al., 1974a; Rosenstein and Hamilton-Miller, 1984).

In an experimental study of dogs with normal renal function, a dose-related ability of AHA[3] to inhibit further struvite urolith growth and to induce struvite urolith dissolution was observed (Krawiec et al., 1984a,b). Administration of AHA at a dosage of 50 to 100 mg/kg of body weight each day caused detectable reduction of urine urease activity, urine pH, and crystalluria, and either inhibited urolith growth (50 mg/kg), or induced urolith dissolution (100 mg/kg). Although administration of AHA at a daily dosage of 25 mg/kg did not cause a detectable reduction in urine pH, it did reduce urease activity and crystalluria and inhibited further urolith growth. These events occurred despite persistent urinary tract infection with urease-producing

---

[3]Lithostat, Mission Pharmacal Company, San Antonio, Texas 78296.

Staphylococcus aureus. The fact that infected dogs treated with AHA had less severe dysuria, bacteriuria, pyuria, hematuria, and proteinuria and had less severe lesions of the urinary tract than positive-control dogs indicates that the drug reduced the pathogenicity of the staphylococci. Reduction in the quantity of ammonia produced by the action of bacterial urease on urea may have minimized the degree of chemically induced damage to tissues of the urinary tract, with an associated reduction in the magnitude of the inflammatory response.

Reversible adverse reactions associated with administration of AHA to human patients include a dose-related hemolytic anemia, gastrointestinal upsets, diminished sense of well being, bone marrow depression, and thrombophlebitis (Griffith, 1978a, 1979; Griffith *et al.*, 1978; 1979; Williams *et al.*, 1984). When AHA was given to dogs in sufficient quantity to dissolve experimentally induced struvite uroliths, a reversible hemolytic anemia and blood dyscrasia occurred (Krawiec *et al.*, 1984a). Prolonged administration of AHA at large doses induced abnormalities in bilirubin metabolism in some dogs. The exact mechanism(s) responsible for these abnormalities was not determined. AHA has been reported to inhibit DNA synthesis and cell division, and has the capacity to chelate metallic ions (Fishbein, 1981). Reduction of the quantity of AHA to a dosage that did not cause adverse reactions eliminated its ability to induce struvite urolith dissolution under the conditions of this study. However, nontoxic doses of AHA were effective in prolonged inhibition of further urolith growth (Krawiec *et al.*, 1984a,b).

In a study performed at the University of Minnesota, oral administration of AHA at a daily dose of 25 mg/kg to pregnant female beagle dogs induced developmental anomalies of the heart, skeletal system, and ventral midline of their pups (Bailie and Osborne, 1984, unpublished data). Cardiac anomalies included atrial septal defects (20%), ventricular septal defects (3%), and atrial and ventricular septal defects (3%). Skeletal anomalies included coccygeal hemivertebrae and fused coccygeal vertebrae (50%), supernumary vertebrae (67%), supernumary ribs (50%), duplicated sternebrae (3%), and lumbar hemivertebrae (3%) (Fig. 28). Defects of the ventral midline of the abdominal wall occurred in 20% of the pups exposed to AHA *in utero*. Other abnormalities observed included retarded growth, high neonatal mortality, and a decreased number of circulating erythrocytes as compared to control dogs. These observations indicate that AHA should not be given to pregnant females.

Two new hydroxamic acids have been evaluated for treatment of infected struvite uroliths (Martelli *et al.*, 1981; Takeuchi *et al.*, 1982).

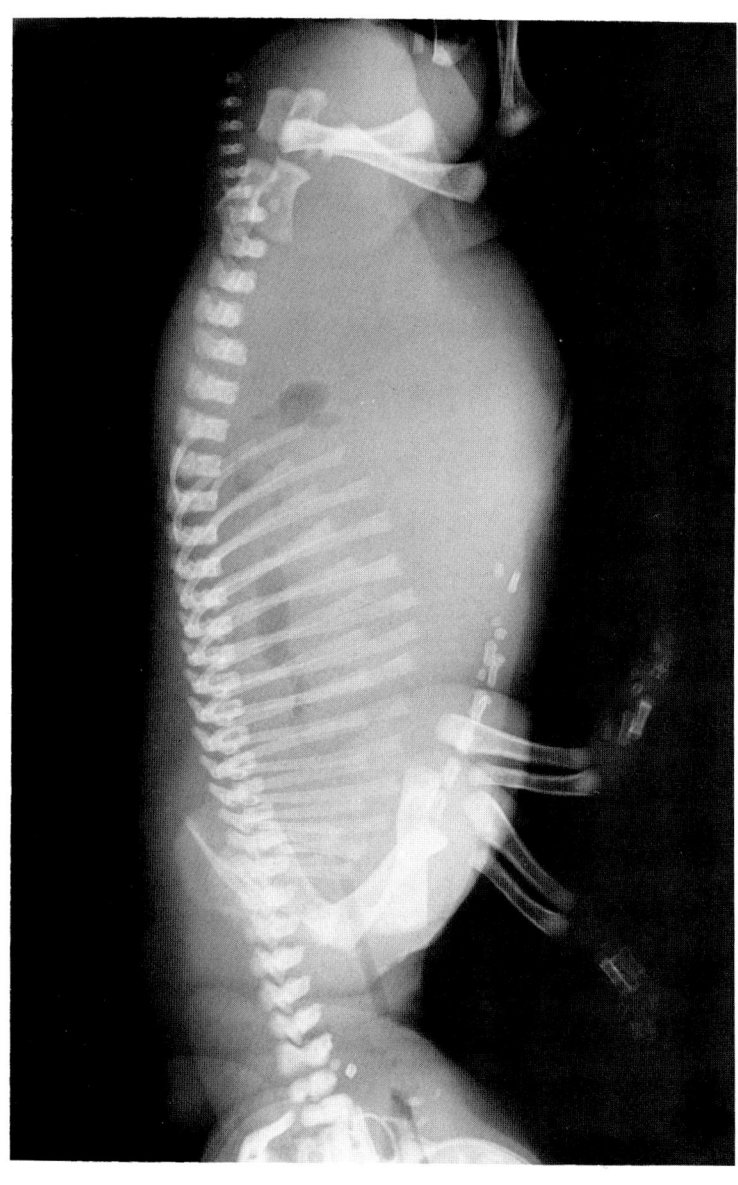

FIG. 28. Radiograph of a female puppy exposed to acetohydroxamic acid *in utero*. Fourteen thoracic vertebrae and 14 pairs of ribs are present. The fifth, sixth, and seventh lumbar vertebrae are flattened dorsoventrally (so-called dorsoventral hemivertebrae), and some sternebrae are duplicated.

Both have been reported to have fewer potential side effects than AHA, although experimental and clinical studies to substantiate these statements have not yet been performed. An organic phosphorus-containing compound called fluorofamide has been reported to be a more potent inhibitor of bacterial urease than AHA (Millner et al., 1982). Preliminary studies of rats and dogs suggest that fluorofamide may be effective in the inhibition of bacterial urease produced in the urinary tract (Millner et al., 1982; Senior et al., 1984).

  d. *Calculolytic Diets.* Following experimental and clinical studies of humans and dogs indicating that inhibition of bacterial urease with a urease inhibitor was effective in the inhibition of struvite urolith growth, and, in some instances, induced struvite urolith dissolution, it was hypothesized that reduction of the urine concentration of urea (the substrate of urease) would provide similar results (Osborne, 1982; Osborne et al., 1982). To test this hypothesis, a calculolytic diet[4] was formulated that contained a reduced quantity of high quality protein (1.6%), and reduced quantities of phosphorus (0.048%) and magnesium (0.006%) (Abdullahi et al., 1984). The diet was supplemented with salt to stimulate thirst and induce compensatory polyuria. Reduction in hepatic production of urea from dietary protein was hypothesized to reduce medullary urea solute concentration and further contribute to diuresis. This calculolytic diet was found to be highly effective in inducing struvite urolith dissolution in five of six experimental dogs, despite persistent infection with urease-producing bacteria (Fig. 29). The uroliths underwent dissolution in about 3.5 months (range was 8 to 20 weeks). The urolith in the remaining dog decreased to less than half of its pretreatment size at the termination of the study, 6 months following initiation of dietary therapy. Urinary tract infections persisted in these dogs until the uroliths dissolved, at which time they underwent remission in three dogs. In the corresponding control group fed a maintenance diet (10% protein, 0.19% phosphorus, and 0.06% magnesium), calculi increased in size by a mean of 5.5 times their pretreatment size (range = 3 to 8 times)(Fig. 29). A urolith developed in the renal pelvis of one of these dogs. Urinary tract infections persisted in control dogs throughout the 6-month study.

  In a related experimental study of sterile struvite uroliths, consumption of the calculolytic diet induced urolith dissolution in a mean of 3.3 weeks (range = 2 to 4 weeks) (Fig. 28) (Abdullahi et al., 1984). In a corresponding control group fed a maintenance diet, uroliths in four dogs dissolved over a mean period of 14 weeks (range = 8 to 20 weeks)

[4]Prescription Diet s/d, Hills Pet Products Inc., Topeka, Kansas 66601.

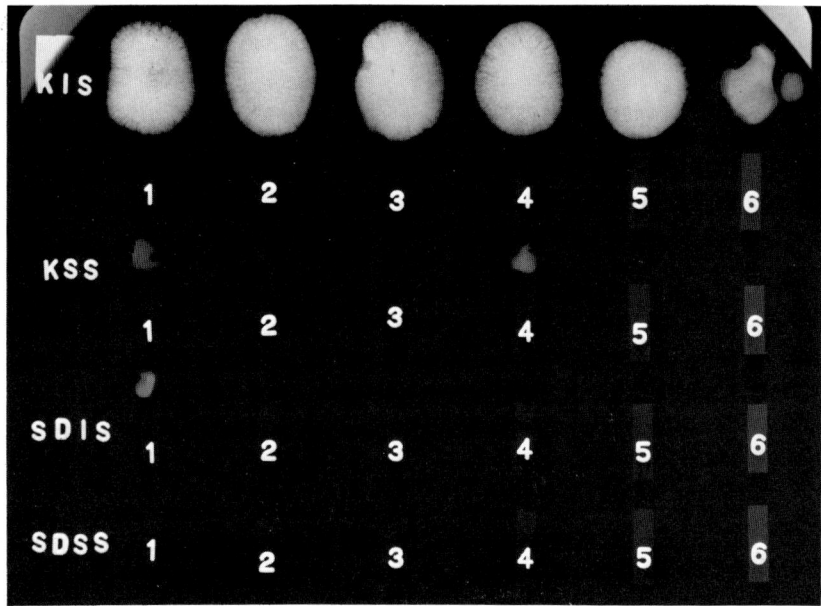

FIG. 29. Radiograph of uroliths removed at necropsy from four groups of six dogs with experimentally induced struvite urocystolithiasis. KIS = control group with transplanted struvite uroliths and staphylococcal urinary tract infections. All stones have increased in size. KSS = control group with transplanted struvite uroliths, but no urinary tract infections. Four of the six uroliths gradually dissolved during the course of study. SDIS = group with transplated struvite uroliths, staphylococcal urinary tract infections, and treatment with a calculolytic diet. Five of six uroliths have dissolved; one urolith is reduced in size. SDSS = group with transplanted struvite uroliths, no urinary tract infections, and treatment with a calculolytic diet. All uroliths dissolved in less than 1 month. (From *Am. J. Vet. Res.*, 1984, **45,** 1508–1529.)

(Fig. 29). In the remaining two control dogs, uroliths were one fifth of their initial size at the termination of the study.

Consumption of calculolytic diets by dogs with experimentally induced staphylococcal urinary tract infections and struvite uroliths was associated with a marked reduction in the serum concentration of urea nitrogen (baseline = 21.8 mg/dl ± 2.9; posttreatment = 3.5 mg/dl ± 2.4), and mild reductions in the serum concentrations of magnesium (baseline = 2.2 mg/dl ± 0.2; posttreatment = 1.8mg/dl ± 0.2), phosphorus (baseline = 4.6 mg/dl ± 0.6; posttreatment 3.8 mg/dl ± 0.8), and albumin (baseline = 3.1 g/dl; posttreatment = 2.1 g/dl ± 0.3). A mild increase in the serum activity of hepatic alkaline phosphatase isoenzyme (baseline = 3.1 mU/ml ± 1.50; posttreatment = 147.7 mU/ml ± 48.1) was also observed. These alterations in serum chemistry values were of no detectable clinical consequence during the 6-month experimental studies, or during clinical studies. However, they indicate that the diet is designed for short-term (weeks to months) dissolution therapy, rather than long-term (months to years) prophylactic therapy. Changes in serum urea nitrogen concentrations may be used as one index of client and patient compliance with dietary recommendations.

In a related experimental study, the struvolytic effect of various combinations of antibiotics (ampicillin given orally at a dosage of 16 mg/kg/day), acetohydroxamic acid (given orally at a dosage of 25 mg/kg/day), and a calculolytic diet was studied in dogs with staphylococcal-induced struvite uroliths (C. A. Osborne and S. U. Abdullahi, 1982, unpublished data). Following 5 months of therapy, four uroliths increased in size and two dissolved in six dogs given ampicillin and a maintenance diet. Four of six uroliths dissolved and two decreased in size in six dogs given ampicillin and a calculolytic diet. All uroliths in six dogs dissolved 6 weeks following the initiation of therapy with a combination of calculolytic diet, ampicillin, and acetohydroxamic acid. The calculolytic effect of the diet used in our studies, and the synergistic effect of antimicrobial agents and urease inhibitors, have been confirmed by other investigators using the same model of struvite urolith formation in dogs (Senior et al., 1984). In the latter study, efficacy of therapy was predicted on the basis of comparison of relative supersaturation of urine with struvite before and after various therapeutic protocols.

When a combination of a calculolytic diet and antimicrobial agents was given to 11 dogs with naturally occurring urease-positive urinary tract infections and urocystoliths presumed to be composed of struvite, similar results were obtained (Osborne et al., 1982, 1984f). Likewise, use of a calculolytic diet to induce dissolution of urocystoliths presumed to be struvite in nine dogs without urinary tract infections has also been effective. The mean time required to induce urocystolith dissolution in these 20 dogs was 2.26 months (range = 2 weeks to 7 months) (Figs. 30–35). The mean urine pH of the 20 patients at the time of diagnosis was 7.6; the mean serum urea nitrogen (SUN) concentration was 19.5 mg/dl. The mean urine pH of these dogs during calculolytic therapy was 6.9; the mean SUN concentration was 7.1 mg/dl. Pretreatment mean serum alkaline phosphatase activity ($\bar{x}$ = 70.5 mŪl) tripled during calculolytic diet therapy ($\bar{x}$=245 mŪl), but rapidly returned to normal values ($\bar{x}$ = 55 mU/ml) following discontinuation of therapy. Likewise mean serum albumin concentration ($\bar{x}$ = 3.3 g/dl) at the time of diagnosis dropped ($\bar{x}$ = 2.58 g/dl) during

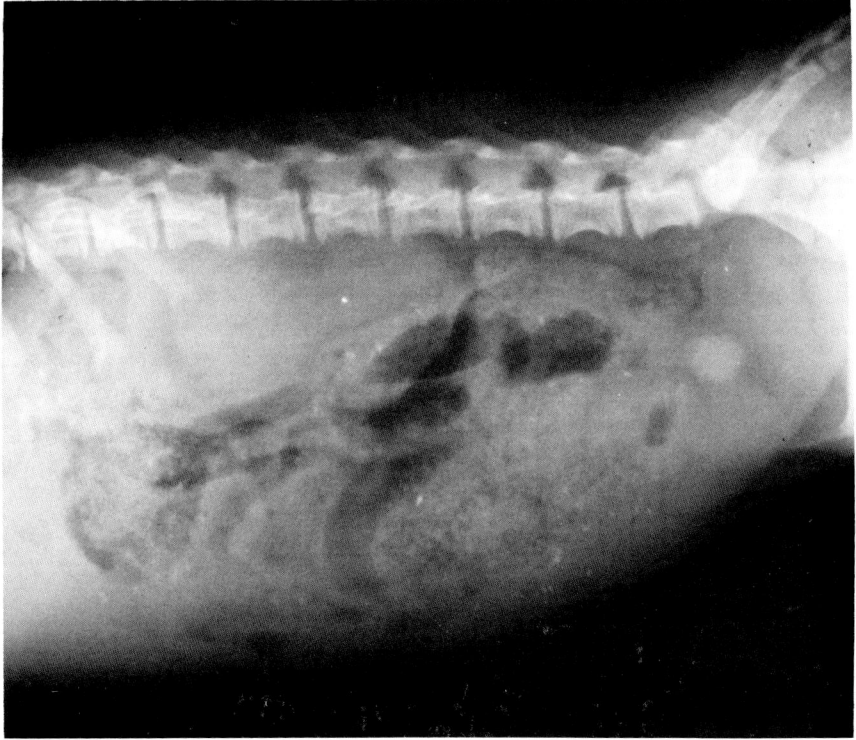

FIG. 30. Survey abdominal radiograph of a 12-week-old female miniature dachshund with a urocystolith presumed to be composed of struvite.

calculolytic therapy, but returned to normal values ($\bar{x}$ = 3.35 g/dl) following cessation of treatment.

Results of clinical and experimental studies revealed that the size and number of uroliths per se do not dictate the probable response to therapy. Likewise, there is no rigid therapeutic time interval after which response is unlikely. As long as uroliths progressively reduce in size at monthly intervals, therapeutic response is satisfactory. If two monthly intervals lapse without any change in urolith size, or if uroliths increase in size and number at any time, the therapeutic protocol should be reevaluated.

Because calculolytic diets stimulate thirst and promote diuresis, the magnitude of pollakiuria in dogs with urocystoliths may increase for a variable time following the initiation of dietary therapy. Pollakiuria and the abnormal odor of urine caused by bacterial degradation of urea usually subside as infection is controlled and uroliths decrease in size. Reduction in ammonia-induced chemical inflammation as a result of ureolysis may also be involved in the remission of these clinical signs.

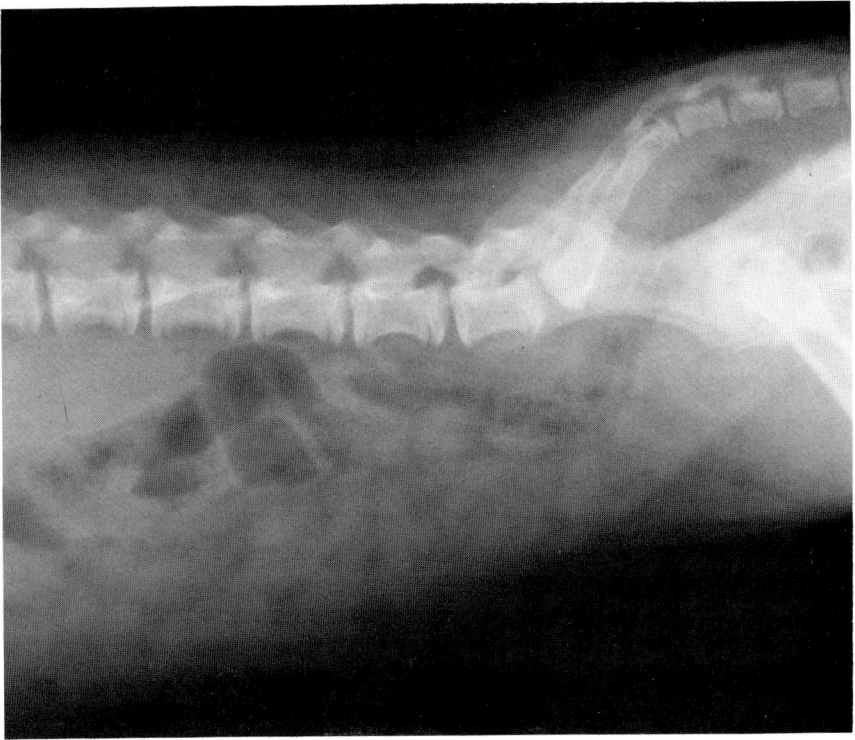

FIG. 31. Survey radiograph of the abdomen of the dog described in Fig. 30 obtained 2 weeks after the initiation of therapy with a calculolytic diet. There are no radiodense structures in the urinary tract.

We have successfully induced dissolution of large bilateral renoliths presumed to be infection-induced struvite in a 6-year-old female basset hound. Although the dog had impaired renal-concentrating capacity (urine specific gravity was 1.016 during clinical dehydration) as a consequence of pyelonephritis, she was not azotemic (SUN = 11 mg/dl; serum creatinine = 0.7 mg/dl) at the time therapy with a calculolytic diet and antimicrobial agents was initiated. This point is emphasized, since dogs with moderate to severe primary renal failure require a greater quantity of dietary protein for anabolism than normal (Polzin et al., 1983). The calculolytic diet used in our studies could induce protein malnutrition if given for prolonged periods to dogs with moderate azotemic primary renal failure.

e. Diuresis. As mentioned in a previous Section (V,L,5), diuresis induced by augmenting water consumption appears to be a logical method to decrease the urine concentration of struvite and other calculogenic substances. However, additional salt is not recommended for

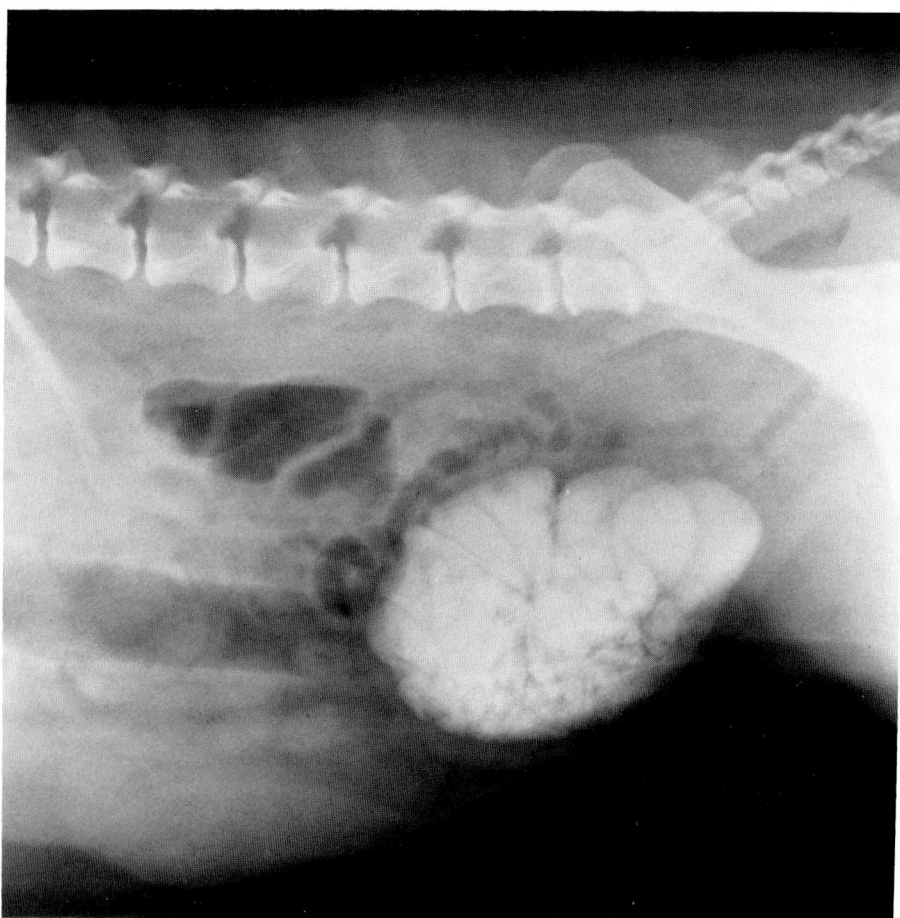

FIG. 32. Survey abdominal radiograph of the abdomen of a 2-year-old female miniature schnauzer with a urease-positive staphylococcal urinary tract infection and urolithiasis (see Figs. 33–35).

dogs fed the calculolytic diet previously described, because the diet has been formulated to contain supplemental sodium chloride. The mean urine specific gravity values of dogs fed the calculolytic diet were 1.008 ± 0.003 as compared to baseline values of 1.028 ± 0.01 (Abdullahi *et al.*, 1984). The mean 24-hr urine volume of dogs fed the calculolytic diet was 549 ml ± 223 ml as compared to baseline values of 352 ml ± 107 ml.

f. Acidification. Because acidification of urine dramatically increases the solubility of struvite, it is an important therapeutic goal. A

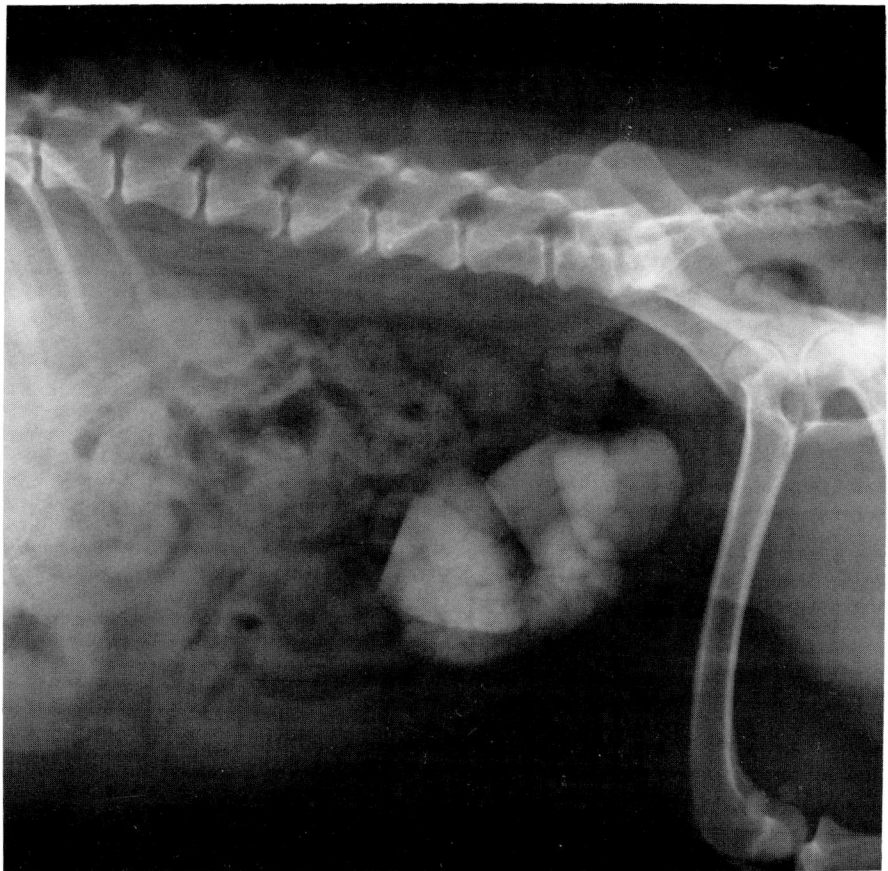

FIG. 33. Survey abdominal radiograph of the dog described in Fig. 32 obtained 9 weeks after the initiation of therapy with a calculolytic diet and orally administered ampicillin.

pH change of only 0.6 units (from 7.4 to 6.8) has been reported to result in a 75% increase in apparent solubility of struvite (Burns and Finlayson, 1982). Since dogs fed a calculolytic diet developed aciduria, however, supplemental use of urine acidifiers is not recommended. The mean urine pH of dogs with experimentally induced staphylococcal urinary tract infections and fed a calculolytic diet was 6.2 ± 0.7 as compared to baseline values of 7.6 ± 0.5. A similar response was observed in clinical trials (mean baseline urine pH 7.6; mean treatment urine pH 6.9).

If urine acidifiers are deemed appropriate, they must be selected and

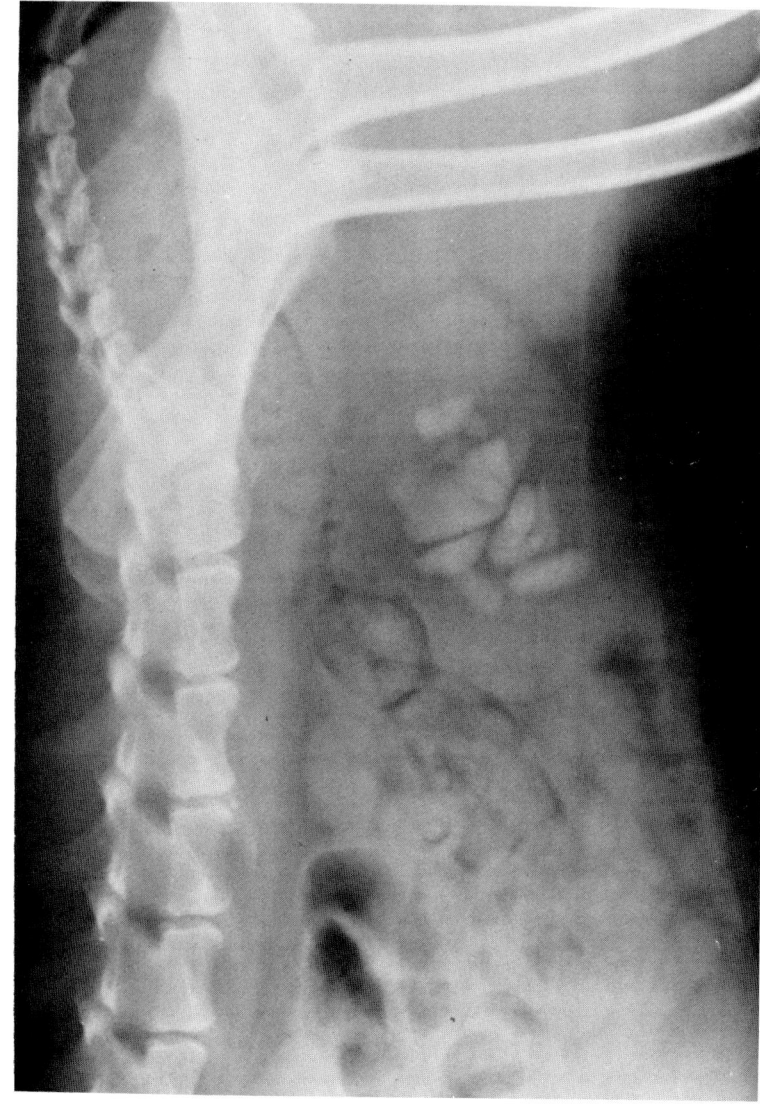

FIG. 34. Survey abdominal radiograph of the abdomen of the dog described in Fig. 32 obtained 21 weeks after the initiation of therapy with a calculolytic diet and orally administered ampicillin.

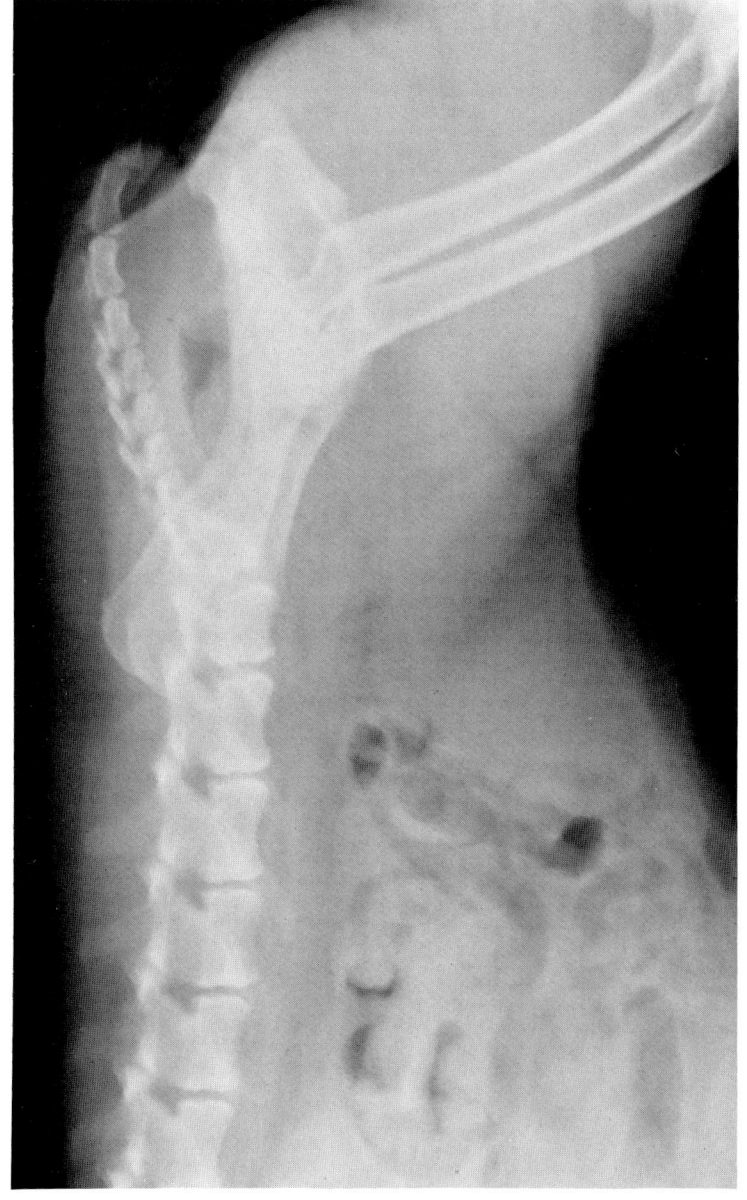

FIG. 35. Lateral survey abdominal radiograph of the abdomen of the dog described in Fig. 32 obtained approximately 7 months following the initiation of therapy. There are no radiodense uroliths in the urinary tract.

administered with appropriate caution. The dosage of urine acidifiers should be adjusted for each patient on the basis of urine pH. The pH of urine obtained a few hours following eating is most likely to be altered by the postprandial alkaline tide. If postprandial urine is acid, therapy is likely to be effective. The most reliable data, however, are obtained by periodically monitoring urine pH throughout the day. Ideally, urine acidifiers should be administered 3 to 4 times per day in order to maintain a consistently acid environment in the urinary tract.

Urinary acidifiers may be ineffective in some patients with urinary tract infections caused by urease-producing bacteria (*Proteus* spp. staphylococci, etc.) because therapeutic dosages may be insufficient to overcome the continuous production of ammonia by bacterial urease (Musher et al., 1974b). Combination therapy with appropriate antimicrobial agents and/or urease inhibitors is recommended.

Acidifiers should not be administered to uremic patients, since they aggravate the severity of metabolic acidosis typically associated with renal failure.

g. Monitoring Response to Therapy. The size of uroliths should be periodically monitored by survey radiography. We recommend radiography at monthly intervals (Figs. 32–35). Survey radiography is usually preferable to retrograde contrast radiography, since use of catheters during retrograde radiographic studies may result in iatrogenic urinary tract infections. Alternatively, intravenous urography may be considered.

Periodic evaluation of urine sediment for crystalluria may also be considered. Struvite crystals should not form if therapy has been effective in promoting formation of urine that is undersaturated with magnesium ammonium phosphate.

Urinary tract infections may persist, despite antimicrobial therapy, in patients with infection-induced struvite uroliths that are consuming the calculolytic diet. However, in most patients the magnitude of bacteriuria is usually reduced substantially (i.e., from $> 10^5$ bacteria/ml of urine to 10^2 or 10^3 bacteria/ml of urine), and the associated inflammatory response progressively subsides. Difficulty in eradication of infection while uroliths persist may be related to the persistence of viable microbes harbored within the stones. Diet-induced diuresis should be considered when formulating dosages of antimicrobial agents that will achieve minimum inhibitory concentrations in urine. Despite persistent bacteriuria during antimicrobial and dietary treatment of infected patients with struvite uroliths, we have had excellent success in inducing urolith dissolution. Concomitant use of calculolytic diets, antimicrobial agents, and acetohydroxamic acid in this situation provided the most effective method of inducing urolith dissolution.

Urine collected by cystocentesis should be quantitatively cultured during therapy, and 5 to 7 days following discontinuation of antimicrobial therapy. It is emphasized that results of urine culture may not be the same as results obtained prior to therapy, or from cultures of the interior of uroliths. Rapid recurrence of urinary tract infections caused by the same type of organism (relapse), or a different type of bacterial pathogen (reinfection) following withdrawal of antimicrobial therapy may indicate residual calculi within the urinary tract, or other abnormalities in local host defense mechanisms that predisposed to urinary tract infections and subsequent urolithiasis.

Since small uroliths may escape detection by survey radiography, we recommend that the calculolytic diet and (if necessary) antimicrobial agents be continued for at least 1 month following radiographic documentation of urolith dissolution.

If uroliths increase in size during therapy, or do not begin to decrease in size after approximately 8 weeks of appropriate medical therapy, alternative methods of management should be considered. Small uroliths that become lodged in the urethra of male or female dogs during therapy may be readily returned to the urinary bladder lumen by urohydropropulsion (Osborne et al., 1983b; Piermattei and Osborne, 1971). Complete obstruction of a ureter or renal pelvis, especially with a concomitant urinary tract infection, is an absolute indication for surgical intervention.

Difficulty in inducing complete dissolution of uroliths by creating urine that is undersaturated with the suspected calculogenic crystalloid should prompt consideration that: (1) the wrong mineral component was identified (Fig. 8), (2) the nucleus of the urolith is of different mineral composition from outer portions of the urolith, and (3) the owner or the patient is not complying with therapeutic recommendations.

h. Prevention of Recurrence. Eradication or control of infections of the urinary tract due to urease-producing bacteria is the most important factor in preventing recurrence of most infection-induced struvite uroliths. If recurrent urinary tract infection persists, indefinite therapy with prophylactic dosages of antimicrobial agents eliminated in high concentration in urine is indicated (Ling, 1983). These include nitrofurantoin, ampicillin, and trimethoprim-sulfa.

In light of the effectiveness of diets in inducing struvite urolith dissolution, dietary modifications to prevent recurrence of uroliths would appear to be logical and feasible. However, further studies must be performed to evaluate the long-term effects of low protein calculolytic diets in dogs before reliable recommendations can be established. Because they induce polyuria, varying degrees of hypoalbuminemia, and mild alterations in hepatic enzymes and morphology, we recommend their long-term use only if patients develop recurrent urolithiasis, despite augmented fluid intake and urine acidification. Diets designed for management of renal failure that contain less salt and more protein may be a viable alternative (Lewis and Morris, 1983; Morris and Doering, 1978), but as yet have not been evaluated by controlled experimental and clinical trials.[5]

Studies to evaluate the effectiveness of acetohydroxamic acid in the prevention of struvite urolithiasis in dogs with persistent urinary tract infections with urease-producing bacteria have been encouraging. Administration of 25 mg of AHA/kg/day to dogs with urinary bladder foreign bodies (zinc disks) and experimentally induced urease-positive staphylococcal urinary tract infections has been effective in preventing urolith formation and minimizing the rate of urolith growth (Fig. 36) (Krawiec et al., 1984b). Acetohydroxamic acid has also been reported to be effective in the prevention of struvite uroliths induced by urease-producing mycoplasma in rats (Lamm et al., 1977).

Caution must be used in deciding whether or not to induce prophylactic diuresis in patients with struvite uroliths induced by recurrent urinary tract infections. Although formation of dilute urine tends to minimize supersaturation of urine with calculogenic crystalloids, it also tends to counteract innate antimicrobial properties of urine (Osborne et al., 1979). Experimental studies performed in cats indicate that diuresis tends to minimize pyelonephritis, but enhances lower urinary tract infections (Lees et al., 1981).

If the urine pH of patients with previous struvite urolithiasis remains alkaline despite antimicrobial and/or dietary therapy, administration of urine acidifiers should be considered.

7. Feline Struvite Urolithiasis

a. Overview. Experimental and clinical studies of feline sterile struvite uroliths have confirmed the feasibility of inducing their dissolution by medical therapy (Lewis and Morris, 1983; Osborne et al., 1984c,e,f,g; Taton et al., 1984). Key components for inducing dissolution of most struvite uroliths in cats appear to be (1) reduction of urine pH to 6.0 or less, and (2) reduction of urine magnesium by consumption of magnesium restricted diets (Table XVI). Although the formation of dilute urine may enhance the rate of urolith disolution, our preliminary results indicate that this factor is not an essential component of medical calculolytic protocols for the treatment of sterile uroliths in cats (Osborne et al., 1984c,f).

[5]Prescription Diet u/d, Hills Pet Products Inc., Topeka, Kansas 66601.

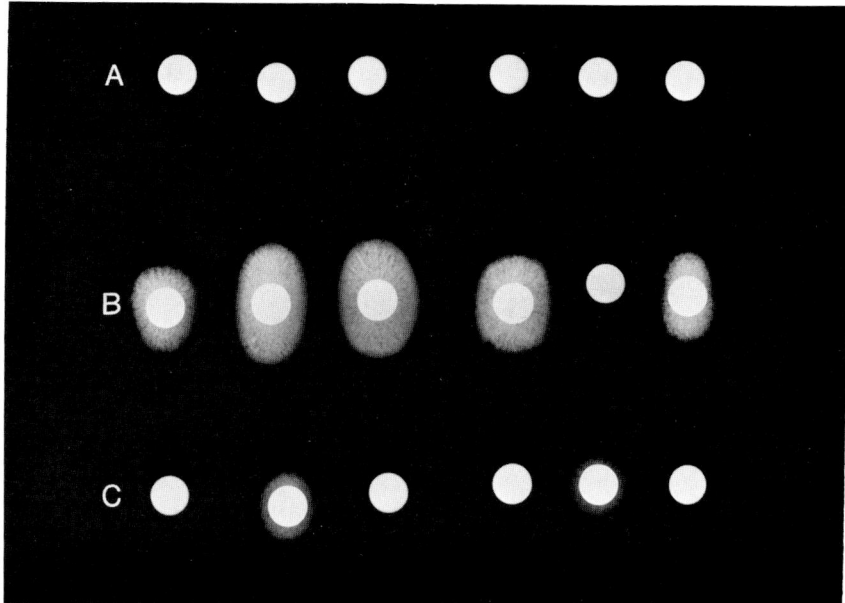

FIG. 36. Radiograph of uroliths removed at necropsy from three groups of six dogs with zinc disk urinary bladder foreign bodies. A = group of dogs with transplanted zinc disks, but no urinary tract infections. There is no evidence of struvite formation around the zinc disks. B = group of dogs with transplanted zinc disks and concomitant staphylococcal urinary tract infections. Struvite formed around five of the six zinc disks. C = group of dogs with transplanted zinc disks, concomitant staphylococcal urinary tract infections, and treatment with acetohydroxamic acid. Small quantities of struvite formed around only two of the six zinc disks. (From *Am. J. Vet. Res.*, 1984, **45**, 1276–1282.)

b. Clinical Studies of Sterile Struvite. In a pilot clinical study of three male and seven female cats with urocystoliths presumed to be composed of sterile struvite, patients were given a high moisture, magnesium-restricted diet[6] supplemented with sufficient DL-methionine (1000 to 1500 mg/day), or a mixture of ammonium chloride and DL-methionine, to induce urine pH values of 6.0 or less. All uroliths dissolved within a mean of 47 days (range = 29 to 100 days) (C. A. Osborne, 1984, unpublished data).

In a follow-up clinical study of eight male and seven female cats fed a high moisture (canned) calculolytic diet,[7] urocystoliths presumed to be composed of sterile struvite dissolved in a mean of 32 days (range = 14

[6]Prescription Diet c/d, Hills Pet Products Inc., Topeka, Kansas 66601.
[7]Prescription Diet Feline s/d, Hills Pet Products Inc., Topeka, Kansas 66601.

TABLE XVI

Summary of Recommendations for Medical Dissolution of Feline Struvite Uroliths

1. Perform appropriate diagnostic studies including complete urinalyses, quantitative urine culture, and diagnostic radiography. Guesstimate urolith composition by evaluation of appropriate clinical data (Table XV)

2. Initiate dietary management designed to reduce the urine concentration of magnesium and create a pH of 6.0 or less. No other food should be fed to patients consuming calculolytic diets. Monitor urine pH 4 for 8 hr after eating. Urine that is acid at this time is likely to be acid throughout the day

3. Although attempts may be made to stimulate thirst-induced diuresis by addition of sodium chloride to the diet, it is not essential. Thirst-induced diuresis may be of benefit to patients with slowly dissolving uroliths

4. Attempt to eradicate or control secondary urinary tract infections with antimicrobial agents. Although control of secondary urinary tract infections is not essential to induce sterile struvite urolith dissolution, it is warranted to prevent damage of tissues of the urinary tract by bacteria and their metabolites

5. Periodically (2 to 4 week intervals), monitor the size of uroliths by survey radiography. Survey radiography is preferable to retrograde contrast radiography to monitor urolith dissolution, since use of catheters during retrograde radiographic studies may result in iatrogenic urinary tract infections. Alternatively, intravenous urography may be considered

6. Periodic evaluation of urine sediment for crystalluria may be considered. Struvite crystals should not form if therapy has been effective in promoting formation of urine that is undersaturated with magnesium ammonium phosphate

7. Continue calculolytic diet therapy for at least 1 month following the radiographic disappearance of uroliths

8. If uroliths increase in size during dietary management, or do not begin to decrease in size after approximately 4 to 8 weeks of appropriate medical management, alternative methods should be considered. Difficulty in inducing complete dissolution of uroliths by creating urine that is undersaturated with the suspected calculogenic crystalloid should prompt consideration that (1) the wrong mineral component was identified (Table III, XV), (2) the nucleus of the urolith is of different mineral composition from other portions of the urolith, and (3) the owner of the patient is not complying with medical recommendations

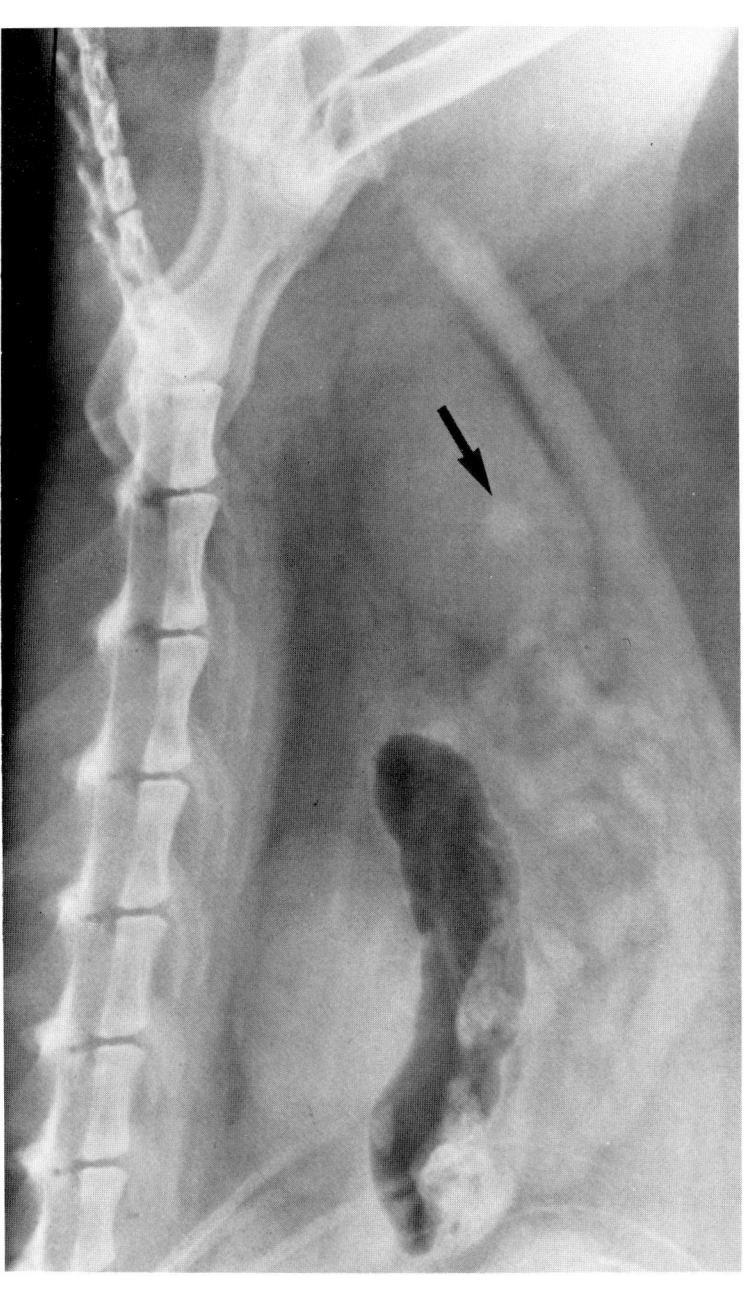

Fig. 37. Survey radiograph of the lateral aspect of the abdomen of a 3-year-old domestic shorthair cat. Note the solitary radiodense urolith in the bladder lumen (arrow).

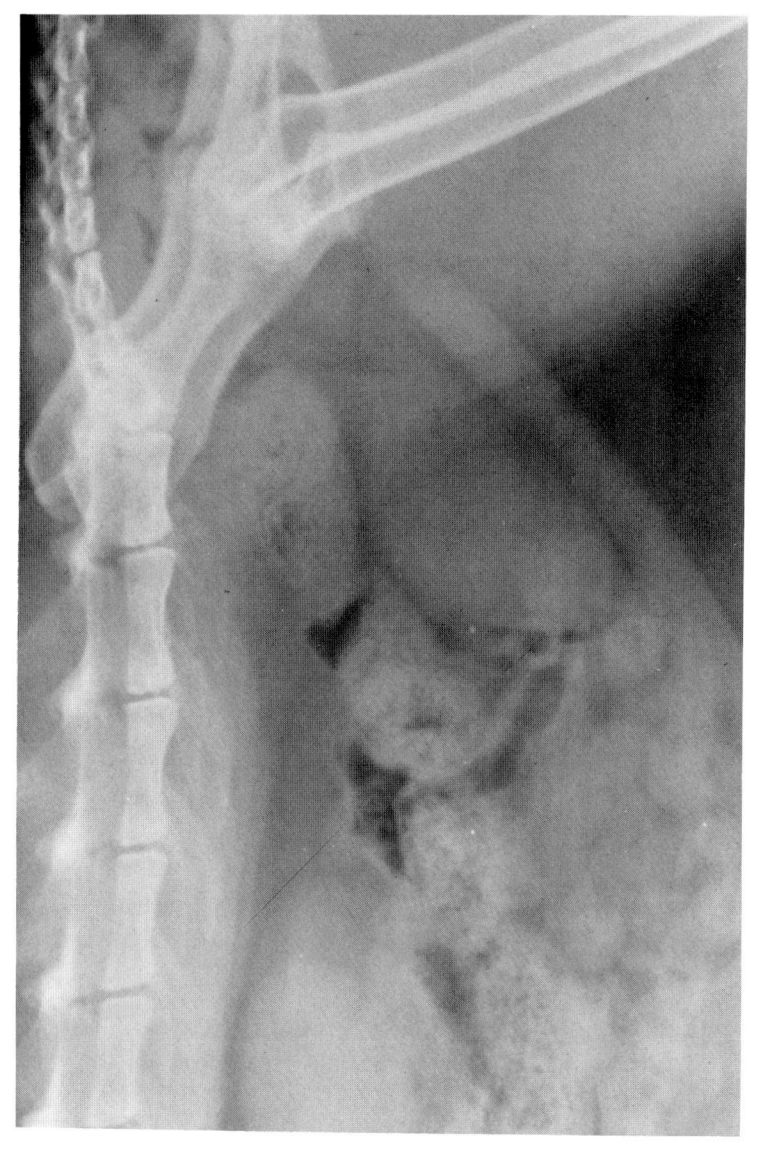

Fig. 38. Survey radiograph of the lateral aspect of the abdomen of the cat described in Fig. 37 obtained 3 weeks following initiation of therapy with a calculolytic diet. There are no radiodense uroliths in the urinary tract.

to 82 days) (Figs. 37 and 38). The high energy diet (720 cal per 15 oz) containing 41.4% dry weight protein was formulated to contain reduced quantities of magnesium (0.058% dry weight), and to promote formation of acid urine (pH ± 6.0). The diet was also supplemented with sodium chloride (0.79% of dry weight sodium) to stimulate thirst and promote diuresis (Osborne et al., 1984e).

Results of these clinical studies confirm that medical dissolution of sterile struvite uroliths in cats is a reasonable alternative to surgery.

c. *Infected Struvite.* Infection-induced struvite uroliths occur in cats, but are less common than sterile struvite uroliths (Osborne et al., 1984a). Although dissolution of infection-induced struvite uroliths is-feasible, our experience with medical management of such patients has been limited. Use of calculolytic diets and appropriate antimicrobial agents is logical. However, we have not yet determined the relative benefit of restricting dietary protein (and, thus, urine urea concentration) in promoting dissolution of infection-induced struvite uroliths in such patients. This point is of considerable significance because of the relatively high protein requirement of cats. We emphasize that the calculolytic diet designed for use in dogs should not be given to cats because of its restricted quantity of protein.

d. *Prevention of Recurrence.* Empirical clinical studies performed at the University of Minnesota Veterinary Teaching Hospital indicate that acidification of urine (pH < 6.0) and consumption of low magnesium diets are effective in preventing recurrence of sterile struvite cystoliths in male and female cats. No attempt was made to determine whether acidification of urine and/or the low magnesium diet were the major factor(s) responsible for the beneficial results.

Prevention of infection-induced struvite uroliths in cats should be based on the same principles as those described for dogs. The key to prevention of recurrence is eradication or control of infection.

M. Medical versus Surgical Management

Detection of uroliths is not, in itself, an indication for surgery. However, along with medical management, surgical intervention has a vital role in therapy of urolithiasis. Surgical candidates include (1) patients with urolith-induced obstruction to urine outflow that cannot be corrected by nonsurgical techniques, especially in patients with concomitant urinary tract infections, (2) patients with uroliths that are refractory to current methods of medical dissolution (e.g., silica, calcium oxalate, calcium phosphate, and probably cystine uroliths), (3) patients with uroliths that are increasing in size and/or number, despite medical therapy designed to inhibit their growth or cause their dissolution (especially if they are causing an obstruction to urine outflow and/or progressive deterioration in renal function, (4) patients with nephroliths and renal dysfunction of such a nature that the time required to induce medical dissolution is likely to be associated with more renal dysfunction than that associated with surgical procedures, (5) patients with anatomic defects of the urogenital tract that predispose to urolithiasis and are amenable to surgical correction at the time uroliths are removed, and (6) patients unable to respond to medical management because of poor client or patient compliance with therapeutic recommendations.

Complete obstruction to urine outflow caused by uroliths in patients with concomitant urinary tract infections should be regarded as a surgical emergency. In this situation rapid spread of infection and associated damage to the urinary tract, especially the kidneys, are likely to induce septicemia and peracute renal failure caused by a combination of obstruction and pyelonephritis.

Unilateral renoliths and/or ureteroliths that have caused outflow obstruction and substantial impairment of function of the associated kidney should be managed by surgical intervention, or (if possible) percutaneous pyelonephrostomy (Osborne *et al.*, 1985; Smith, 1982). Medical therapy designed to induce urolith dissolution during a period of several weeks in patients with poorly draining kidneys is unlikely to be effective, since the urolith(s) will not be continually bathed with newly formed urine modified to induce litholysis. The same concept applies to urethroliths that cannot be removed by nonsurgical methods.

Combined use of surgical removal of struvite uroliths followed by medical calculolytic protocols may be of value in some patients. Examples include patients in which uroliths or fragments of uroliths remain following surgery, and patients with struvite crystalluria of a character and magnitude that indicate rapid recurrence is likely. In this circumstance, meticulous procedure should be utilized in repairing surgical incisions in dogs, since canine calculolytic diets are protein restricted.

Acknowledgments

Supported in part by grants from the American Association of Feline Practitioners; the Iams Company, Lewisberg, Ohio; The Minnetonka Kennel Club, Minnetonka, Minnesota; Mark L. Morris Associates, Topeka, Kansas; The Morris Animal Foundation, Denver, Colorado; The Paralyzed Veterans Association, Washington, D.C.; Ralston Purina Company, St. Louis, Missouri; and Urolithiasis Laboratory, Houston, Texas.

References

Abdullahi, S. U., Osborne, C. A., Lenininger, J. R., Fletcher, T. F., and Griffith, D. P. (1984). *Am. J. Vet. Res.* **45**, 1508–1519.
Alken, P. (1982). *Urol. Clin. North Am.* **9**, 145–151.
Backman, U., Danielson, B. G., Felstrom, B., Johnasson, G., Ljunghall, S., and Wilkstrom, B. (1981). *In* "Urolithiasis: Clinical and Basic Research" (L. H. Smith, W. G. Robertson, and B. Finlayson, eds.), pp. 67–69. Plenum, New York.
Bartone, F. F., and Johnston, J. H. (1977). *J. Urol.* **118**, 76–79.
Bartos, K. D., and Palmore, W. P. (1981). *Abstr. Annu. Meet. Conf. Res. Workers Anim. Dis. 62nd*, p. 25.
Birch, D. F., Fairley, K. F., and Pavillard, R. E. (1981). *Kidney Int.* **19**, 58–64.
Bohonowych, R. O., Parks, J. L., and Greene, R. W. (1978). *J. Am. Vet. Med. Assoc.* **173**, 301–303.
Boistelle, R., Abbona, F., Berland, Y., Grandvuillemin, M., and Olmer, M. (1984). *Urol. Res.* **12**, 79.
Boyce, W. H., and Garvey, F. K. (1956). *J. Urol.* **76**, 213–227.
Boyce, W. H., and King, J. S. (1963). *Ann. N.Y. Acad. Sci.* **104**, 563–578.
Boyce, W. H., King, J. S., and Fiedler, M. L. (1962). *J. Clin. Invest.* **4**, 1180–1189.
Brande, A. I., and Siemienski, J. (1960). *J. Bacteriol.* **80**, 171–179.
Brodey, R. S. (1955). *J. Am. Vet. Med. Assoc.* **126**, 1–9.
Brown, N. O., Parks, J. L., and Greene, R. W. (1977a). *J. Am. Vet. Med. Assoc.* **170**, 415–418.
Brown, N. O., Parks, J. L., and Greene, R. W. (1977b). *J. Am. Vet. Med. Assoc.* **170**, 419–422.
Bunce, G. E., Saacke, R. G., and Mullins, J. (1980). *Exp. Mol. Pathol.* **33**, 203–210.
Burns, J. R., and Finlayson, B. (1982). *J. Urol.* **128**, 426–428.
Burns, J. R., and Guathier, J. F. (1984). *J. Urol.* **132**, 455–456.
Burr, R. G. (1977). *Invest. Urol.* **15**, 180–182.
Carbone, M. G. (1965). *J. Am. Vet. Med. Assoc.* **147**, 1195–1200.
Carson, C. C., and Malek, R. S. (1982). *J. Urol.* **127**, 977–978.
Castaneda-Zuniga, W. R., Miller, R. P., and Amplatz, K. (1982). *Urol. Clin. North Am.* **9**, 113–119.
Chaussy, C., and Schmiedt, E. (1983). *Urol. Clin. North Am.* **10**, 743–750.
Chow, F. H. C., Hamar, D. W., and Udall, R. H. (1973). *Proc. Soc. Exp. Biol. Med.* **144**, 912–916.
Chow, F. C., Dysart, I., Hamar, D. W., Lewis, L. D., and Rick, L. J. (1976). *Feline Pract.* **9**, 51–55.
Chow, F. C., Duch, D. S., and Hamar, D. W. (1983). *In* "Comparative Aspects of Nutritional and Metabolic Diseases" (J. C. Woodward and M. Bruss, eds.), pp. 41–60. CRC Press, Boca Raton, Florida.
Chute, R., and Suby, H. I. (1940). *J. Urol.* **44**, 590–595.
Cifuentes Delatte, L. (1983). *In* "Stones: Clinical Management of Urolithiasis" (R. A. Roth and B. Finlayson, eds.), pp. 21–52. Williams and Wilkins, Baltimore, Maryland.
Cifuentes Delatte, L., and Soriano, F. (1984). *Urol. Res.* **12**, 30.
Clark, W. T. (1974a). *Vet. Rec.* **95**, 204–206.
Clark, W. T. (1974b). *J. Small Anim. Pract.* **15**, 437–444.
Clark, W. T. (1976). *J. Small Anim. Pract.* **17**, 575–581.
Coe, F. L. (1978). "Nephrolithiasis: Pathogenesis and Treatment." Yearbook Publ., Chicago, Illinois.

Coe, F. L., and Favus, M. J. (1981). *In* "The Kidney" (B. M. Brenner and F. C. Rector, eds.), Vol. 2, 2nd ed. Saunders, Philadelphia, Pennsylvania.
Conway, N. S., Maitland, A. I., and Rennie, J. B. (1949). *Br. J. Urol.* **21,** 30–38.
Cornelius, C. E., and Bishop, J. A. (1961). *J. Urol.* **85,** 842–848.
Davalos, H. F. (1943). *J. Urol.* **49,** 639–645.
Dedmond, R. E., and Wrong, O. (1962). *Clin. Sci.* **22,** 19–32.
de la Pena, A., and de la Pena, E. (1944). *J. Urol.* **52,** 108.
Delisle, G. T. (1977). *J. Bacteriol.* **130,** 1390–1392.
Delluva, A. M., Markley, K., and Davies, R. E. (1968). *Biochim. Biophys. Acta.* **151,** 646–650.
Drach, G. W. (1983). *Urol. Clin. North Am.* **10,** 709–717.
Dretler, S. P., and Pfister, R. C. (1983). *Annu. Rev. Med.* **34,** 359–366.
Droller, M. J., and Freiha, F. S. (1977). *J. Am. Med. Assoc.* **237,** 1467–1468.
Duch, D. S., Hamar, D. W., Chow, F. C., and Lewis, L. D. (1978). *Biochem. Med.* **19,** 236–245.
Elliot, J. S. (1954). *J. Urol.* **72,** 331–336.
Elliot, J. S., Quande, W. L., Sharp, R. F., and Lewis, L. (1958). *J. Urol.* **80,** 269–271.
Elliot, J. S., Sharp, R. F., and Lewis, L. (1959). *J. Urol.* **80,** 366–368.
Emerick, R. J. (1969). *South Dakota Farm Home Res.* **20,** 19–23.
Feit, R. M., and Fair, W. R. (1979). *J. Urol.* **122,** 592–594.
Feldman, S., Putcha, L., and Griffith, D. P. (1978). *Invest. Urol.* **15,** 498–501.
Finco, D. R., and Barsanti, J. A. (1984). *Vet. Clin. North Am.* **14,** 529–536.
Finco, D. R., Rosin, E., and Johnson, K. H. (1970). *J. Am. Vet. Med. Assoc.* **157,** 1225–1228.
Finlayson, B. (1974). *Urol. Clin. North Am.* **1,** 181–212.
Finlayson, B. (1977). *In* "Calcium Metabolism in Renal Failure and Nephrolithiasis" (D. S. David, ed.), pp. 337–382. Wiley, New York.
Fishbein, W. N. (1981). *In* "Urolithiasis: Clinical and Basic Research" (L. H. Smith, W. G. Robertson, and B. Finlayson, eds.), pp. 209–214. Plenum, New York.
Fishbein, W. N., and Daly, J. E. (1970). *Proc. Soc. Exp. Biol. Med.* **134,** 1083–1090.
Fleisch, H. (1978). *Kidney Int.* **13,** 361–371.
Fleisch, H., and Russel, R. G. G. (1977). *In* "Calcium Metabolism in Renal Failure and Nephrolithiasis" (D. S. David, ed.), pp. 293–336. Wiley, New York.
Ford, D. K., and McDonald, J. (1967). *J. Bacteriol.* **93,** 1509–1512.
Fowler, J. E. (1984). *J. Urol.* **131,** 213–215.
Friedlander, A. M., and Braude, A. I. (1974). *Nature (London)* **247,** 67–69.
Garcia de la Pena, E., and Cifuentes Delatte, L. (1981). *In* "Urolithiasis: Clinical and Basic Research" (L. H. Smith, W. G. Robertson and B. Finlayson, eds.), pp. 935–942. Plenum, New York.
Gill, W. B., Jones, K. W., and Ruggiero, K. J. (1982). *J. Urol.* **127,** 152–154.
Gillespie, J. H., and Timoney, J. F. (1981). "Hagan and Bruner's Infectious Disease of Domestic Animals," 7th ed., pp. 226–237. Cornstock Pub. Assoc., Cornell Univ. Press, Ithaca, New York.
Goulden, B. E. (1968). *Vet. Rec.* **83,** 509–514.
Grant, A. M. S., Baker, L. R. I., and Neuberger, A. (1973). *Clin. Sci.* **44,** 377–384.
Grant, R. B., Penner, J. L., Hennessy, J. N., and Jackowski, B. J. (1981). *J. Clin. Microbiol.* **13,** 561–565.
Grenabo, L., Brorson, J. E., Hedelin, H., and Pettersson, S. (1984). *Urol. Res.* **12,** 30.
Griffith, D. P. (1978a). *Kidney Int.* **13,** 372–382.
Griffith, D. P. (1978b). *In* "Nephrolithiasis: Pathogenesis and Management" (F. L. Coe, ed.), pp. 203–228. Yearbook Publ., Chicago, Illionois.

Griffith, D.P. (1979). *Urol. Res.* **7,** 215–221.
Griffith, D. P. (1982). *Kidney Int.* **21,** 422–430.
Griffith, D. P., and Klein, A. S. (1983). *Int. Perspect. Urol.* **6,** 210–227.
Griffith, D. P., and Musher, D. M. (1973). *Invest. Urol.* **11,** 228–233.
Griffith, D. P., and Musher, D. M. (1975). *Urology* **5,** 299–302.
Griffith, D. P., Bragin, S., and Musher, D. M. (1976). *Invest. Urol.* **13,** 351–353.
Griffith, D. P., Gibson, J. R., Clinton, C. W., and Musher, D. M. (1978). *J. Urol.* **119,** 9–15.
Griffith, D. P., Moskowitz, P. A., and Carlton, C. W. (1979). *J. Urol.* **70,** 25–29.
Griffith, D. P., Moskowitz, P. A., and Feldman, S. (1981). *In* "Urolithiasis: Clinical and Basic Research" (L. H. Smith, W. G. Robertson, and B. Finlayson, eds.), pp. 199–208. Plenum, New York.
Hallson, P. C., and Rose, G. A. (1979). *Lancet* **1,** 1000–1002.
Hansen, N. M., Felix, R., and Bisaz, S. (1976). *Biochim. Biophys. Acta* **451,** 549–559.
Hardy, R. M., Osborne, C. A., Cassidy, F. C., and Johnson, K. H. (1972). *Vet. Med. Small Anim. Clin.* **67,** 1205–1211.
Harwood, E. J. (1982). *Lab. Anim.* **16,** 314–318.
He, J., Liu, G. D., and Shen, S. J. (1984). *Urol. Res.* **12,** 94.
Hedelin, H., Brorson, J. E., Grenabo, L., and Pettersson, S. (1984). *Urol. Res.* **12,** 30.
Hinman, F. (1979). *J. Urol.* **121,** 700–705.
Jackson, O. F. (1972). *Vet. Rec.* **91,** 292–293.
Johnson, L. W. (1981). *In* "Current Veterinary Therapy: Food Animal Practice" (J. L. Howard, ed.), pp. 1037–1041. Saunders, Philadelphia, Pennsylvania.
Johnston, G. R., Feeney, D. A., and Osborne, C. A. (1982). *Compend. Contin. Educ.* **4,** 931–946.
Kallfelz, F. A., Bressett, J. D., and Wallace, R. J. (1980). *Feline Pract.* **10,** 25–35.
Kaspar, L. V., Poole, C. M., and Norris, W. P. (1978). *Lab. Anim. Sci.* **28,** 545–550.
Kenney, G. E., and Cartwright, F. D. (1977). *J. Bacteriol.* **132,** 144–150.
Keutel, H. J., and King, J. S. (1964). *Invest. Urol.* **2,** 115–122.
Keyser, L. D. (1945). *J. Urol.* **54,** 194–210.
Kimberling, C. V., and Arnold, K. S. (1983). *Vet. Clin. North Am.* **5,** 637–655.
Kinter, L. B., McDonald, J., Beeuwkes, R., and Gittes, R. (1982). *J. Urol.* **128,** 1077–1080.
Kirby, R., Crane, S., and Schaer, M. (1983). *J. Am. Vet. Med. Assoc.* **178,** 827–828.
Klausner, J. S., and Osborne, C. A. (1979). *J. Am. Vet. Med. Assoc.* **174,** 1100–1104.
Klausner, J. S., Osborne, C. A., O'Leary, T. P., and Griffith, D. P. (1977). *Sci. Proc. Annu. Gaines Vet. Symp. 27th,* pp. 25–37. (Gaines Dog Research Center, White Plains, New York.)
Klausner, J. S., Osborne, C. A., O'Leary, T. P., Gebhart, R. N., and Griffith, D. P. (1980a). *Am. J. Vet. Res.* **40,** 712–719.
Klausner, J. S., Osborne, C. A., O'Leary, T. P., Muscoplat, C. M., and Griffith, D. P. (1980b). *Invest. Urol.* **18,** 127–132.
Klausner, J. S., O'Leary, T. P., Kitchell, B. E., and Osborne, C. A. (1985). *J. Am. Vet. Med. Assoc.* (in press).
Kobashi, K., Kumaki, K., and Hose, J. (1971). *Biochim. Biophys. Acta* **227,** 429–441.
Kornberg, H. L., Davies, R. E., and Wood, D. R. (1954a). *Biochem. J.* **56,** 355–363.
Kornberg, H. L., Davies, R. E., and Wood, D. R. (1954b). *Biochem. J.* **56,** 363–372.
Krajden, S., Fuksa, M., Lizewski, S., Barton, L., and Lee, A. (1984). *J. Clin. Microbiol.* **19,** 541–542.
Krawiec, D. R., Osborne, C. A., Leininger, J. R., and Griffith, D. P. (1984a). *Am. J. Vet. Res.* **45,** 1266–1275.

Krawiec, D. R., Osborne, C. A., Leininger, J. R., and Griffith, D. P. (1984b). *Am. J. Vet. Res.* **45**, 1276–1282.
Lamm, D. L., Johnson, S. A., Friedlander, A. M., and Gittes,R. F. (1977). *Urology* **10**, 418–421.
Lees, G. E., Osborne, C. A., Stevens, J. B., and Ward, G. E.(1981). *Am. J. Vet. Res.* **42**, 825–833.
Lesher, R. J., and Jones, W. A. (1978). *J. Clin. Microbiol.* **8**, 344–345.
Levenson, S. M., Crowley, L. V., Horowitz, R. E., and Malm,O. J. (1959). *J. Biol. Chem.* **234**, 2061–2062.
Lewi, H. J. E., White, A., Hutchinson, A. G., and Scott, R.(1984). *Urol. Res.* **12**, 107–109.
Lewis, L. D. (1981). *Sci. Proc. Annu. Meet. Am. Anim. Hosp.Assoc.*, pp. 273–284.
Lewis, L. D. (1983). *Sci. Proc. Annu. Meet. Anim. Hosp.Assoc.*, pp. 319–323.
Lewis, L. D., and Morris, M. L. (1983)."Small Animal Clinical Nutrition." pp. 8–1 to 8–40. Mark Morris Associates,Topeka, Kansas.
Lewis, G. A., Schuster, G. A., and Cooper, R. A. (1983). *Urology* **22**, 401–403.
Ling, G. V. (1983). *In* "Current Veterinary Therapy" (R. W. Kirk, ed.), Vol. 8, pp. 1051–1055. Saunders, Philadelphia, Pennsylvania.
Ling, G. V., and Hirsh, D. C. (1983). *In* "CurrentVeterinary Therapy" (R. W. Kirk, ed.), Vol. 8, pp. 1048–1051. Saunders, Philadelphia, Pennsylvania.
MacLaren, D. M. (1968). *J. Pathol. Bacteriol.* **96**, 45–56.
MacLaren, D. M. (1969). *J. Pathol.* **97**, 43–49.
McDonald, M. I., Lamm, M. H., Birch, D. F., Darcy, A. F., Fairley,K. F., and Pavillard, E. R. J. (1982). *J. Urol.* **128**, 517–519.
Malek, R. S., and Boyce, W. H. (1977). *J. Urol.* **117**, 336–341.
Marberger, M. (1983). *Urol. Clin. North Am.* **10**, 729–742.
Marquardt, H., and Nagel, R. (1977). *Urology* **9**, 627–629.
Martelli, A., Bull, P., and Brunocilla, E. (1982). *J. Urol.* **128**, 1130–1132.
Meyer, J. L., and Angino, E. E. (1977). *Invest. Urol.* **14**, 347–350.
Millner, O. E., Anderson, J. A., Appler, M. E., Benjamin, C. E., Edwards, J. G., Humphrey, D. T., and Shearer, E. M. (1982). *J. Urol.* **127**, 346–350.
Mitchell, R. S. (1979). "Mineral Names. What Do They Mean?" Van Nostrand-Reinhold, New York.
Moore, S., and Gouldand, G. (1975). *Br. J. Urol.* **47**, 489–494.
Morris, M. L., and Doering, G. G. (1978). *Canine Pract.* **5**, 53–59.
Morrissey, J. F., Ochoa, M., Lotspeich, W. D., and Wterhouse, C. (1963). *Ann. Intern. Med.* **58**, 159–166.
Musher, D. M., Griffith, D. P., Tyler, M., and Woelfel, A. (1974a). *Antimicrob. Agents Chemother.* **5**, 101–105.
Musher, D. M., Saenz, C., and Griffith, D. P. (1974b). *Antimicrob. Agents Chemother.* **5**, 106–110.
Nemoy, N. J., and Stamey, T. A. (1971). *J. Am. Med. Assoc.***215**, 1470–1476.
Nielsen, I. M. (1956). *J. Urol.* **75**, 602–613.
Noronha, R. F. X., Gregory, J. G., and Duke, J. J. (1979). *J. Urol.* **121**, 478–479.
Osborne, C. A. (1982). *Sci. Proc. Am. Anim. Hosp. Assoc.*, pp. 211–212.
Osborne, C. A., and Klausner, J. S. (1978). *Sci. Proc. Annu. Meet. Am. Anim. Hosp. Assoc. 45th* pp. 569–620.
Osborne, C. A., and Stevens, J. B. (1981). "Handbook of Canine and Feline Urinalysis." Ralston Purina, St. Louis, Missouri.
Osborne, C. A., Klausner, J. S., and Lees, G. E. (1979).*Vet. Clin. North Am.* **9**, 587–609.

Osborne, C. A., Klausner, J. S., Krawiec, D. R., and Griffith, D. P. (1981). *J. Am. Vet. Med. Assoc.* **179**, 239–244.

Osborne, C. A., Abdullahi, S. U., Leininger, J. R., Polzin, D. J., Hauer, N. E., Klausner, J. S., Hardy, R. M., Kuzma, A. B., and Gidlund, C. J. (1982). *Minn. Vet.* **22**, 14–17.

Osborne, C. A., Abdullahi, S. U., and Johnston, C. R. (1983a). In "Current Veterinary Therapy" (R. W. Kirk, ed.), Vol. 8., pp. 1076–1081. Saunders, Philadelphia, Pennsylvania.

Osborne, C. A., Abdullahi, S. U., Klausner, J. S., Johnston, G. R., and Polzin, D. J. (1983b). *J. Am. Vet. Med. Assoc.* **182**, 47–50.

Osborne, C. A., Johnston, G. R., Polzin, D. J., Kruger, J. M., Bell, F. W., Poffenbarger, E. M., Feeney, D. A., Stevens, J. B., and McMenomy, M. (1984a). *J. Am. Hosp. Assoc.* **20**, 17–32.

Osborne, C. A., Johnston, G. R., Polzin, D. J., Kruger, J. M., Poffenbarger, E. M., Bell, F. W., Feeney, D. A., Goyal, S., Fletcher, T. F., Newman, J. A., Stevens, J. B., and McMenomy, M. F. (1984b). *Vet. Clin. North Am.* **14**, 409–438.

Osborne, C. A., Johnston, G. R., Polzin, D. J., Kruger, J. M., Poffenbarger, E. M., Bell, F. W., Feeney, D. A., Goyal, S., Fletcher, T. F., Newman, J. A., Caywood, D. D., and McMenomy, M. F. (1984c). *Proc. 7th Kal Kan Symp.*, pp. 107–124. (Kal Kan Foods Inc., Vernon, California.)

Osborne, C. A., Clinton, C. W., Brunkow, H. C., Frost, A. P., and Johnston, G. R. (1984d). *Vet. Clin. North Am.* **14**, 481–491.

Osborne, C. A., Kruger, J. M., Polzin, D. J., Johnston, G. R., Poffenbarger, E. M., Bell, F. W., Goyal, S., Newman, J. M., Fletcher,T. F., Levine, S. H., Jenkins, D. M., McCarthy, R. J., O'Keefe, D.A., and McMenomy, M. F. (1984e). *Minn. Vet.* **24**, 22–32.

Osborne, C. A., Abdullahi, S. U., Polzin, D. J., Leininger, J. R., and Kruger, J. M. (1984f). *Proc. 7th Kal Kan Symp.* pp.52–79. (Kal Kan Foods Inc., Vernon, California.)

Osborne, C. A., Polzin, D. J., and Abdullahi, S. U. (1984g). In "Textbook of Small Animal Surgery" (D. Slatter, ed.). Saunders, Philadelphia, Pennsylvania.

Osborne, C. A., Polzin, D. J., Klausner, J. S., and Kruger, J. M. (1984h). *Vet. Clin. North Am.* **14**, 617–640.

Osborne, C. A., Polzin, D. J., Feeney, D. A., and Caywood, D. D. (1985). In "A Textbook of Small Animal Surgery" (I. M. Gourley and P. B. Vasseur, eds.). Lippincott, Philadelphia, Pennsylvania (in press).

Pak, C. Y. C. (1976). In "The Kidney" (B. C. Brenner and F. C. Rector, eds.), 2nd ed., Vol. 2, pp. 1376–1398. Saunders, Philadelphia, Pennsylvania.

Pak, C. Y. C. (1978). "Calcium Urolithiasis: Pathogenesis, Diagnosis, and Management." Plenum, New York.

Parsons, C. L., Stauffer, C., Mulholland, S. G., and Griffith, D. P. (1984). *J. Urol.* **132**, 365–366.

Pettersson, S., Brorson, J. E., Grenabo, L., and Hedelin, H. (1983). *Lancet* **1**, 526–527.

Piermattei, D. L., and Osborne, C. A. (1971). *J. Am. Vet. Med. Assoc.* **159**, 1755–1757.

Polache, C., Berman, H., and Frondel, C. (1951). "Dana's System of Minerology," Vol. 2., 7th ed. Wiley, New York.

Pollack, S., and Wagner, B. M. (1976). *Vet. Med. Small Anim. Clin.* **71**, 1693–1696.

Polzin, D. J., Osborne, C. A., Hayden, D. W., and Stevens, J. B. (1983). *J. Am. Vet. Med. Assoc.* **183**, 980–986.

Prien, E. L. (1974). *Urol. Clin. North Am.* **1**, 231.

Pyrah, L. N. (1979). "Renal Calculus." Springer-Verlag, Berlin and New York.

Resnick, M. I. (1983). *Urol. Clin. North Am.* **10**, 585–766.

Rich, L. J., and Kirk, R. W. (1968). *Am. J. Vet. Res.* **29**, 2149–2156.

Rich, L. J., and Norcross, N. L. (1969). *Am. J. Vet. Res.* **30**, 1001–1005.
Rich, L. J., Dysart, I., and Chow, F. C. (1974). *Feline Pract.* **4**, 44–47.
Robertson, W. G., and Peacock, M. (1982). *In* "Scientific Foundations of Urology" (G. D. Chisholm and D. I. Williams, eds.), 2nd ed., pp. 267–278. Heinemann Medical Books, London.
Robertson, W. G., Peacock, M., and Nordin, B. E. C. (1971). *Clin. Sci.* **40**, 365–374.
Rocha, A. H., and Santos, L. C. S. (1969). *J. Med. Microbiol.* **2**, 372–376.
Rose, A. G., and Sulaiman, S. (1982). *J. Urol.* **127**, 177–179.
Rosenstein, I. J. M., and Hamilton-Miller, J. M. T. (1984). *Crit. Rev. Microbiol.* **11**, 1–12.
Rosenstein, I. J. M., Hamilton-Miller, J. M. T., and Brumfitt, W. (1981). *Infect. Immun.* **32**, 32–37.
Roth, R. A. (1976). *Surg. Clin. North. Am.* **56**, 753–766.
Rous, S. N., and Turner, W. R. (1977). *J. Urol.* **118**, 902–904.
Russell, J. M., Harrison, L. H., and Boyce, W. H. (1981). *J. Urol.* **125**, 471–474.
Sayed, I. A., and Kenney, G. E. (1978). *J. Bacteriol.* **134**, 967–972.
Schwille, P. O., Scholz, D., and Paulus, M. (1979). *Invest. Urol.* **16**, 457–462.
Scott, R. (1975). *Urology* **6**, 667–675.
Scott, W. W., Huggins, C., and Selman, B. C. (1943). *J. Urol.* **50**, 202–209.
Senior, B. W. (1979). *J. Med. Microbiol.* **12**, 1–8.
Senior, B. W., Bradford, N. C., and Simpson, D. S. (1980). *J. Med. Microbiol.* **13**, 507–512.
Senior, D. G., Thomas, W. C., Gaskin, J. M., and Finlayson, B. (1984). *Urol. Res.* **12**, 39.
Sheldon, C. A., and Smith, A. D. (1982). *Urol. Clin. North Am.* **9**, 121–130.
Shepard, M. C., and Lunceford, C. D. (1965). *J. Bacteriol.* **93**, 265–270.
Shepard, M. C., and Lunceford, C. D. (1967). *J. Bacteriol.* **93**, 1513–1520.
Shepard, M. C., and Lunceford, C. D. (1978). *J. Clin. Microbiol.* **8**, 566–574.
Shepard, M. C., Lunceford, C. D., Ford, D. K., Purcell, R. H.,Taylor-Robinson, D., Razin, S., and Black, F. T. (1974). *Int. J. Syst. Bacteriol.* **24**, 160–171.
Singh, M., Chapman, R., Tresidder, G. C., and Blandy, J. (1973). *Br. J. Urol.* **45**, 581–585.
Sinno, K., Boyce, W. H., and Resnick, M. I. (1979). *J. Urol.* **121**, 662–664.
Smith, A. D. (1982). *Urol. Clin. North Am.* **9**, 1–196.
Smith, A. D., and Lee, W. J. (1983). *Urol. Clin. North Am.* **10**, 719–727.
Smith, L. H. (1974). *Urol. Clin. North Am.* **1**, 241–260.
Smith, L. H., Boyce, W. H., Finlayson, B., Lassiter, W. E., Meyer, J. L., Pak, C. Y. C., Stamey, T. F., and Thomas, W. C.(1978). "Urolithiasis. Research Needs in Nephrology and Urology,"Vol. 5., pp. 1–32. U.S. Dept. of Health, Education, and Welfare. Bethesda, Maryland.
Sorensen, D. K. (1980). *In* "Bovine Medicine and Surgery" (H. E. Amstutz, ed.), pp. 841–845. Amer. Vet. Pub. Inc.,Santa Barbara, California.
Spector, A. R., Gray, A., and Prien, E. L. (1976). *Invest. Urol.* **13**, 387–389.
Stamey, T. A. (1980). "Pathogenesis and Treatment of Urinary Tract Infections." Williams and Wilkins, Baltimore, Maryland.
Stapleton, F. B., Roy, S., Noe, N., and Jenkins, G. (1984).*New Engl. J. Med.* **310**, 1345–1348.
Stegmayr, B., and Stegmayr, B. (1983). *Scand. J. Urol.Nephrol.* **17**, 197–203.
Stone, E. A. (1984). *Vet. Clin. North Am.* **14**, 77–92.
Suby, H. I., and Suby, R. M. (1947). *J. Urol.* **57**, 995–1000.
Summerskill, W. H. J., Thorsell, F., and Feinberg, J. H. (1968). *Gastroenterology* **54**, 20–27.
Sutherland, J. W. (1981). *J. Urol.* **126**, 573–575.
Sutherland, R. W. (1954). *Br. J. Urol.* **26**, 22–45.

Sutor, D. J. (1972). In "Urolithiasis: Physical Aspects" (B. Finlayson, ed.), pp. 43–60. Nat. Acad. Sci., Washington D.C.
Sutor, D. J., and Wooley, S. E. (1970). Res. Vet. Sci. **11,** 298–299.
Sutor, D. J., Percival, J. M., and Doonan, S. (1978). Clin. Chim. Acta **89,** 273–278.
Takeuchi, H., Okada, Y., Kobashi, L., and Yoshida, O. (1982). Urol. Res. **10,** 217–219.
Takeuchi, H., Takayama, H., Konishi, T., and Tomoyoshi, T. (1984). J. Urol. **132,** 67–69.
Tannen, R. L. (1983). Med. Clin. North Am. **67,** 781–798.
Taton, G. F., Hamar, D. W., and Lewis, L. D. (1984). J. Am. Vet. Med. Assoc. **184,** 437–443.
Taylor-Robinson, D., Czonka, G. W., and Prentice, M. J. (1977). Q. J. Med. **46,** 309–326.
Thompson, R. B., and Stamey, T. A. (1973). Urology **2,** 627–633.
Thornhill, J. A. (1977). In "Current Veterinary Therapy" (R. W. Kirk, ed.), Vol. 7., pp. 1087–1097. Saunders, Philadelphia,Pennsylvania.
Udall, R. H., and Jensen, R. (1958). J. Am. Vet. Med. Assoc. **133,** 514–516.
Udall, R. H., Deem, A. W., and Maag, D. D. (1958). Am. J. Vet. Res. **19,** 825–829.
Vermeulen, C. W., and Goetz, R. (1954). J. Urol. **72,** 761 –769.
Weaver, A. D., and Pillinger, R. (1975). Vet. Rec. **97,** 48–50.
Werness, P. G., Bergert, J. H., and Smith, L. H. (1981). In "Urolithiasis: Clinical and Basic Research" (L. H. Smith,W. G. Robertson, and B. Finlayson, eds.), pp. 17–21. Plenum, NewYork.
White, E. G., and Porter, P. (1969). In "Textbook of Veterinary Clinical Pathology" (W. Medway, J. E. Prier, and J.S. Wilkinson, eds.), pp. 132–151. Williams and Wilkins, Baltimore, Maryland.
Wickham, J. E. A. (1976). In "Scientific Foundations of Urology" (D. I. Williams and G. O. Chisholm, eds.), Vol. 1.,pp. 323–329. Yearbook Publ. Chicago, Illinois.
Williams, J. J., Rodman, J. S., and Peterson, C. M. (1984). New Engl. J. Med. **311,** 760–764.
Wojewski, A., and Zajaczkowski, T. (1973). Int. Urol. Nephrol. **5,** 249.

The Relative Importance of Enteric Pathogens Affecting Neonates of Domestic Animals

SAUL TZIPORI[1]

Attwood Institute for Veterinary Research, Department of Agriculture, Westmeadows, Victoria, Australia

I.	Introduction	104
II.	Rotaviruses	105
	A. Characteristics of Rotavirus	105
	B. *In Vitro* Cultivation	106
	C. Gene Coding Assignment	107
	D. Genetic and Antigenic Diversity	108
	E. Group A Rotaviruses	109
	F. Other Rotavirus Groups	116
	G. Development of Rotavirus Vaccines	119
III.	Enterotoxigenic *E. coli* (ETEC)	125
	A. Pathogenic Mechanisms	126
	B. Control of ETEC Diarrhea	137
	C. Postweaning Diarrhea (PWD)	148
IV.	*Cryptosporidium*	158
	A. Cryptosporidiosis in Animals	159
	B. Human Cryptosporidiosis	160
	C. Diagnosis of *Cryptosporidium* Infection	164
	D. New Advances in Laboratory Studies	165
	E. Control of Cryptosporidiosis	166
V.	*Clostridium perfringens* Type C	168
	A. Characteristics of the Disease	168
	B. Characteristics of the Organism	169
	C. Mechanisms of Diarrhea	170
	D. Diagnosis	171
	E. Control	171
VI.	Calf Diarrhea	172
	A. Epidemiology	172
	B. Infections Specific to Calves	175

[1]Present Address: Microbiology Department, Royal Childrens Hospital, Parkville, Victoria, Australia.

VII.	Piglet Enteritis	179
	A. Epidemiology	179
	B. Infections Specific to Piglets	183
VIII.	Diarrhea in Foals	186
	A. Rotavirus Diarrhea	186
	B. *Streptococcus durans*	188
	C. *Cl. perfringens* Type C	189
	D. Other Enteropathogens	191
IX.	Concluding Remarks	192
	References	193

I. Introduction

The etiology of diarrhea and the mechanisms by which enteropathogens cause disease have been the subject of intense global research in the last decade. This research led to the identification of a considerable number of enteric pathogens previously unrecognized or ill defined. These developments, coupled with newly acquired molecular biological tools, provided an unprecedented opportunity for development of sensitive and rapid diagnostic tests, better definition of mode of action of virulence attributes, and opened new horizons for development of control measures.

Some organisms although host specific are found in a great number of species of animals, e.g., rotavirus and enterotoxigenic *Escherichia coli* (ETEC). Others, like *Cryptosporidium,* lack host specificity and readily cross the species barrier causing disease in some and subclinical infections in others. A few infections that are significant only to young animals of a particular species include coccidiosis in pigs and enteropathogenic *E. coli* (EPEC) in humans. The first part of this article (Sections II–V) analyzes information relating to pathogens shared by more than one animal species, while Sections VI–VIII discuss the epidemiology of diarrhea and infections that are specific to piglets, calves, and foals. Wherever appropriate, the significance of corresponding infections in humans is also discussed in some detail. This is essential, since in diarrheal diseases, more so than in any other scientific field, a considerable portion of the available knowledge is complementary, and is largely a consequence of collaborative and comparative studies between the medical and the veterinary fields, as is evident throughout this article.

The literature regarding coronavirus infections in bovine and swine will not be reviewed in this article. It should not be seen to indicate that they are not significant. On the contrary, coronavirus infections in calves, and transmissible gastroenteritis (TGE) infection in swine, particularly in parts of North America, are probably the most important causes of economic loss associated with enteric infections for both species (Morin et al., 1983; L. J. Saif, personal communication). Apart from epidemiological observations, they will not be dealt with for two reasons: (1) as neither occurs in Australia the author is not familiar with them, and (2) unlike other areas of perhaps lesser significance, progress in research on enteric coronavirus in domestic animals has been slow. It may reflect a sad reality that, with a lack of medical interest due to the absence of a similar disease in humans, research on these important infections is less vigorous than it ought to be.

II. Rotaviruses

The significance of these viruses, although recognized in the late 1960s (Mebus et al., 1969), only became a subject for extensive research with the discovery that these viruses cause diarrhea in humans (Bishop et al., 1973; Flewett et al., 1973; Kapikian et al., 1974; Middleton et al., 1974). Research on rotaviruses essentially provided a new impetus into investigations of other infections of the gastrointestinal tract. There are now a considerable number of reviews and chapters in books on the biology of rotaviruses and the diseases they cause in humans and animals to which the reader is referred (Flewett and Woode, 1978; Holmes, 1979; McNulty, 1978). A comprehensive analysis of the most pertinent information relating to the morphology, genome, capsid proteins, antigenic determinants, viral replication and genetics, and biology of rotaviruses has been published (Holmes, 1983) and is highly recommended.

In this section only recent developments in genetics and cultivation as they relate to the understanding of virus serotyping and serogrouping will be considered. The emergence of a complex serotyping among these viruses, and the effect it has on development of prototype vaccines and future vaccines will also be discussed.

A. CHARACTERISTICS OF ROTAVIRUS

The particles are icosahedral, measuring 65–75 nm in diameter, have 2 concentric layers of capsid and contain a genome of 11 segments of double-stranded RNA (dsRNA). These characteristics place this group firmly within the family Reoviridae (Mathews, 1979). They infect mature, small intestinal enterocytes of mammals and birds (Flewett and Woode, 1978; Holmes, 1979; McNulty, 1978) and their infectivity of cells resides with the outer capsid (Bridger and Woode, 1976; Elias, 1977), except possibly in the case of murine rotavirus or EDIM (Thouless *et al.*, 1977). Rotaviruses were thought to share a common virus capsid antigen (Flewett and Woode, 1978; McNulty, 1978). Recently, however, viruses that are morphologically and biologically indistinguishable from rotavirus but do not share a common antigen have been detected in animals and humans, and have been referred to as either atypical rotaviruses, or pararotaviruses.

B. *In Vitro* Cultivation

Apart from several cell culture-adapted rotaviruses, mostly of bovine origin, the majority of strains recognized up to the late 1970s were noncultivable. The slow process of research on the epidemiology, serotyping, genetics, immunology, and development of vaccines was directly related to the difficulties encountered in propagating these fastidious viruses in cell culture.

In an attempt to enhance plaque formation in the Rhesus monkey kidney cell line MA-104 by the Nebraska calf diarrhea virus (NCDV), Matsuno *et al.* (1977) applied trypsin and DEAE-dextran. The incorporation of trypsin into cell culture medium was subsequently shown to promote viral propagation *in vitro* of otherwise noncultivable viruses of bovine (Babiuk *et al.*, 1977), porcine (Theil *et al.*, 1977), and avian origin (McNulty *et al.*, 1979). This method is now widely used and is very highly successful for routine cultivation of wild types of rotavirus. Adaptation of human rotaviruses to cell culture is more difficult and requires, in addition to trypsin, rolling of cultures for several subcultures before they become established (Sato *et al.*, 1981; Urasawa *et al.*, 1981). Trypsin acts directly on the virus, not on the host cells (Barnett *et al.*, 1979) and this effect is due to specific cleavage of one of the outer capsid proteins (Espejo *et al.*, 1981), which appears to facilitate uncoating of the virus inside the cell (Clark *et al.*, 1981).

Another interesting strategy to circumvent the difficulties in cultivation, particularly of human rotaviruses in cell culture, was achieved through adaptation by reassortment. The segmented nature of rotavirus genome has been shown to allow a high frequency of gene reassortment during coinfection *in vitro* (Matsuno *et al.*, 1980) and *in vivo* (A. J. Herring and S. Tzipori; S. Tzipori and M. Smith, unpublished data). This led Greenberg *et al.* (1981) to try to rescue noncultivable human rotaviruses by reassorting them with cultivable *ts* mutants of bovine rotavirus UK strain. In this manner, the genes of the noncultivable human rotavirus that restricted growth *in vitro* were replaced by the corresponding genes from the tissue-culture-adapted *ts* UK bovine rotavirus, while retaining their human serotype specificity. This method was subsequently extended to study 50 additional human rotavirus strains collected over 16 years (Greenberg *et al.*, 1982).

Further analysis of these gene reassortments by Kalica *et al.* (1981) has identified the sixth gene segment as being responsible for the common antigen or subgroup specificity, detected by ELISA, immunofluorescence (IF), and immune adherence hemagglutination assay (IAHA). The ninth gene segment, on the other hand, was said to be associated with serotypes detected by plaque reduction neutralization (PRN) test. The fourth RNA segment appears to be responsible for restriction of cultivation of noncultivable human rotaviruses in cell culture (Greenberg *et al.*, 1982).

C. Gene Coding Assignment

Like other members of the Reoviridae family, rotaviruses possess isometric capsids of two protein layers which enclose the genome. The proteins encoded by each of the 11 RNA segments have been determined for UK bovine virus (McCrae and Faulkner-Valle, 1981) and for the simian rotavirus SA11 (Dyall-Smith and Holmes, 1981; Kantharidis *et al.*, 1983; Smith *et al.*, 1980). Of the 11 segments, 7, 8, and 9 are of particular interest from the point of view of serotyping.

Segments 7, 8, and 9, which run closely together on polyacrylamide gel electrophoresis, are often difficult to resolve, and the order of migration of these genes varies among viral strains (Dyall-Smith *et al.*, 1983). One of these gene segments encodes for the major glycosylated outer shell structural protein, which is responsible for serotypic specificity as recognized by neutralizing antibody (Bastardo *et al.*, 1981; Kalica *et al.*, 1981; Thouless, 1979), while the other two encode nonstructural proteins (Arias *et al.*, 1982; Dyall-Smith and Holmes, 1982).

In the simian rotaviruses SA11 and human Wa, serotype specificity is determined by segment 9 (Dyall-Smith *et al.*, 1983; Kalica *et al.*, 1981), while in the UK bovine rotavirus it is encoded by segments 8 or 9 (Greenberg *et al.*, 1981). This correlates with the major outer shell glycoprotein assignment to gene 9 of SA11 and to gene 8 of UK bovine rotavirus (McCrae and McCorquodale, 1982) and the neutralizing activity of antibody produced to this glycoprotein.

Cloning and nucleotide sequencing of RNA gene segments encoding viral proteins responsible for group or subgroup antigenic determinants, serotypic specificity, and other viral characteristics are of vital importance. Studies have concentrated mainly on sequencing gene segments 7, 8, and 9 of the simian SA11 and UK bovine rotaviruses (Dyall-Smith *et al.,* 1983; Elleman *et al.,* 1984). Comparisons between strains will provide the molecular and structural basis for the nature and diversity of these viruses. This will also assist with determining the nature and degree of attenuation of viral strains used for vaccines as compared with the parent strains.

As mentioned earlier, there is a considerable variation in the gene order of RNA segments when separated by electrophoresis and there is often an inversion in order of migration between segments 10 and 11 of human rotavirus having "long" and "short" electrophoretic patterns (Holmes, 1983). Gene mapping, using Northern blot hybridization on dsRNA segments from different virus strains, has been used to identify corresponding segments (Dyall-Smith *et al.,* 1983). When the UK bovine rotavirus gene 7 sequence, for instance, was compared with the corresponding gene segment 8 of the SA11 simian rotavirus, they were found to be identical in size and the arrangement of the proposed coding and noncoding regions, with 88% homology in nucleotide sequence (Dyall-Smith *et al.,* 1983). This is interesting when considering that the UK bovine and the SA11 simian rotaviruses were isolated from two different species of animal, from geographically remote countries (South Africa and the United Kingdom, respectively), and 16 years apart, yet the gene and predicted amino acid sequences of the two corresponding RNA segments are highly conserved; this is indicative of a gene coding for a nonstructural protein which is not subjected directly to the host immune system (Dyall-Smith *et al.,* 1983).

Analysis of viral genomes by hybridization studies is likely to be of considerable importance in the future, as comparisons between similar and dissimilar serotypes can be made in order to examine the degree of sequence relatedness or diversity between corresponding segments.

D. GENETIC AND ANTIGENIC DIVERSITY

Early serological studies showed that rotaviruses derived from various sources were antigenically related. How closely related, or even identical they were was not realized until 1977 when Thouless *et al.* (1977) demonstrated 4- to 8-fold differences in what might have been the first neutralization test, between homologous and heterologous noncultivable rotavirus isolates of bovine, human, porcine, equine, murine, lapine, and ovine origin. While extensive and meaningful serological studies were difficult until appropriate routine *in vitro* cultivation techniques became available, the existence of genetic diversity among isolates was recognized much earlier. Migration patterns of the 11 dsRNA segments in polyacrylamide gel electrophoresis were shown to differ between rotaviruses present in feces obtained from different animals and humans (Kalica *et al.*, 1978; Rodger and Holmes, 1979; Verly and Cohen, 1977). The technique was found to be particularly useful for distinguishing between different rotavirus strains for epidemiological studies (Rodger *et al.*, 1981), as it is more discriminating than serology (Holmes, 1983).

The migration pattern of the genome in polyacrylamide gel has been a useful tool for a multiplicity of purposes: it has been found useful for detection of mixed infections in a population, or even in individual animals, with two or more electropherotypes. The migration profile is often used to distinguish between viruses that belong to the same serotype: it was suggested that subgroupings of human rotaviruses can also be distinguished by their segment migration patterns (Kalica *et al.*, 1981). Genomes that gave short electrophoretic patterns are found to belong to subgroup 1, while the long patterns correlate with subgroup 2. Their correlation, however, may be only coincidental as it has been shown that subgroup antigen depends on segment 6 rather than segment 11 (Holmes, 1983).

The technique has been found very useful, together with serology and one-dimensional terminal fingerprints of the RNA segments, in the assignment of atypical rotaviruses to groups B and C.

The recognition of serotypic diversity among rotaviruses, promoted largely as a result of *in vitro* cultivation, is a recent development, particularly among animal rotaviruses. The extent and significance of this diversity will have to be assessed at some later date when more information will become available. Nevertheless, it is fair to say that those that are clinically the most important at present have been identified.

E. Group A Rotaviruses

Most clinically significant strains in terms of prevalence in animal and human populations belong to Group A. The existence of groups B and C and possibly others, known otherwise as atypical rotaviruses, will be discussed separately.

Within group A there are now two, possibly more, subgroups which are distinguishable despite their common antigen and demonstrated by broad serological tests capable of recognizing the group antigen. These include ELISA, IF, IAHA, and complement fixation (CF) tests.

On the other hand, rotaviruses are also divided into different serotypes which are demonstrated by specific neutralizing antibody. The most common tests used for serotyping are PRN (Bohl et al., 1984; Hoshino et al., 1983a), and neutralization of cytopathic effect (NT) (Murakami et al., 1983; Ojeh et al., 1984); both tests are commonly used on cell culture-adapted rotaviruses. Neutralization detected by the fluorescent focus reduction test (Ojeh et al., 1984; Woode et al., 1983) is a useful technique applied to strains unadapted to cell culture.

Subgroup and serotype specificities relate to different antigens located in inner and outer shells respectively, a distinction made only recently by Kapikian et al. (1981). It should be pointed out that any of the serological tests listed with regard to detection of subgroup antigens can potentially be made specific to recognize serotype specificity by using hyperimmune sera, or monoclonal antibody directed against the outer shell viral proteins.

The existence of different serotypes among human rotavirus strains had been recognized long before attempts were made to identify serotypes among animal strains. Serotyping at present is being carried out by different research groups at different geographical locations and, at this stage, correlation between the designated serotypes is not complete. Correlation between human serotypes designated by various groups is more advanced than in the veterinary field. Four distinct serotypes are at present recognized among human strains (Wyatt et al., 1983). The existence of different rotavirus serotypes has now been recognized in pigs (Bohl et al., 1984), calves (Murakami et al., 1983; Ojeh et al., 1984; Snodgrass et al., 1984c; Woode et al., 1983), foals (Hoshino et al., 1983a, b), and birds (McNulty et al., 1980).

1. Porcine Rotavirus

Two serotypes have recently been identified by Bohl et al. (1984) in the United States. Porcine rotavirus serotype 1, represented by the cell culture-adapted Ohio State University (OSU) strain, was found to be distinct from bovine, simian, canine, and human serotypes 1 and 3 by PRN test. Porcine rotavirus serotype 2, which was more difficult to propagate in cell culture, is represented by the strain Gottfried (G). The G strain is closely related to the canine and simian and, to a lesser extent, human serotype 3. There was no evidence of cross-protection between porcine serotype 1 and serotype 2 in gnotobiotic piglets. A serological survey indicated that more than 95% of 349 herds examined in the United States had antibodies to porcine serotype 1. The existence and frequency of porcine serotype 2 elsewhere have not yet been reported.

2. Bovine Rotavirus

Two distinct serotypes have been identified in Japan (Murakami *et al.*, 1983) and in the United States (Woode *et al.*, 1983) and three in the United Kingdom (Ojeh *et al.*, 1984; Snodgrass *et al.*, 1984c). In each of these studies, bovine rotavirus serotype 1 was assigned to the most prevalent type, all of which cross-reacted with the NCDV (Lincoln strain). It is reasonable to assume, therefore, that the three assigned serotypes 1 should possess similar serotypic specificity. The assigned serotypes 2 in the three studies had been neither compared nor tested against a common type, and, therefore, they may or may not be serologically related.

Murakami *et al.* (1983) used the neutralization test to distinguish between serotypes 1 and 2. They had also recognized a tentative third serotype, on the basis of partial one-way cross-reaction using hyperimmune sera raised in guinea pigs. Calves experimentally inoculated with either serotype 1 or 2 produced postinfection, specific, neutralizing antibodies against the homologous type only. Woode *et al.* (1983) also isolated bovine rotavirus in cell culture that did not fall into either serotype 1 or 2, which indicated the existence of possibly one or more additional serotypes. Protection in gnotobiotic calves occurred only with the homologous serotype. Snodgrass *et al.* (1984c) showed that there was no passive cross-protection between their serotypes 1 and 2 in gnotobiotic lambs that had been fed heterologous hyperimmune sera produced in rabbits. In contrast, some protection was afforded against infection with homologous viruses.

Murakami *et al.* (1983) found that, with the exception of a few, most of the 66 sera obtained from 6 herds in Japan contained neutralizing antibodies against serotypes 1 and 2, and both types were also almost evenly isolated from feces of infected calves (Table I), indicating an equal distribution and degree of virulence. On the other hand, Snodgrass *et al.* (1984c) have examined sera from 47 cows from 11 herds and found widespread antibodies to their serotypes 1 and 2, but an isolation rate of 91 and 1%, respectively from the feces of infected calves (Table I). This perhaps indicates that the UK bovine rotavirus serotype 2, while as prevalent, is less virulent. The distribution of neutralizing antibodies among the rotavirus serotypes 1 and 2 in the United States has not been reported.

Neutralizing antibodies against three different serotypes which are unrelated to the three bovine serotypes, and which closely resemble or are identical to human rotavirus serotypes 1 (Wa), 2 (DS-1), and 3 (P strain), have also been measured in 47 cows from 11 herds in the

TABLE I

THE DISTRIBUTION OF ROTAVIRUS STRAINS BETWEEN ASSIGNED BOVINE ROTAVIRUS SEROTYPES

Country (authors)	Serotype 1 (%)	Serotype 2 (%)	Serotype 3 (%)	Total number of isolates tested
United Kingdom (Snodgrass et al., 1985)	94[a]	1	5	85
Japan (Murakami et al., 1983)	50[a]	43	7[b]	14
United States (Woode et al., 1983)	89[a]	7	4[b]	73

[a]Cross-react with NCDV.
[b]Or untyped.

United Kingdom (Snodgrass et al., 1984c). This provides evidence that there may be additional serotypes circulating in the bovine species to which corresponding viral strains have not been isolated.

Woode et al. (1983) have concluded from analysis of polyacrylamide gel comigration, that segment 9 probably codes for NT-specific antigens of bovine rotavirus and proposed that the rate of comigration of segment 9 may be used to predict particular serotypes. Snodgrass et al. (1984c) observed no particular relationship between migration patterns and serotypes, although the comigration of one representative of serotype 1 together with serotype 2 induced differences in the migration rate of segment 9. It would have been of interest had they compared the migration rate of segment 9 among the 11 strains belonging to serotype 1 to see whether they would have comigrated as one band.

3. Equine Rotaviruses

Hoshino and co-workers have identified two distinct equine serotypes that are designated H-1 (Hoshino et al., 1983a) and H-2 (Hoshino et al., 1983b) and were originally isolated in the United Kingdom. Presumably they were not assigned to serotypes 1 and 2 because the prevalence of these serotypes in the equine population had not been determined; it is desirable whenever possible to nominate serotypes according to their prevalence, as has been the case with bovine and porcine rotaviruses. Cross-protection between H-1 and H-2 was not reported. H-1 strain was found to be serologically identical to the porcine serotype 1 (OSU), but electropherotypically distinct, indicating that, although both share the same serotype antigen, they are different viruses. H-1 was also serotypically distinct from four human serotypes,

TABLE II

REPRESENTATIVE ROTAVIRUS STRAINS RECOGNIZED AS DISTINCT SEROTYPES AMONG HUMAN AND ANIMAL STRAINS

Species of origin	Distinct serotype	Known subgroup	Representative strain	Source
Human	1	2	Wa	Wyatt et al. (1983)
	2	1	DS-1	
	3[a]	2	P,YIP No.43	
		N[b]	CMH No. 53	
	4	2	St. Thomas 4	
Porcine	1[c]	1	OSU	Bohl et al. (1982)
	2	2	G	
Bovine	1	1	NCDV, UK	Snodgrass et al. (1984a);
	2	?	678(UK),KK-3(Jap), B223(US)	Murakami et al. (1983); Woode et al. (1983)
	3	?	(Not nominated)	
Equine	1[c,d]	1	H-1	Hoshino et al. (1983a);
	2[a,d]	N[b]	H-2	
Simian	1[a,d]	1	SA11,MMO18006	Hoshino et al. (1983b)
Canine	1[a,d]	1[b]	CU-1	
Chicken	1[d]	N[b]	CH 1	McNulty et al. (1980)
Turkey	1[d]	N[b]	Ty 1	
	2[d]	?	Ty 3	

[a]Serologically related.
[b]N, neither serogroup 1 or 2.
[c]Serologically related.
[d]Not assigned to a serotype group (see text).

NCDV (bovine serotype 1), and canine and simian rotaviruses (Table II). However, H-1 was antigenically somewhat related to the canine CU-1 and NCDV in one-way fashion by the hemagglutination inhibition (HI) test. H-2, on the other hand, is serotypically similar to the two simian and the canine rotaviruses, and human serotype 3 using the PRN and HI tests. As expected, H-2 did not cross-react using PRN and HI with NCDV, OSU, and human serotypes 1 (Wa), 2 (DS-1), and 4 (St. Thomas-6). H-1 and H-2, in addition to belonging to two distinct serotypes, also appear to differ in their subgroup specificity.

Table II lists the number of serotypes and the nominated representative strain(s) known for each of the animal species and humans. The table demonstrates that serotype specificity is not a characteristic that is exclusive to a single host, presumably because gene encoding for proteins carrying neutralizing epitopes have the potential to reassort independently of other biological characteristics.

4. Minor Antigenic Variations

Antigenic drift has also been noted among serotypes; some strains show a degree of antigenic divergence from particular serotypes (Murakami et al., 1983; Snodgrass et al., 1985; Woode et al., 1983) and others fall between existing serotypes (Hoshino et al., 1984). Whether they ought to be designated as subtypes or distinct serotypes poses a problem which may be resolved when more isolates are analyzed.

Kalica et al. (1981) analyzing 16 simian × bovine (UK) reassortments have found that rotaviral hemagglutination (HA) and neutralization are functions encoded by two different gene products: gene 4 encodes viral hemagglutinin, and gene 8 or 9 encodes a major neutralizing protein. Greenberg et al. (1983), however, have demonstrated, by analyzing a series of monoclonal antibodies directed against two surface proteins of simian rotavirus, that both viral HA and NT properties can be mediated by antibodies to gene 4 as well as to gene 8 or 9 products. They have also shown that both viral HA and a major NT protein exhibit distinct type specificity. For example, simian and canine rotaviruses have been shown to be indistinguishable from each other by PRN and HI tests using monoclonal antibodies directed against gene 8 or 9 products; however, a cross-reactivity between the two has not been detected by PRN and HI tests using monoclonal antibodies against the gene 4 product. Therefore, although the quantitative nature and quantitative distribution of two biologically distinct antibodies in polyclonal hyperimmmune sera employed in this study are not known, this may introduce additional serotype diversity, as relationships among rotaviruses studied by PRN tests would be different from those examined by HI tests (Greenberg et al., 1983).

While rotavirus strains appear to be fairly host specific (Tzipori et al., 1981), one may speculate that the existence of a vast pool of electropherotypes and the ease with which the segmented genome of these different electropherotypes reassort with one another provide a source for potential new virus recombinants arising from coinfections that might well cross the species barrier. It has been demonstrated *in vitro* that new reassortments may emerge from coinfection that retain the same infectivity but have altered serotype specificities. The detection in bovine sera antibodies reactive against human serotypes by Snodgrass et al. (1984c) is suggestive.

5. The Host Response to Antigenic Variation

In early neutralization tests which were carried out with either postinfection sera or with hyperimmune sera that had preexisting antibodies against other rotaviruses, the demonstration of 4- to 8-fold differences was regarded as being significant enough to distinguish between serotypes. With improved techniques, culture-adapted viruses were used to produce hyperimmune sera by repeatedly injecting specific pathogen free (SPF) animals or animals that were known to be free of antibodies. At least 20-fold differences of NT between homologous and heterologous 2-way cross-neutralization reactions are now thought to be required to differentiate between two serotypes (Gaul et al., 1982; Hoshino et al., 1983a,b, 1984; Ojeh et al., 1984; Woode et al., 1983). Postinfection sera compared with hyperimmune sera discriminate poorly between strains, even when they are derived from gnotobiotic animals and despite having lower homologous titers.

The issue of whether serotypic specificity of the immune response can confer protection against heterotypic challenge is far from settled. There are two ways in which to assess the available data concerning the above question: measurement of the specificity of the antibodies and cross-protection experiments.

Cows injected with a single rotavirus serotype responded heterotypically to five different serotypes to which they had previously been exposed, but failed to respond against two other serotypes to which they had no previous exposure (Snodgrass et al., 1984c). Similar responses were demonstrated by the same investigators using rabbits experimentally infected at intervals with five different serotypes. With each vaccination the rabbits responded heterotypically against the serotypes used for vaccination, but not against two serotypes with which the rabbits were not vaccinated. This suggests that repeated exposure of animals to different rotavirus serotypes results in acquisition of antibodies specific to each serotype to which the animal has previously been exposed, and this exposure does not broaden to include serotypes to which the animal has no previous experience. Broad protection by colostrum, which has been demonstrated in pigs (Bridger and Brown, 1981; Lecce *et al.*, 1976) and presumably occurs in other species, is then a reflection of repeated infections with different serotypes of rotavirus, and in part this broad response can be maintained by infection with a single serotype. In contrast to the above findings, sera of gnotobiotic animals experimentally infected with three human serotypes recognized the heterologous virus in two cases, and primary rotavirus infection in infants was reported to have stimulated antibody response to two serotypes (Wyatt *et al.*, 1982). With regard to heterotypic cross-protection experiments in gnotobiotic animals there is evidence in some instances which suggests that different serotypes from the same species of animal will not protect against each other, as mentioned earlier (Bohl *et al.*, 1982; Snodgrass *et al.*, 1984c; Woode *et al.*, 1983), yet a heterologous protection was reported in gnotobiotic newborn calves injected *in utero* with a bovine rotavirus, against a Wa-like human rotavirus (Wyatt *et al.*, 1979). Colostrum-deprived piglets vaccinated with RIT4237, a strain derived from NCDV, were also protected against challenge with human rotavirus strains of subgroups 2 and 3 (Zissis *et al.*, 1983). Evidence of sequential episodes of rotavirus gastroenteritis in humans by different subgroups or serotypes (Fonteyne *et al.*, 1978; Rodriguez *et al.*, 1978) or even the same serotypes (Lambert *et al.*, 1983; Simmon *et al.*, 1981) must add further to the complexity.

Whether a heterotypic response does or does not depend on previous experience may be related to the extent of diversity or relatedness of the group and subgroup antigens and, therefore, in some instances it will be shown to depend on previous exposure and in other instances perhaps not. In any case, one can assume that vaccination of an adult animal with the most prevalent serotype will induce antibodies not only against the homologous one, but against, at the very least, serotypes to which the animal has had previous experience (Gaul *et al.*, 1982; Snodgrass *et al.*, 1984c) and, at best, even against serotypes to which the animal has no previous experience but which share the same group antigen.

F. OTHER ROTAVIRUS GROUPS

The identification of agents morphologically indistinguishable from rotaviruses, but unrelated serologically, suggests the existence of one or more subgenera. Such viruses have now been detected in pigs (Bohl *et al.*, 1982; Bridger *et al.*, 1982), calves (Chasey and Davies, 1984;

Snodgrass *et al.*, 1984a), lambs (Snodgrass *et al.*, 1984a), humans (Dimitrov *et al.*, 1983; Nicolas *et al.*, 1983; Rodger *et al.*, 1982), and chickens (McNulty *et al.*, 1981). Studies on these agents, which have been termed pararotaviruses, atypical rotaviruses, or rotavirus-like agents, have only begun and their distribution and clinical significance is not yet clear, although the fact that they have escaped attention despite extensive research on enteric viruses may indicate that they are either uncommon or are largely of low virulence. Because their significance is not clear, interest in them is taxonomic at present.

One of the factors which distinguish atypical rotaviruses (ARV) from common, or group A, rotavirus strains (Pedley *et al.*, 1983) is that they do not share a common or group antigen (Group A antigen) which has been an important characteristic of rotavirus strains until the discovery of ATV. Allowing for minor intra and interspecies variation, Group A rotavirus strains have a characteristic RNA electrophoretic fractionation pattern on polyacrylamide gel (Lourenco *et al.*, 1981; Schnagl *et al.*, 1981). Genome profile analysis of ARV showed that they possess the 11 discrete genome segments characteristic of rotaviruses, but with a profile clearly distinct from that commonly observed in Group A (Bohl *et al.*, 1982; Bridger *et al.*, 1982; Chasey and Davies, 1984; Rodger *et al.*, 1982).

The third significant difference between Group A and ARV may be demonstrated by the one-dimensional terminal fingerprint technique (Clarke and McCrae, 1981). Application of the terminal fingerprint technique to some of group A has shown that each genome has a region of 30 to 40 nucleotides at each terminus whose fingerprint is uniquely conserved for that segment and which can be used for identification purposes (Clarke and McCrae, 1983).

Because of the segmental monocistronic nature of rotaviruses it was proposed (Pedley *et al.*, 1983) that differences between Group A and ARV could reflect one of two possible levels of genome variation, one associated with marked differences in the segment encoding the major inner core group antigens, the other associated with differences involving major biological characteristics. The biology, however, of ARV, as far as can be ascertained from the available data, is largely indistinguishable from that of Group A. They induce diarrhea of varying severity when given to young gnotobiotic experimental animals and they infect mature enterocytes of the small intestine causing villous atropy (Askaa and Bloch, 1984; Snodgrass *et al.*, 1984a). Diarrhea was consistently produced in gnotobiotic piglets aged up to 19 days and death in piglets less than 5 days old (Bohl *et al.*, 1982). Two strains were isolated that differed in their electropherotypes (C strain and S strain), did not share a serological relationship with the OSU strain and did not exhibit cross-protection in gnotobiotic piglets. The two ARV strains, C and S, which cross-reacted serologically with one another, were difficult to propagate in cell culture (Bohl et al., 1982). Another pig ARV isolated in Denmark was, however, readily propagated in cell culture. It was distinct from the strain reported above (Askaa and Bloch, 1984).

Pedley et al. (1983) have divided these ARV into Groups B and C on the basis of (1) lack of cross-reactivity by IF, (2) analysis of dsRNA genome fractionation in polyacrylamide gel, and (3) one-dimensional terminal fingerprint. They were able to demonstrate that three isolates from pigs, one ARV isolated in the United Kingdom (Bridger, 1980), another from the United States (Bohl et al., 1982), and the OSU representing the common Group A antigen did not cross-react with one another by direct IF performed on gut sections of infected piglets and using postinfection sera. Consequently, Pedley et al. (1983) have assigned Group B to the UK ARV (strain NIRD-1) and Group C to the USA ARV (strain Cowden), each representing a distinct group antigen. The genome electrophoretic profile analysis, and the one-dimensional terminal fingerprint analysis were also consistent with the serological division into two distinct additional groups.

Further data to support this division of ARV into at least Groups B and C was provided by Snodgrass et al. (1984a), who had applied IF and genome profile analysis to four newly isolated strains of ARV which included, in addition to two new strains from pigs, one each from calves and lambs. These investigators divided, by direct or indirect means using the criteria of indirect IF applied to gut sections and postinfection sera, the ARV into Groups B and C, consolidating the findings of Pedley et al. (1983). The ARV strains identified to date, and their proposed distribution between Groups B and C are summarized in Table III. So far, all six ARV strains of human origin seem to fall into Group C, ovine and bovine into Group B, and porcine into Groups B and C respectively. Snodgrass et al. (1984a) have also confirmed serologically the suggestion made by Pedley et al. (1983) that Group D should be assigned to ARV strains isolated from chickens (McNulty et al., 1981) which failed to react with Groups A, B, and C. A new human strain of ATV isolated recently from two epidemics of diarrhea in adults in China may yet form a new group (Tao et al., 1984).

It appears that interspecies and virulence diversity, electrophoretic mobility, and antigenic variations with the groups, are likely to be characteristic of Groups B and C, as they are of Group A. It remains to be determined whether each of the new groups may be further divided

TABLE III

A Tentative Assignment of ARV Strains into Groups Distinct from Common Group A Rotaviruses

ARV	Strain	Source
Group B		
1 Porcine	NIRD-1	Bridger et al. (1982)[a]
2 Ovine	E1101	Snodgrass et al. (1984)[a]
2 Bovine	DAS22, D531	Snodgrass et al. (1984)[a]
2 Bovine	NA[b]	Chasey and Davies (1984)[c]
Group C		
1 Human	NA[b]	Rodger et al. (1982)[d]
3 Human	HM, JM, LK	Snodgrass et al. (1984)[a]
1 Porcine	Cowden	Bohl et al. (1982)[a]
1 Porcine	D238	Snodgrass et al. (1984)[a]
1 Porcine	NA[b]	Chasey and Davies (1984)[c]
1 Human	NA[b]	Dimitrov et al. (1983)[d]
1 Human	NA[b]	Nicolas et al. (1983)[d]
1 Porcine	Belgium strain	Pedley et al. (1983)[a]
Group D		
1 Chicken	132	McNulty et al. (1981)[d]

[a]Assigned by Pedley et al. (1983).
[b]Not assigned.
[c]Suggested by the author.
[d]Suggested by Snodgrass et al. (1984a).

into subgroups and serotypes. The division of rotaviruses into a number of separate antigenic groups is shaping up to a complex, parallel to that of influenza viruses (Ritchey et al., 1976). Cross-hybridization analysis between RNAs of viruses from different groups is, however, required before the tentative division into distinct groups can be finally substantiated.

G. Development of Rotavirus Vaccines

Rotavirus infection, although widespread in various animal populations, is a major cause of diarrhea in children and economically is of concern to the cattle industry. Hence, efforts to develop preventive measures have been directed against the infection in calves and, more recently, in humans.

Newborn calves are at risk from rotavirus infection during the first 2 weeks of life and protection against clinical diarrhea is associated with the presence of a certain amount of specific antibodies against the virus in the gut lumen, either excreted by the calf following active immunization, or passively acquired from continuous consumption of specific antibodies present in the milk. Cows may often have high levels of colostral antibodies, but the level in the milk is much lower and tends to decline further within a short time after parturition (Acres and Babiuk, 1978; Saif et al., 1984; Snodgrass et al., 1982).

The development of rotavirus vaccines against diarrhea in calves followed traditional lines. First, live attenuated-modified virus was given orally to newborn calves (Mebus et al., 1973) but this was superseded by parenteral vaccination with modified live, or inactivated virulent virus that was given to the pregnant dam (Snodgrass et al., 1980). Passive protection to the newborn calf was further improved by parenteral vaccination followed by intramammary infusion (Saif et al., 1983, 1984). A comprehensive analysis of the literature on the development of bovine rotavirus vaccines has been published (Saif and Smith, 1984).

This section will highlight some of the findings reported by these authors and examine the prospect of application of new technology to the development of future vaccines.

1. Vaccination of Calves

Early attempts to provide protection against rotavirus diarrhea were directed to induce active immunization via oral inoculation of the newborn calf with live attenuated virus. Viruses which have a segmental genome, such as rotaviruses, are subjected to a high degree of genetic reassortment (Greenberg et al., 1982) which in turn facilitates the establishment of attenuated viral strains. However, the basis for attenuation, curiously termed "genetic roulette" (Chanock, 1982), of currently used live vaccines and the nature and number of mutations required for attenuation are unknown.

It is not clear whether attenuated rotaviruses such as NCDV or, for that matter, strains that cause only subclinical infections, do so because: they only multiply in a limited number of cells, or are localized to a particular region in the gut, or infection does not result in the destruction of epithelial cells, or the efficiency of attachment and penetration into epithelial cells is compromised and only a few cells become affected at any one time.

While vaccination of calves with attenuated virus appeared to have provided protection against challenge with a rotavirus under experimental conditions in colostrum-deprived calves (Mebus et al., 1973; Woode et al., 1978) under field conditions, its efficiency was questionable (Acres et al., 1977; de Leeuw et al., 1980). The failure of the oral vaccine was attributed to interference from maternal antibodies (Burki et al., 1983; de Leeuw et al., 1980), possibly the degree of attenuation (Saif and Smith, 1984), and the time interval between oral vaccination and the development of protective immunity. This time interval, which may also relate to the degree of attenuation, was suggested when it was shown that calves were protected against challenge 7 days after vaccination, but not 3 or 5 days (Woode et al., 1978). Protection that occurs in less than 3 days is more likely to be mediated by interference (interferon for instance) rather than by specific antibodies (de Leeuw et al., 1980). Specific antibodies appear in jejunal fluid 2–12 days after infection of calves with a virulent rotavirus (Bachmann et al., 1984) but whether antibody levels in jejunal fluid measured 2 days after vaccination are sufficiently high to protect against infection is questionable. In addition to maternal interference, there are technical problems associated with vaccinating calves within hours after birth, particularly in beef cattle.

2. Vaccination of the Dam

An alternative to active immunization is to enhance maternal lactogenic immunity by vaccination of the pregnant dam to provide passive protection to the young calf against enteric infections. A commercial modified live rotavirus–coronavirus vaccine appeared in 1979 in the United States which required one parenteral injection without an adjuvant. This preparation was subsequently shown to neither significantly increase the titer of specific antibodies against rotaviruses in serum and mammary secretions (Myers and Snodgrass, 1982; Saif et al., 1983), nor did it provide sufficient protection to calves against artificial challenge (Saif et al., 1983).

There are inherent problems in assessing the efficiency of vaccines which mediate their protection to the calf by lactogenic immunity. This is because of the large number of variables and their complex interaction involved in achieving an optimal level of immunity (Saif and Smith, 1984), which can be measured either in terms of the specific antibody response in mammary secretions following vaccination, or, more significantly, the quality of protection this kind of immunity is likely to confer on the calf during the neonatal period.

When considering the quantity of mammary secretions the following parameters are important: the specific antibody titers achieved after vaccination in the colostrum and milk; their maintenance for at least 2–3 weeks after parturition; and the isotypic subclass most appropriate in the milk for protection. These relate to the titer of the virus vaccine used, whether it is live or inactivated (Saif et al., 1983), the type of adjuvant included (Hess et al., 1982), the parenteral route of administration, and the number of, and interval between, injections as they relate to parturition. The total volume of the vaccine probably plays some role. This has been demonstrated for other vaccines (Tzipori and Spradbrow, 1978) but not yet for rotavirus. When assessing vaccines in terms of protection of the calf against clinical rotavirus diarrhea, the following are important considerations: the nature of the challenge (artificial or natural), size, and virulence and the serotype of the virus used (Saif and Smith, 1984), as they relate to the amount and time of consumption of milk. There must be a marked difference between suckled calves and those that receive their protection as a supplement in milk or milk replacer. Artificial challenge often consists of a large, single viral dose given at a time considered to be appropriate by the investigator. Natural exposure, while it may be of a smaller dose than artificial, is continuous and at some point it can coincide with physiological or other events not well understood which may facilitate establishment of infection.

From analysis of the studies reported to date in relation to passive immunity (Saif et al., 1983) it was clear that serum and mammary secretions of rotavirus antibody were increased after two parenteral injections with virulent inactivated or live modified virus, as compared with unvaccinated dams. The most effective were those given in combination with oil–adjuvant in one or two doses prior to parturition (Dauvergne et al., 1983; Hartmann et al., 1982; Snodgrass et al., 1980; van Opdenbosch et al., 1981). However, whether the higher level of lactogenic immunity achieved in these studies was sufficiently protective against clinical illness is not as clear. Dauvergne et al. (1983) and Eichhorn et al. (1983) observed a reduction in incidence of rotavirus shedding, or diarrhea, or both in calves suckling vaccinated cows. In another study, the onset of diarrhea in suckling calves challenged artificially at 7 days of age was significantly delayed but the severity of diarrhea was not influenced (Snodgrass et al., 1980). Yet rotavirus diarrhea was almost completely eliminated in suckled calves exposed to natural challenge (D. R. Snodgrass, personal communication). Fortification of passive immunization of the pregant dam, with active immunization of the newborn calf with presumably attenuated rotavirus did not appear to have had the beneficial effect of reducing the incidence of diarrhea attributed to infection with rotavirus (Mann, 1983). Extremely high colostral and milk rotavirus specific antibody titers were achieved by combined parenteral vaccination and intramammary infusion of pregnant cows with a modified live derivative of

NCDV bovine rotavirus. Cows were given a 40 ml vaccine, containing 20 ml of 10^8 PFU/ml, emulsified in an equal volume of incomplete Freund adjuvant injected half into each hip before drying-off 8–10 weeks before parturition. A total of 20 ml of the above mixture was infused 2 weeks later into the four quarters of the involuted mammary gland (Saif et al., 1983). This extremely high, live adjuvanted rotavirus vaccine induced specific antibodies in colostrum and milk which were mainly associated with isotype IgG_1, at least 100-fold higher than the control, and to a lesser extent IgG_2, IgA, and IgM (Saif et al., 1984). The use of the parenteral–intramammary route by Saif et al. (1983) was based on the hypothesis that a peripheral stimulus may lead to migration of sensitized cells to the gland and subsequent intramammary presentation of antigens might then result in further expression of the clone of cells, effectively increasing antibody levels in mammary secretions (Watson and Lascelles, 1975). Feeding calves a 1% of pooled colostrum supplement from such vaccinated cows conferred both clinical protection and prevented rotavirus shedding against artificial challenge with a homologous virulent rotavirus. Calves fed 0.1% supplement colostrum had delayed onset and shorter duration of diarrhea and rotavirus shedding as compared with feeding 1% control colostrum. Calves which were completely protected from challenge resisted a second challenge 2 weeks later.

Often, despite clinical protection conferred by feeding colostrum, animals may become subclinically infected and may, therefore, resist a second challenge upon withdrawal of the colostrum supplement. This was observed in calves (Saif et al., 1983), lambs (Snodgrass and Wells, 1976), and piglets (Bridger and Brown, 1981). Other animals were shown to be protected while supplement feeding continued, but developed mild diarrhea or viral shedding upon withdrawal of the colostrum (Bridger and Brown, 1981; Saif et al., 1983).

Effective protection against rotavirus infection in calves appears to be associated with IgG_1 (Saif et al., 1984; Snodgrass et al., 1980), rather than IgA which is the major isotype responsible for porcine mucosal immunity in the gut of pigs and of other monogastric animals. Unlike monogastric species, the predominant isotype in mammary secretions of ruminants is IgG_1 (Saif and Smith, 1984) and this contention is further supported by the apparent resistance of IgG_1 to certain proteolytic enzymes (Brock et al., 1977), a characteristic of secretory IgA in other species. Stimulation of active immunity of the gut by infection is, however, associated predominantly with IgA, as it is with other species which appear largely in the mucosa of the proximal small intestine (Vonderfecht and Osburn, 1982).

When assessing the efficiency of protection of a vaccine against experimental challenge, the use of homologous rotavirus was considered essential (Saif and Smith, 1984) because of the existence of two (Murakami et al., 1983; Ojeh et al., 1984; Woode et al., 1983) and possibly more (Snodgrass et al., 1984c) distinct bovine rotavirus serotypes which do not cross-react by neutralization, or even cross-protect against each other. However, as suggested by some (Gaul et al., 1982) and demonstrated by Snodgrass et al. (1984c) this may not be critical. As discussed earlier, vaccination with one serotype leads to heterotypic response to all serotypes to which the animal has had previous experience. Studies with influenza have shown that antibody response to specific hemagglutinins of unrelated subtypes was enhanced by previous injections with heterotypic viruses with common internal antigens, possibly by T helper cells which recognize specific hemagglutinins (Russell and Liew, 1979). If this supposition of heterotypic immunity depending on complete virus as antigen can be confirmed, conventional tissue culture-derived vaccines may have a considerable advantage over potential vaccines based on single proteins.

3. Human Vaccines

Rotavirus vaccine against diarrhea in humans is also at an early stage; the most promising candidate, it seems, is the NCDV derivative strain RIT 4237 mentioned earlier (Zissis et al., 1983), which has been used as an oral vaccine in a controlled trial against natural rotavirus infection in children. Of 86 human infants vaccinated orally with a single dose, only 2 developed rotavirus diarrhea in an epidemic with rotavirus subgroup 2 in Finland, as compared with 18 of 92 placebo recipients, thus providing a protection rate of 88% (Vesikari et al., 1984). Vaccination was not associated with clinical symptoms or shedding of the vaccine virus in stools.

A similar method of passive protection to that described for calves was applied to children at risk; feeding IgA-rich colostrum containing human rotavirus neutralizing antibodies produced by injecting pregnant cows with human rotavirus has reduced the incidence of rotavirus diarrhea (Ebina et al., 1983).

4. Future Vaccines

Avenues that are available and which, no doubt, will be utilized in future vaccines against rotavirus diarrhea in humans and bovines include the production of subunit vaccines by the use of hybrid-DNA technology; isolated viral genes responsible for the production of surface antigen components have been cloned in *E. coli* in relation to proteins of foot and mouth disease virus (FMDV) (Kleid et al., 1981) and the hepatitis B virus surface antigen (Edman et al., 1981). These kinds of preparations obviously offer *infinite* possibilities. However, one drawback with this system which may prove crucial for construction of rotavirus vaccines is that no glycosylation occurs in bacterial systems (Norrby, 1983).

Immunization with synthetic polypeptides can now also be exploited with the availability of genetic information provided by the combined utilization of hybridomas producing virus specific antibodies (which can help identify the appropriate structural antigenic determinants), hybrid-DNA technology, and nucleic acid sequencing methods.

Synthetic peptides representing different surface virus structures capable of eliciting neutralizing antibody can be used to induce immunity against viral infections. Such synthetic peptides, which are poor immunogens, have to be combined with various proteins. Synthetic peptides as a form of future vaccines are even more attractive, considering the existence of distinct rotavirus serotypes, as short synthetic polypeptides specific for each type could be combined to give polytypic vaccines.

III. Enterotoxigenic *E. coli* (ETEC)

Although some *E. coli* were suspected to be enteric pathogens as early as 1885, (Escherich, 1885) it was not until the introduction of a serotyping scheme (Kauffman, 1947), and through epidemiological studies, that certain serogroups were firmly established as enteropathogens.

E. coli causes a wide range of enteric infections in humans and animals. In the veterinary field *E. coli* exerts its most serious effect on young pigs, causing a number of disease syndromes (Moon, 1974) of which only diarrhea or colibacillosis caused by enterotoxigenic strains (ETEC) will be discussed. In calves and other small ruminants ETEC is the only significant group, although infections with non-ETEC have also been described (Chanter et al., 1984; Moon et al., 1979).

In humans, strains of *E. coli* are associated with three different disease entities (Gross, 1983), categorized by Levine et al. (1983) into groups on the basis of their degree of invasiveness of the host mucosa: (1) mucosal adhesion by ETEC, (2) mucosal adherence and brush border dissolution caused by enteropathogenic *E. coli* (EPEC), and (3) mucosal invasion and intraepithelial cell proliferation characterized by shigella-like diarrhea caused by enteroinvasive *E. coli* (EIEC).

Strains of *E. coli* associated with a disease category tend to fall into particular serogroups, and those that cause ETEC diarrhea in humans are distinct from those that cause diarrhea in animals. The mechanisms by which ETEC cause diarrhea in susceptible animal species and man are similar, and have been understood for quite some time. However, the nature of the virulence factors involved, their characteristics, and similarities and differences between and within species of animals were not well understood until recently. This was brought about by application of new technology which not only helped resolve these issues, but overcame major technical difficulties which, until now, had hampered the development of proper diagnostic procedures. With the identification of other relatively "new" enteric pathogens, epidemiology of colibacillosis in animals has become more meaningful and can now be put into proper perspective. How this new volume of knowledge can be best applied to production of new efficient vaccines will also be discussed.

A. PATHOGENIC MECHANISMS

For ETEC to be enteropathogenic they must possess at least two properties. They must be able to proliferate in the small intestine, which they do first by adhering to the epithelium. While proliferating there, they must produce enterotoxin(s) which causes the secretion of fluid from the body into the alimentary tract, causing diarrhea. The ability to colonize the small intestine and to produce toxin are plasmid-borne characteristics (Smith and Huggins, 1978). Other non-plasmid-determined characteristics, such as the capsular K antigen and which appear to be essential for some pig and calf strains to express their full enteropathogenicity (Hadad and Gyles, 1982; Nagy *et al.*, 1976, 1977), have been reported.

1. Attachment to the Mucosa

The significance of a need for attachment of bacteria to mucosal surfaces was recognized long ago on theoretical grounds (Freter *et al.*, 1961; Smith and Hall, 1967) when colonization of mucosal surfaces was demonstrated histologically, and when the particular immunity was correlated with inhibition of adhesion (Freter, 1969). During the early 1970s there was a surge of interest in the subject of mechanisms by which bacteria colonize a mucosal surface. In 1971 Smith and Linggood first showed that the plasmid-encoded fimbrial antigen designated K88 was an essential virulence factor for the majority of strains of *E. coli* causing diarrhea in piglets, and they suggested that K88 mediated the adhesion of these *E. coli* to the mucosal surface of the small intestine of piglets. This suggestion was confirmed by Jones and Rutter (1972), who subsequently demonstrated that, in piglets from certain litters, K88-producing *E. coli* were unable to adhere to the intestinal brush borders (Sellwood et al., 1975). The "nonadhesive" pig phenotype was inherited in an autosomal recessive fashion and conferred relative resistance to *E. coli* diarrhea (Rutter et al., 1975). These classical experiments illustrated the importance of mucosal adhesion as a prerequisite for bacterial proliferation and the development of diarrhea. At the same time Orskov et al. (1975) described K99, a fimbrial surface antigen analogous to K88, which mediates mucosal adhesion and diarrhea in calves and lambs.

All colonizing factors so far identified in animal and human ETEC strains are fimbriated, that is they form pili or hairlike protein organelles on the surface of the bacteria. The degree of expression of these pili varies greatly among strains *in vivo* and *in vitro*, which creates difficulties for their detection by electron microscopy or identification by culture and serology.

Pilus antigens are thought to be host specific. They are, however, associated with strains causing diseases in specific hosts, rather than due to the presence of specific receptors on the host enterocytes; evidence will be presented that, at least under *in vitro* conditions, some of these colonizing factors can attach specifically to receptors of more than one host. At least four antigenetically distinct colonizing factors designated K88, K99, 987P, F41 and, possibly, a fifth one (Aning et al., 1983) have been identified, each of which attaches *in vivo* to specific brush border receptors on enterocytes of the small intestine of piglets. K99 and F41 are also associated with diarrhea in calves and lambs, while, in humans, fibriae designated CFA/I, CFA/II, E8776 (Levine, 1983), and CFA/III have been described (Darfeuille et al., 1983). The genes which encode for these pili are located on transmissible plasmids which frequently encode for enterotoxins as well.

These pili are preferentially expressed when the strains are grown on solid agar rather than in broth, and are not expressed when the cultures are incubated at 18 to 22°C. Bacteria bearing these surface pili cause mannose-resistant hemagglutination (MRHA) of erythrocytes of certain animal species and are characteristic for each. This provides a simple screening test and is used for diagnosis.

In animals, K88, K99, and to a lesser extent 987P have been studied most extensively. K99 and 987P are reported to be able to proliferate only in the posterior portion of the small intestine, in contrast to K88 which colonizes the entire small intestine. This is undoubtedly important in determining the severity of diarrhea produced by ETEC, because the anterior small intestine is much more susceptible to the action of enterotoxins than the ileum (Smith, 1980). This, however, is not due to lack of receptors for K99 and 987P in the anterior small intestine, rather it is related to their inefficiency in binding to the anterior portion, which has a considerably higher flow rate and is subjected to greater pH extremes and proteolysis as compared with the slower moving ingesta at the posterior part. It can be demonstrated by *in vitro* tests that there is no difference in the number of bacteria with K99 that adhere to brush border preparations from the anterior jejunum as compared with ileum (S. Tzipori, unpublished data). Furthermore, colonization of the anterior small intestine by K99 strains is occasionally noted in a proportion of piglets when large numbers are examined (S. Tzipori, unpublished data). In *in vitro* studies using brush border membranes from newborn piglets K88 adheres more strongly than K99. It has also been shown that intestinal epithelial cells from calves and pigs develop an innate resistance to K99 adhesion *in vitro* with increasing host age, while susceptibility to K88 remains lifelong (Runnels *et al.*, 1980).

The role of capsular polysaccharide in promoting colonization of the small intestine has been noted (Hadad and Gyles, 1982; Smith and Huggins, 1978; Sojka *et al.*, 1978). In one experiment a bovine strain with K99, but lacking the capsular polysaccharide (acapsular mutant), failed to colonize the small intestine of calves. In contrast mutants which contained the capsular polysaccharide, but were without K99, proliferated and colonized the posterior portion of the small intestine, although to a lesser extent than did the parent strain, which contained both capsule and K99 (Hadad and Gyles, 1982). It is evident that removal of K99 antigen from wild calf and lamb strains significantly reduces their efficiency as pathogens and, in particular, their colonizing ability. It was suggested that the K99 pili and the polysaccharide capsule act in concert to anchor the bacteria to epithelial cells.

Certain bovine *E. coli* strains produce, in addition to K99, a second adhesive antigen which also exhibits MRHA (Morris *et al.*, 1980). The two adhesive antigens are immunologically distinct, one being cationic (K99) and the second, now referred to as F41, being anionic. F41 adhesive activity was associated with the presence of fimbriae (Morris *et al.*, 1982). Recently, ETEC strains were isolated from piglets in the United States (Moon *et al.*, 1980) and in the United Kingdom (Morris *et al.*, 1983) with an adhesive antigen that was serologically related only to F41, suggesting that F41 may be either produced together with K99 by some strains of *E. coli,* e.g., the bovine strain B41, or alone, e.g., the pig strain $3P^-$ (Moon *et al.*, 1980).

Histological or IF demonstration of bacterial attachment to the microvillous surface of the small intestine is probably the most direct method of determining etiology. The advantage of IF is that it can be made specific enough to identify any particular colonizing factor; it also indicates the extent of colonization, and is rapid if performed on cryostat sections (Bertschinger et al., 1972; Francis, 1983). Although it is the quickest and most direct technique, IF does have drawbacks: it is comparatively labor-intensive, it requires sophisticated equipment, only a few samples can be processed, and necropsy of animals is a prerequisite. Commonly though, K99 in calves and lambs, or K99, K88, and 987P in piglets can be detected by slide agglutination or ELISA by using specific hyperimmune sera raised against the adhesin antigens. Often, demonstration of adhesin antigen or LT can be carried out directly on fecal specimens (Mills et al., 1983). Agglutination tests require overnight culture, and, for K99, incubation in a specialized medium is recommended to enhance the expression of the pili (Guinée et al., 1980).

Initially, demonstration of colonizing factors by immunological methods was not simple because of the difficulties associated with obtaining pilus antigens free of other bacterial components and in sufficient quantity to produce hyperimmune sera (Guinée et al., 1980). Recombinant DNA techniques are now employed to obtain reagents of high quality for immunological assays and vaccines. There are at least three serological variants of K88 antigen (K88ab, K88ac, and K88ad) and the genetic determinants that encode for K88ac and K88ab were identified and cloned, respectively (Mooi et al., 1979; Shipley et al., 1981). Methods are now available to construct laboratory strains which express high levels of variant K88 on the cell surface, and thus, are ideal candidates for vaccines, while other mutants can be made to secrete high levels of adhesive antigens into the culture supernatant and thus facilitate purification of these antigens.

The presence of *E. coli* adhesive antigens can also be demonstrated in the *in vitro* brush border adhesion test in which brush borders are prepared from the small intestine of animals that may be potential hosts for the organism, and in which it may cause diarrhea. The adhesion of bacteria to the brush border membranes may be an indication of the production of pilus antigens. The *in vitro* adhesion test is also the only available method to determine the K88 phenotypic character of young individual pigs for epidemiological studies or for research. In our laboratory an adhesion test for binding porcine brush border membrane to *E. coli* with K88 antigen was developed using the ELISA technique (Chandler et al., 1985). Microtiter plates are coated with K88 *E. coli* and reacted with small intestinal scrapings containing brush border material. Adhesion of membrane material to immobilized K88 was detected by rabbit anti-pig brush border IgG followed by urease-labeled sheep anti-rabbit IgG conjugate. This test enables rapid testing of a large number of intestines and may be used for the identification of resistant phenotypes in a population.

The *in vitro* adhesion test, which was used so elegantly to demonstrate correlation between certain adhesins and pathogenicity, does not apply to all cases. There are instances where bacteria fail to adhere *in vivo*, yet attachment *in vitro* is evident; conversely, failure to adhere *in vitro* does not rule out colonization *in vivo*. Studies have shown that a receptor specific for K88 pilus antigens is present on brush border membranes prepared from young or adult horses, as demonstrated by the *in vitro* adhesion test; the affinity of K88 *E. coli* to equine brush border membranes was as strong as that observed for porcine membranes (Tzipori *et al.*, 1984a). The specificity of the receptor for K88 in the equine brush border was demonstrated as follows: K88 pili, when reacted with equine brush border membrane, competitively inhibited the adhesion of K88 *E. coli*, while K88 *E. coli* previously reacted with K88 antibodies failed to adhere to the equine brush border membranes. However, despite the evidence for the presence of a receptor, ETEC strains with K88 failed to become established in the small intestine when fed in moderate doses to newborn foals. One foal, which was given a large dose (5×10^{10} bacteria), did develop diarrhea; necropsy showed scattered foci of bacterial colonization restricted to the mid region of the small intestine (Tzipori *et al.*, 1984a). It is unlikely that a receptor specific for K88 evolved on the brush borders of absorptive cells to facilitate bacterial attachment. It is more likely that organisms have acquired mechanisms for attachment to an existing receptor which, presumably, has a specific physiological function common to a number of species of animals. It is evident, therefore, that it is not sufficient to have an adhesive antigen that corresponds to a receptor on the brush border for ETEC to induce diarrhea; the bacteria must also be ecologically adapted to proliferate in the small intestine of the particular species of animal. Certain *E. coli* serotypes tend to be associated more commonly with some species of animal.

Adhesion reactions *in vitro* are an oversimplification of the process of colonization *in vivo;* there are other intervening forces which influence colonization, including chemotactic attraction of bacteria to mucus gel, penetration of, and trapping within the mucus gel, adhesion to receptors in the mucus, adhesion to the epithelial cell surface, and multiplication of the mucus-associated bacteria (Freter, 1981). The value of the *in vitro* test is questionable because there is more than one basic mechanism by which bacteria may associate with the mucosa, numerous intervening reactions in the mucosal microenvironment modify the various steps leading to association, and mucosal association may sometimes be detrimental to bacteria (Freter, 1981).

There is some evidence that enterotoxin production is essential for the bacteria, even with a colonizing factor, to proliferate and become established, particularly in the anterior portion of the small intestine. Studies on the pathogenicity of *E. coli* in rabbits suggest that toxin liberation is required to initiate changes at the mucus gel–brush border junction that facilitate attachment of the organism to the gut wall (Takeuchi *et al.*, 1978). A mutant of K88 *E. coli* in the absence of toxin production colonized poorly and then only the lower small intestine of piglets as compared with its ETEC-parent strain (Tzipori *et al.*, 1983a). The role of enterotoxins demonstrated in well-recognized enteropathogenic bacteria such as *Yersinia enterocolitica* (Robins-Browne *et al.*, 1979), *Salmonella typhimurium, Campylobacter* spp. (Ruiz-Palacious *et al.*, 1983), *Aeromonas* spp. (Sanyal *et al.*, 1975), and *Clostridium perfringens* (Borriello *et al.*, 1984), while not clear, may well be to facilitate their establishment in the gut by inducing changes in the lumen and at the mucosal surface.

Mucoprotein receptor sites for K88 can be shown to be predominantly located in the brush borders of the mucous membrane. Similar K88 receptor sites have been located on the surface of globules of fat in sows' milk and may act to inhibit the adherence of K88 organisms to pig enterocytes (Porter and Linggood, 1983). As with K88 receptors on the brush border membrane, those on the fat globules are also genetically controlled; bacterial adhesion to washed milk fat globules caused the globules to agglutinate. It has been suggested that lactating sows can be typed according to their fat globular receptor phenotype (Atroshi *et al.*, 1983). Bijlsma *et al.* (1982) screened pigs for their phenotype with the three K88 variants, K88ac, KK88ab, and K88ad, in the *in vitro* adhesion test and identified at least five different phenotypes ranging from susceptibility to all three to complete resistance to all of them.

2. Enterotoxin Production

After ETEC colonize the mucosa they liberate enterotoxins whose action on the mucosa is manifested clinically as diarrhea. Strains can produce one or more enterotoxins, divided broadly into a heat-labile toxin (LT) and a heat-stable toxin (ST). A comprehensive review of the biology of bacterial toxins, and their membrane receptors in the gut by Eidels *et al.* (1983) is highly recommended for additional information.

a. *Heat Labile Toxin (LT)*. LT consists of two polypeptide subunits: subunit A has a molecular weight of about 25,000 and has the ability to stimulate adenylate cyclase activity; subunit B has a molecular weight of about 11,500 and forms aggregates of five monomers which are able to adsorb to the Y-1 adrenal cells used in LT tests (Gross, 1983). This toxin resembles cholera toxin (CT) in a number of ways, e.g., its immunological characteristics and biological action, and, besides being similar in subunit structure and mechanisms of action, they possess a large degree of sequence homology. In both toxins the B subunit is responsible for binding to the G_{M1} ganglioside of the epithelial cells of the small intestine, while subunit A stimulates adenylate cyclase activity, thereby increasing the concentration of intracellular cyclic AMP in the cells. Cyclic AMP inhibits the absorption of Na^+ and hence of Cl^- and water, in the villous cells. In crypt cells cAMP exerts a direct secretory effect by increasing Na^+ secretion and consequently, causing loss of Cl^- and water. The result is secretion into the lumen of the proximal small intestine of electrolyte-rich fluid which will appear clinically as watery diarrhea. Interestingly, unlike LT, whose gene is located on a transmissible plasmid, the gene for CT is borne on the bacterial chromosome (Robins-Browne, 1980).

Production of LT by *E. coli* has mainly been assayed on cultures of mouse Y-1 adrenal cells (Donta *et al.*, 1974), or Chinese hamster ovary cells (Guerrant *et al.*, 1974). These methods are still widely used to detect the presence of LT. However, they require cell culture facilities which often are not readily available in small diagnostic laboratories. Detection of LT by immunological or genetic methods is an alternative. A direct ELISA method for LT which requires the use of cholera antitoxin prepared in guinea pigs and enzyme-labeled goat anti-guinea pig serum has been described (Yolken *et al.*, 1977). Other immunological tests have also been described, including a radioimmunoassay (Greenberg *et al.*, 1977). Of the immunological tests, the simplest and probably most commonly used today, is the G_{M1}-ELISA. Discovery of the fact that the G_{M1} ganglioside binds LT and CT led to the development of a ganglioside ELISA for detecting these toxins. Wells in microtiter plates are coated with G_{M1} ganglioside and the test samples then added. Bound toxin is detected by adding guinea pig cholera antitoxin followed by enzyme-labeled goat anti-guinea pig serum (Sack *et al.*, 1980). Alternatively, LT antitoxins raised in rabbits and labeled anti-rabbit IgG can be used instead of cholera antitoxin (Back *et al.*, 1979; Svennerholm and Holmgren, 1978).

Additional LT tests described more recently include the Biken test

(Honda et al., 1982), the rapid latex particle agglutination test (LPAT) (Finkelstein and Yang, 1983), a staphylococcal coagulation test (Brill et al., 1979), and the gene probe (Moseley et al., 1982).

The Biken test is a simple gel immunodiffusion test originally developed using CT antitoxin, but which was subsequently modified with LT antisera. The chief disadvantage of this test is that results are obtained after 3–4 days.

The LPAT was recently introduced and is suitable for the rapid recognition of LT-producing colonies of *E. coli*. The test appears to be simple and economical to perform; it is directly applicable to colonies on a variety of commonly used enteric diagnostic isolation media and the results are available in minutes. The LAPT test, which was devised to detect LT of human *E. Coli* strains (Finkelstein and Yang, 1983), was found to be suitable for detecting LT of porcine *E. coli* strains (Finkelstein et al., 1983). Comparison of purified anti-LT indicated a high degree of cross-reactivity in this test between LT of human and porcine strains. The staphylococcal coagulation test involves the coating of *Staphylococcus aureus,* with antiserum against highly purified LT as the reagent used to detect LT in cell lysates of bacterial colonies grown on agar. The test procedure can be completed in 90 min. In the original test (Brill et al., 1979), CT antitoxin was used to detect LT, but the test was subsequently modified by using LT antitoxin with reported increased sensitivity (Honda et al., 1983; Ronnberg and Wadstrom, 1983). Radiolabeled, specific fragments from enterotoxin genes may be used as "probes" to detect homologous DNA sequences in *E. coli*. This way, the gene coding for LT may be detected in ETEC strains or in feces, which is a distinct advantage, obviating the need for culture, but it requires radiolabeled, cloned gene probes and several days to develop autoradiograms. Another serious drawback is that it only detects the existence of a portion of the LT gene, not necessarily the production and secretion of active toxin.

b. *Heat Stable Toxin (ST)*. The *E. coli* STs bear no antigenic cross-reactivity to *E. coli* LT. There is more than one ST: the methanol-soluble ST_a is active in infant mice and in neonatal piglets, but not weaned pigs, whereas the methanol-insoluble *E. coli* ST_b is active in weaned pigs and rabbits, but not in infant mice (Eidels et al., 1983; Gross, 1983). *E. coli* strains may produce ST_a, or ST_b, or both (Burgess et al., 1978). Furthermore, ST produced by strains isolated from various host species may differ both in molecular weight and amino acid sequence. ST_a is found in strains of human and animal origin, while ST_b strains are usually of porcine origin.

ST does not affect the concentration of cAMP, but instead stimulates the activity of guanylate cyclase, causing an increase in cGMP. This takes place only in intestinal epithelial cells and not in a variety of other tissues and cell lines, suggesting that a unique toxin receptor exists on intestinal cells. The mechanism by which increased cGMP leads to a net secretion of water and electrolytes is not well understood, but the action of ST appears to be mainly antiabsorptive; it lacks the secretory activity of LT and CT (Newsome et al., 1978).

E. coli ST_a and ST_b are immunologically and genetically distinct. ST_a has been the most extensively investigated; it is a heat-stable (100°C up to 30 min), small protein with a molecular weight of approximately 2000 (Eidels et al., 1983). Human and porcine ST_as are immunologically cross-reactive (Giannella et al., 1981).

The complete amino acid sequences of two human and one porcine ST_a have been determined. There is a large degree of amino acid sequence homology among the human ST_as and between them and the porcine ST_a. Thus, the difference in host susceptibility between different ST_a-producing strains is likely to be due to virulence factors other than ST_a, e.g., colonization factors. There is evidence which suggests that the receptor for E. coli ST_a is distinct from E. coli LT (Eidels et al., 1983).

By means of the DNA hybridization technique, using cloned ST_a genes from different sources as probes, it has been shown that two subclasses of ST_a exist. These two subclasses, which have been referred to as ST human and ST porcine or bovine, have been shown by DNA sequencing studies to share 69% DNA homology (Moseley et al., 1983). Genes encoding for the ST_b toxin have been cloned and found to share little homology to ST_a genes (Levine et al., 1983).

Injections of enterotoxin preparations into ligated ileal loops of rabbits, pigs, calves, and dogs cause accumulation of fluid. In these tests ST is distinguished from LT by its stability to heat and its rapidity of action. The infant mouse test is the most widely used (Dean et al., 1972). In this test the infant mice are given an injection of culture supernatant (often stained with methylene blue) through the abdominal wall directly into milk-filled stomachs. After 4 hr the mice are killed and the intestine examined for dilatation due to accumulated fluid. The intestines are then removed and the ratio of gut weight to remaining body weight determined as an effective measure of accumulated fluid. The test only works for ST_a.

ST_b causes distention of the jejunal loops of pigs, but not of mice. The role of ST_b of ETEC in piglet diarrhea has not yet been determined, largely because studies of ST_b infections have been hampered by the difficulty of examining specimens in pig ileal loops. Experimentally at least, isolates with ST_b alone were reported to have failed to cause diarrhea in experimentally infected piglets (Moon et al., 1980).

Until recently the nonimmunogenic nature of ST had prevented development of more convenient immunological tests, but antiserum to purified ST_a has now been prepared by coupling the toxin to a bovine serum albumin carrier (Frantz and Robertson, 1981). The antiserum has been used to develop a RIA. The gene encoding for ST_a has been shown to be distinct from that of ST_b (Lee et al., 1983). DNA hybridization assays, employing a radio-labeled fragment of DNA encoding for ST_b (Echeverria et al., 1984), and for ST_a and LT (Patamaroj et al., 1983), were used as probes to determine the prevalence of the three enterotoxins in pig ETEC strains isolated in Thailand. While the DNA hybridization probe for ST was shown to be sensitive for detecting ST-producing colonies in primary cultures of feces, the technique is complex, requiring radiolabeled gene probes and several days to develop autoradiograms. This restricts its use to research studies of epidemiology of ETEC strains. An assay for the detection of ST_a, based on the observation that guanylate cyclase is activated by this toxin in membranes of intestinal mucosa, was developed (Waldman et al., 1984). The assay was said to be rapid, quantitative, permitting a large number of samples to be assayed, and about 10-fold more sensitive than the suckling mouse bioassay. An ELISA test which detects ST_a was described by Klipstein et al. (1984). They used a synthetically produced ST_a to raise hyperimmune antisera in goats. The minimum amount of ST_a detectable by this method was 140 pg/ml, which is an amount 285-fold smaller than that detectable by the suckling mouse assay. The test was sensitive to human and porcine ST. Concomitant use of both ST and LT ELISA tests, as suggested by these investigators, should provide a rapid, simple, and sensitive method for identifying ETEC strains.

Escherichia coli strains, particularly those of porcine origin, may have LT, ST_a, or ST_b in different combinations but the frequency of each type is not known. A collection of 96 *E. coli* animal strains, at the National Animal Disease Centre, from various countries including the United States, was examined for the production of enterotoxins (Finkelstein et al., 1983). Thirty-five strains produced LT only, 10 produced LT and ST, and 46 produced ST only, of which 25 produced ST_a, 18 ST_b, and 3 produced $ST_a + ST_b$. It was not clear which ST among the 10 LT and ST strains, was the more common. The DNA hybridization assay mentioned earlier was applied to identify ETEC in pigs with diarrhea on farms in Thailand. ETEC were identified in 40% of diarrheic litters aged less than 10 days. The great majority being ST_a

producers (79%) and one or two producing LT/ST or LT alone (Patamaroj et al., 1983). Only 9% of ETEC were ST_b producers. The great majority (32%) were in ETEC isolated from weaned piglets (Echeverria et al., 1984).

3. Serogroup and Enterotoxigenicity

ETEC from cattle and pigs are divided into two classes according to their serogroup, the type of enterotoxins they produce, and their *in vivo* enterotoxigenicity. Class 1 comprises a limited number of ETEC strains from pigs characterized as hemolytic and nonmucoid, belonging to classical serotypes (Gyles et al., 1971). Some strains produce only ST, whereas others produce both LT and ST, which are detected by stimulation of fluid secretion in jejunal loops in pigs aged 6 to 8 weeks (Smith and Gyles, 1970). Class 2 are ETEC strains which dilate intestinal segments of piglets younger than 2 weeks of age (Moon and Whipp, 1970). In contrast to Class 1 porcine ETEC, porcine Class 2 ETEC are nonhemolytic and mucoid, belonging to O serogroups 8, 9, 20, 64, and 101 and do not dilate jejunal loops in older pigs. Bovine ETEC strains have several features in common with porcine Class 2 ETEC, which include possession of O antigens 8, 9, 20, and 101, the pilus antigen K99, and production of ST_a. They tend to be mucoid (Harnett and Gyles, 1983). Among 34 porcine isolates of O groups 9, 20, 64, 101, and X46, 26 were ETEC and 8 produced no toxins. Twelve belonged to Class 1, producing both ST_a and ST_b, and 14 to Class 2 producing ST_a only. Eight bovine strains behaved as porcine Class 2 ETEC. All strains from both porcine Class 1 and Class 2 and bovine strains induced fluid accumulation in ligated intestines of neonatal calves (Harnett and Gyles, 1983). These authors demonstrated a correlation among porcine isolates between the O serogroup and the type of enterotoxin the bacteria liberated. On the other hand, there does not appear to be such correlation between the O serogroup and pilus antigen; O20 and O64 can have either K88 (Tzipori et al., 1980b) or K99 (Tzipori et al., 1984a), both serogroups belong to Class 2 ETEC.

Porcine ETEC strains belonging to Class 2 have been associated mainly with diarrhea in piglets aged from a few hours to a few days (Tzipori et al., 1980a; 1982a). Experimentally, the serogroups O20 and O64 bearing K88 pilus antigen and O8 bearing K99 induced severe diarrhea in newborn gnotobiotic piglets, but when piglets were infected at 7 days of age, only O serogroup 64 caused diarrhea; O20 caused mild diarrhea in only half the number of piglets, while O8 strain caused no illness at all. The contrast in enteropathogenicity between O20 and O64 is interesting, considering that both produced

ST_a toxin and both possessed the $K88_{ac}$ pilus antigen. IF has indicated that colonization with O64 was more extensive suggesting that, as with K99 (Hadad and Gyles, 1982; Nagy et al., 1976; Smith and Huggins, 1978), the O and/or K antigens may play some role in bacterial colonization of K88 strains.

As with animal ETEC, strains that cause enterotoxigenic diarrhea in humans tend to belong to particular serogroups which differ from those associated with EPEC or EIEC. Infections with ETEC in regions of good nutrition and hygiene are uncommon, although they may cause outbreaks of diarrhea among infants in hospital nurseries. ETEC infections of humans, unlike those of domestic animals, can cause diarrhea in adults; indeed ETEC are one of the most common causes of travelers' diarrhea (Gross, 1983). In 1975 some 2000 staff and visitors at a national park in the United States developed diarrhea caused by E. coli 06 which produced ST and LT (Rosenberg et al., 1977). Other outbreaks in adults were described in Japan (Kudoh et al., 1977).

B. Control of ETEC Diarrhea

1. Development of ETEC Vaccine

Prevention by vaccination has emerged in the last decade as the most promising measure for control of ETEC diarrhea in piglets and calves. This has become more urgent with the emergence of widespread resistance of bacteria to commonly used antimicrobial agents. Interest in vaccination has also intensified as a result of increased knowledge of intestinal immunity, and recognition of various types of antigens responsible for *E. coli* enteropathogenicity. The identification of other pathogens causing diarrhea in young animals in the meantime has also helped define the limitations of vaccination against *E. coli* as the sole measure for control of diarrhea.

One of the early indications that feeding viable cultures of ETEC to sows before farrowing may control diarrhea in suckling piglets was reported in 1967 by Stevens and Blackburn. Kohler (1974) subsequently demonstrated protection against challenge in gnotobiotic piglets given colostrum from sows fed live ETEC during pregnancy, Although vaccination of pregnant animals with live virulent organisms in order to protect suckled piglets (Kohler et al., 1975) was arguably not a practical solution to the problem, it did nevertheless point out that protection by vaccination of the dam was a feasible proposition.

There are two types of vaccines available at present; those that utilize whole bacterial cells and those that rely on purified bacterial components.

a. Whole Cell Bacterial Vaccines. There are two types of whole cell bacterial vaccines available commercially at present.

i. Combined oral parenteral vaccine. Workers in the United Kingdom have shown that daily oral vaccination of pregnant sows with extract of heat-inactivated *E. coli* serotype O149:K91:K88ac during the second half of pregnancy, coupled with an intramuscular injection on day 95, induced better protection against challenge with the same strain in their suckled piglets than did two intramuscular injections. Analysis of specific antibodies in the colostrum coincided with very high levels of IgM against the serogroup O149. In contrast, two intramuscular injections induced moderate levels of IgG antibodies directed against pilus antigen K88 and O149 in colostrum, and provided poorer protection against challenge than did the combined oral parenteral vaccine. Protection following combined oral parenteral immunization, it seems, was achieved by stimulation of IgM antibodies against O149 rather than against K88 (Porter and Linggood, 1983). Protection attributed largely to antibodies against the somatic antigen, to the exclusion of capsule, pilis, enterotoxins, and flagella. particularly when whole organisms were used (as reported in these studies), is not clear. It is certainly not the role; Moon and Runnels (1984), using the same oral–parenteral vaccination schedule but with *E. coli* somatic O101 antigen, failed to demonstrate O antigen-induced protection against challenge in piglets. In contrast, they showed that some protection resided with capsular K antigens. Similarly, an attempt to protect calves with O antigen vaccine was unsuccessful (Myers, 1978). Oral–parenteral vaccination reported by Porter *et al.* (1977) appears to promote a "plasmid-curing" phenomenon, which is manifested by loss of K88 and, therefore, the capacity of challenge *E. coli* to adhere, rendering the bacteria nonpathogenic. This was demonstrated in suckled piglets fed oral vaccine to protect them against postweaning diarrhea (PWD) and in pregnant sows. In both cases, when orally vaccinated animals were challenged with K88-bearing *E. coli* they excreted the strain, but it was lacking K88. This plasmid-curing phenomenon was further demonstrated *in vitro* by incubating K88 *E. coli* with a 10% immune fraction of colostrum. Plasmid curing does not appear to relate to antibodies directed against K88 or O149, but was suspected to be associated with antibody specific to ST antigen and is found in the IgG fraction. In addition, antibody produced in response to one O serotype is capable of eliminating K88 plasmids from another unrelated serotype (Porter and Linggood, 1983). Intagen (BOCH Silcock) is a commercial vaccine based on the combined oral–parenteral, and is widely used in Europe and the United Kingdom.

ii. Parenteral vaccines. The majority of currently available commercial vaccines, however, are based on two parenteral injections given 5 to 6 weeks and 2 to 3 weeks prior to parturition, respectively. This method may not be quite as efficient as the combined oral–parenteral, but vaccines are cheaper and easier to administer. They tend to stimulate primarily IgG antibodies. They contain an inactivated mixture of the several common serotypes known to be associated with diarrhea, incorporated with a suitable adjuvant. Provided vaccines contain sufficient antigenic mass combined with an appropriate adjuvant, they will boost specific antibody response in the serum and colostrum of the dam (Logan and Meneely, 1981). While these vaccines can be shown to be protective to suckled piglets under experimental conditions their assessment under field conditions is often more difficult. Ciosek *et al.* (1983) compared the efficiency of four multivalent vaccines including two commercial vaccines widely used in Europe (NOBI-VAC LT-K88, Intervet International; and Gletvax, Wellcome) and two locally produced, and showed that only one of the locally produced and the NOBI-VAC conferred some protection against diarrhea in piglets. The quality of these vaccines depends not only on the quantity of bacterial antigens but the type. For instance, the inclusion of K88 in any such vaccine is important. Antibodies against K88 tend to be more bactericidal by preventing colonization of the mucosal surface, whereas vaccines containing little or no K88 tend only to reduce proliferation of challenge bacteria in the small intestine (Nagy *et al.,* 1979). Vaccine efficiency may decrease over a period of time. Porcovac (Hoechst), an inactivated vaccine in aluminum hydroxide and prepared from 11 serotypes including K88 antigens, was reported to provide a measure of control of diarrhea when used on a large scale vaccination program in the United Kingdom, Sweden, Italy, and the Federal Republic of Germany (Daerr *et al.,* 1980). A report 2 years later, which examined the cause of diarrhea among piglets suckling sows vaccinated with Porcovac as compared with nonvaccinated, showed higher incidence of infection with either K99 ETEC or ETEC lacking K88, K99, or 987P (Soderlind *et al.,* 1982), further evidence that, under the pressure of continuous vaccination, a shift in the ETEC population may occur.

b. Vaccines Based on Purified Bacterial Components. A new generation of vaccines based on the use of purified, highly concentrated, bacterial components has emerged. They require a relatively small number of antigenic determinants to still be effective against the widest range of ETEC affecting piglets. This is in contrast to the use of killed whole-cell bacteria which may include up to a dozen or so different serotypes. The use of pili as sources of vaccines to prevent diarrhea caused by ETEC has been established for quite sometime (Jones and Rutter, 1974; Morgan *et al.,* 1978; Nagy *et al.,* 1978). Parenteral vaccination of pregnant animals with purified pili stimulates the production of pilus-specific antibodies in serum and in colostrum (Isaacson *et al.,* 1980). Protection of suckled piglets against challenge with ETEC bearing the same pili occurs even in the absence of O:K antigen homology between the vaccine organisms and the challenge organisms (Isaacson, 1981). Now that methods for production, purification, and concentration of pilus antigens are available, construction of vaccines containing the major pilus antigens known to be associated with ETEC is the next step.

Vaccines containing the three major pilus antigens are now available, and the incorporation of a fourth pilus antigen, F41, has been reported (To, 1984). Multivalent vaccines containing all four pilus antigens would seem to provide the widest protection against ETEC known to cause diarrhea in the pig population at present. It would seem a natural progression that recombinant DNA technology be applied to produce these pili in large quantities (Anon., 1982).

c. Genetically Engineered Pilus Vaccines. E. coli bacterin EcoBac, containing K88, K99, and 987P subunits genetically engineered when given twice parenterally to pregnant sows, increased levels of specific antibodies against the three pilus antigens in serum and colostrum. This in turn coicided with marked protection of piglets against challenge with ETEC as compared with piglets suckled by unvaccinated sows (Simonson *et al.,* 1984). Protection was less effective during the first day of life. Increased levels of antibodies were detected in all three major classes of immunglobulins but IgG was by far the most prominent, as is to be expected with parenteral vaccination.

The following experiments were conducted in our laboratory to evaluate the protective value of a multipilus vaccine. Cells containing recombinant DNA plasmids coding for *K88ac, K88ab,* and *K99* genes as sources of fimbrial antigens were used. These cells were grown in 10-liter fermenters and the fimbriae were harvested by 60°C treatment of the cells. The cellular supernatant was then concentrated and dialyzed through membrane filters with a nominal molecular weight cutoff of 100,000. The fimbrial antigen concentration was measured by immunoassay and the three antigens mixed in equal amounts in 1 ml of saline; and equal volume of adjuvant was then added (S. Clark, unpublished data).

Vaccination of pregnant sows with two parenteral injections resulted in substantial increases in levels of specific pilus antibodies in serum and colostrum of sows, and in serum of suckled piglets. Antibody titers coincided with protection against challenge with a mixture of three ETEC strains containing corresponding pilus antigens. The challenge strains used included O149:K91:H10:K88ac, O141:K85ab:-K88ab; and O64:KNS:K99. To optimize the vaccine we examined the effect of route of administration, dose–response relationship, protection as it related to time of challenge after birth, the optimum interval between the two parenteral injections, and the efficiency of various adjuvants (S. Tzipori, S. Clark, and M. Smith, unpublished data). Table IV compares two routes of administration. Oral feeding of gelatin capsules containing the vaccine over 5 consecutive days appeared to have contributed little to the antibody response after the parenteral vaccination, although protection was the same as that of piglets suckling sows which received two parenteral injections. Although serological data are provided only for K88ac, a similar relationship was obtained for K88ab and K99. Necropsies performed on piglets within 48 hr of challenge revealed that challenge bacteria had not adhered to the mucosa of the small intestine and that appreciable numbers of bacteria were detected only in the colon. One of the control sows gave birth to piglets of mixed phenotype, half being genetically

TABLE IV

Antibody Response and Protection against Challenge[a] within 24 hr in Piglets Suckling Sows Vaccinated 6 and 3 Weeks before Farrowing with Genetically Engineered Pilus Antigens[b]

Route of vaccination	Number of sows	Number of piglets		K88ac IgG antibody titer[c] in	
		Born	With diarrhea (dead)	Colostrum	Piglets' serum
Two parenteral	3	28	0	499	236
Parenteral + oral[d]	3	29	0	174	94
Placebo	2	22	21(5)	33	23

[a]Challenge included a mixture containing 10^8 of each O149:K88ac, O141:K88ab, and O64:K99.

[b]K88ac, K88ab, and K99 mixed with aluminum gel adjuvant.

[c]Geometric means of absorbance values. (Similar results were obtained for K88ab and K99 antibodies.)

[d]Oral vaccine was given in gelatin capsules on five consecutive days, each containing equal dose to one parenteral without adjuvant.

TABLE V

Dose Response Relationship between Vaccination of Sows 3 and 6 Weeks before Farrowing in Terms of Antibody Response and Protection against Challenge within 12 hr[a]

Number of sows	Concentration[b] pilus type	Number of piglets		K88ac IgG antibody titer[c] in	
		Born	With diarrhea	Colostrum	Piglets' serum
2	100 µg	22	0	7260	1670
2	10 µg	23	1 (4%)	2151	494
2	1 µg	22	8 (36%)	489	152
2	Placebo	21	21 (100%)	136	30

[a]Challenge included a mixture containing 10^8 of each O149:K88ac, O141:K88ab, and O64:K99.
[b]Concentration of each of the three pilus types in 1 ml of vaccine mixed with equal volume of oil adjuvant.
[c]Geometric means of absorbance values. (Similar results were obtained for K88ab and K99 antibodies.)

resistant to K88; these piglets had diarrhea which was caused primarily by K99 ETEC. In piglets that were genetically susceptible, interestingly enough, the small intestine was colonized by K88 or K99 ETEC with little overlap, as determined by bacterial counts and by staining the mucosa by the peroxidase–antiperoxidase (PAP) technique. Experiments in gnotobiotic piglets have shown that, in mixed infections with O149:K88 and O64:K99, the K88 predominated, colonizing the entire small intestine while colonization of K99 was patchy and restricted to small segments in the ileum.

Table V demonstrates a linear relationship between the amount of pilus antigens (µg/vaccine for each of the three) and antibody response represented by K88ac, measured in sows' colostrum and in the serum of their respective suckled piglets 48 hr after birth. There is a good correlation between pilus antibody titers and the degree of protection. Piglets challenged at birth, before consumption of colostrum, were the most susceptible (Table VI). They remained so for at least 12 hr after birth, indicating that colostrum consumption during this period is not great in at least some of the piglets. By 72 hr they were better protected.

The interval between the two parenteral injections was found to be important. A comparison between intervals of 3, 5, 7, and 9 weeks showed that 7 weeks and above was superior to 3 or 5 weeks. This is contrary to the recommended practice of a 2–4 weeks interval between

TABLE VI

Relationship between Time of Challenge after Birth and Incidence of Diarrhea in Piglets Suckling Sows Vaccinated with either 10 μg/Pilus of Vaccine plus Oil Adjuvant or Placebo

Sows vaccinated with	Number of piglets		
	Born	Challenged	With diarrhea
10 μg	19	At birth	4 (21%)
	23	12 hr old	2 (9%)
Placebo	9	At birth	9 (100%)
	22	12 hr old	21 (95%)
	11	72 hr old	4 (36%)

injections. These results are somewhat similar to those obtained for *Cl. perfringens*, type C by Ripley and Gush (1983) who, in fact, recommended priming at service. The type and the amount of adjuvant, as with any other vaccine, play a significant role in the level of antibody obtained after vaccination. Oil-based adjuvants were, in our experiments, the most efficient; aluminum hydroxide gel and saponin were no better than saline. The difference in levels of antibodies following vaccination using oil-based adjuvant (Table V), or gel (Table IV), is apparent, but not in terms of protection which, partly, is also due to the difference in the time of challenge after birth.

d. Prevention of ETEC Diarrhea in Calves. Protection by vaccination of cows against ETEC diarrhea in calves is less complex than that of piglets and, as mentioned earlier, oral vaccination in ruminants is not considered as an alternative; there are only a few serotypes which cause diarrhea in calves, and they all fall into strains that have K99 pilus antigen and liberate ST_a. The period of susceptibility of calves to ETEC diarrhea lasts only 1 or 2 days after birth (Smith and Hall, 1967; Tzipori *et al.*, 1981), which is an added advantage, considering that levels of immunoglobulins in cows milk fall rapidly after parturition. In addition, the cow–calf relationship is one to one and is more intimate than in pigs. This ensures that there is a better chance that, if boosted, specific antibodies present in the colostrum will get to the newborn calf. Because of these factors it has been easier to demonstrate the efficiency of bacterial vaccines against ETEC diarrhea. As with porcine vaccines there are whole-cell bacterins (Acres *et al.*, 1979; Contrepois *et al.*, 1978; Myers, 1980), with partially purified K99 antigen (Contrepois *et al.*, 1978; Nagy, 1980), or purified K99 antigen

(Acres *et al.,* 1979). A correlation has been shown between K99 colostral titers in cows and the severity of diarrhea experienced by their experimentally challenged suckled calves (Acres *et al.,* 1982). Similar results were obtained from studies on vaccines against ETEC in ovines using either inactivated whole-cell bacterins (Gregory *et al.,* 1983) or K99 pilus antigen (Altmann and Mukkur, 1983).

e. Factors Affecting Vaccine Efficiency. The efficiency of enteric viral and bacterial vaccines is readily demonstrated experimentally. However, under field conditions more often than not their efficiency is questionable. There are a number of reasons for this failure: (1) The organisms causing diarrhea in the field are not as well defined as those used experimentally. There may be a number of them acting sequentially or simultaneously. (2) Vaccine quality varies greatly, as has been shown by some investigators, and their determinant antigens may be different from those causing diarrhea, e.g., vaccines with K88ac may not be highly protective against ETEC with K88ab and K88ad. (3) Pressure of continuous vaccination may result in a shift in bacterial populations or a change in virulence determinants; in a major piggery where vaccination was applied to combat diarrhea caused by O64:K88 the O64 ETEC were found to have acquired K99 within 2 years (S. Tzipori, unpublished observations). It has been suggested that the new variant K88ad may have arisen in response to the pressure of the hosts' immune reaction to the K88 *E. coli* population as a result of introducing parenteral vaccination containing K88 antigen (Guinée and Jansen, 1979). (4) Partial failure is probably more to do with the fact that not all piglets receive high enough levels of colostral antibody within a certain period. This is to some extent independent of the levels achieved by vaccination. It has been shown that the amount of immunoglobulins consumed is influenced by birth order, litter weight, and litter size (Yaguchi *et al.,* 1980). Logan and Meneely (1981), who examined the effect of various commercial vaccines on colostrum and antibodies absorbed by suckled piglets, showed that considerable variation of antibody titers existed between piglets. Nine percent of piglets suckling vaccinated sows had virtually no antibodies in their circulation, which may be one of the reasons vaccination has not been totally successful in controlling diarrhea. Therefore, it is not sufficient that sows have high titers of antibodies in their colostrum, efforts must also be made to ensure that all the piglets suckle within a short time after birth to be adequately protected. In establishments with a high level of contamination, piglets may become infected before they have consumed adequate colostrum. Therefore, high levels of hygiene in the immediate surroundings of the sow may be important.

Ideal vaccines should be those that provide the widest possible protection, be safe, cheap to produce, and easy to administer. Vaccines consisting of the major pilus antigens affecting pigs produced by recombinant DNA technology are likely to be the vaccines of the future. However, effective immunity against ETEC diarrhea is likely to result more from a combination of antibody-mediated defense mechanisms, both antipilus antibodies and antitoxins acting together, than from a single activity. Studies by Svennerholm and Ahren (1982) have shown synergy between antibodies to certain somatic antigens and antienterotoxin, which together provided protection against homologous and heterologous strains of *E. coli*. The addition of LT, which has now been cloned, to such vaccines will undoubtedly increase their efficiency. Immunization with porcine LT has already been shown to significantly increase the level of LT antitoxin in the colostrum and to provide protection against ETEC (Dobrescu and Huygelen, 1976; Dorner *et al.*, 1980). Similar results were obtained with vaccination of sows with procholeragenoid, a heat-treated CT (Furer *et al.*, 1982). It remains to be determined whether inclusion of ST enterotoxins will further improve vaccine efficiency. Although vaccination of pregnant sows with ST coupled with bovine IgG conjugate failed to protect suckled piglets against infection with ST-producing strains of *E. coli* (Moon *et al.*, 1983), it may have synergistic effects when combined with other somatic antigens.

2. Other Methods for Control of ETEC

Means for control of ETEC diarrhea other than vaccination have been proposed by scientists over the years, but few will be mentioned. These include (1) selection and breeding of pigs genetically resistant to K88 adhesion, (2) feeding of lactobacilli or *Streptococcus faecium,* (3) treatment with appropriate bacteriophages, and (4) treatment with monoclonal antibodies.

a. Selection for Resistance to K88. In areas where K88 ETEC diarrhea is the predominant cause, prevention by breeding should be considered. In Australia, in the absence of TGE and epidemic diarrhea virus (a coronavirus unrelated to TGE), and where coccidiosis has only been detected on two occasions (R. Culter and R. Jones, unpublished data; S. Tzipori, unpublished data), and *Cl. perfringens* type C has not been reported, ETEC, and K88 ETEC in particular, remain the major cause of diarrhea. In our laboratory, a program was initiated which included development of an immunoassay as a means to distinguish between pig phenotypes (Section III, A,1), and a breeding program has also been instituted which will incorporate resistance to K88 as a characteristic to be included in the selection of animals for breeding.

b. Lactic Acid-Producing Bacteria. The usefulness of probiotics as a means of preventing enteric disease is not settled. For every report demonstrating antidiarrheal effect with lactobacillus therapy, there is one that has failed. The rationale for treating intestinal infections with agents producing lactic acid stems from a longstanding belief that these organisms inhibit or interfere with the growth of enteric pathogens by altering the intestinal milieu. *S. faecium* is a lactic acid-producing organism which, in addition, is thought to interfere with ETEC by adhering to the mucosa, thus competing with *E. coli* for binding sites. Other mechanisms are also thought to be involved. Experiments in gnotobiotic piglets demonstrated that piglets challenged with S. faecium and ETEC experienced less diarrhea and recovered earlier as compared with piglets infected with ETEC alone (Underdahl *et al.*, 1982). These authors suggested a regime of daily feeding of newborn piglets with this bacterium for the first 7 days of life, thus colonizing the small intestine and reducing the effects of ETEC infection, or alternatively, to be incorporated into weaner diet as a feed additive to control PWD.

c. Deployment of Bacteriophage. A novel approach for control that has been described is the deployment of phages to treat bacterial enteric infections of domestic animals. Preliminary experiments have shown that a specific phage was found to be more effective in controlling generalized experimental infections in mice with *E. coli* strains than antibiotics (Smith and Huggins, 1982). Using a complement of two phages given shortly after experimental inoculation of colostrum-deprived calves with ETEC B44, Smith and Huggins (1983) demonstrated protection against clinical diarrhea and death, because the degree of destruction of the infecting *E. coli* strain by phages was sufficient to prevent the bacteria becoming established in sufficiently high numbers in the small intestine. Clinical response to treatment with the phages was poorer when treatment was delayed until diarrhea commenced. Treatment with one phage caused a mutant of *E. coli* B44 of reduced virulence, but resistant to the first phage to develop. The second phage was used to eliminate the mutant. The phages were as active against adhering organisms as they were against organisms in the lumen. Similar strategies were applied to piglets and lambs.

The advantages of phage treatment over antibiotics according to Smith and Huggins (1983) are that only one dose is needed, unlike antibiotic treatment; resistant mutants which emerge tend to be of reduced virulence (attributed to loss of capsular K antigen), and that there is little danger of susceptible animals contracting disease from infected animals. Presumably the mutants of reduced virulence that emerge from phage-treated bacteria would proliferate in the population and provide active protective immunity. One disadvantage of deployment of bacteriophages is the narrow range of their activity, and phages will need to be found that will attack points which are more widely spread among enteropathogenic *E. coli*.

d. Treatment with Monoclonal Antibodies. Monoclonal antibody specific for K99, when given orally, was shown to reduce the severity of clinical diarrhea in calves experimentally infected with ETEC (Sherman *et al.*, 1983). Calves were fed the antibody before challenge, which suggests a prophylactic rather than a therapeutic role. Such reagents can be useful as a supplement to feeding hyperimmune colostrum, particularly in herds and at times of extremely high incidence of the infection. Treatment of piglets with monoclonals produced against K99, K88, and 987P to control diarrhea is also being considered by a few commercial companies.

e. Prevention of Postweaning Diarrhea (PWD). Control or reduced incidence of PWD may be achieved by formulation of suitable diets. Breeding of genetically resistant pigs is of particular relevance as PWD diarrhea is predominantly precipitated by K88-bearing *E. coli*.

Vaccination as a means for control has been described. Intagen, the inactivated combined oral parenteral vaccine, has been administered to suckled piglets (Porter *et al.*, 1974). Piglets were fed oral vaccine from 10 days before and up to the time of weaning while suckling the sow. After challenge, excretion patterns between vaccinated and placebo-receiving piglets were taken as a measure of protection. The phenomenon of "K88 plasmid-curing" was noted in these experiments (Porter and Linggood, 1983).

Rijke *et al.* (1983) have observed a difference in immune response to vaccination against PWD between piglets suckling immunized, and nonimmune sows. However, a proper vaccination schedule made it possible to immunize piglets from both immune and nonimmune sows against PWD.

While O149:K88 appears to be the predominant ETEC associated with PWD worldwide, there are exceptions. In one report a strain, O149:K91, causing PWD lacked the K88 antigen, although it was capable of adhering to the mucosa of the small intestine. Vaccination of suckling piglets in a herd with PWD caused by this organism using a formalized autogenous *E. coli* decreased the morbidity and mortality; continued oral and parenteral vaccination gave the best results (Svendsen, 1979). Timing of vaccination after birth appears to be sig-

TABLE VII

Antibody Response to Piglets to Two Parenteral Injections with Three Pilus Antigens Produced by Recombinant DNA Technology[a]

Method of rearing	Number of piglets	Age of piglets (in days) at			Range of K88ac antibody titers[b]
		First vaccination	Second vaccination	Bleeding	
Suckled	9	8	20	26	2560–5120
	9 (cont)[c]	8	20	26	40
	4	14	20	26	360–2560
SPF	3	8	20	26	1280–5120
	3	8	—	20	40–160
	3 (cont)[c]	8	20	26	<20

[a] Measured in serum at weaning of conventionally suckled or specific-pathogen-free (SPF) piglets.

[b] Similar results were obtained for K88ab and K99 antibodies (geometric means of absorbance values).

[c] Received placebo instead of 100 μg/pilus antigen/ml/pig mixed with oil adjuvant.

nificant; vaccination with LT K88 vaccine at 5–10 days of age, repeated about a week before weaning gave the best results, but this regime required at least 3 weeks between injections. We have attempted to contain vaccination to the 3–4 week preweaning period using triple pilus antigen vaccine derived by recombinant DNA technology, as described earlier. Table VII indicates that higher titers of K88ac resulted from two parenteral vaccinations given 8 and 20 days after birth, as compared with 14 and 20 days, respectively. Similar titers were obtained in experiments using SPF animals which indicated that, at 8 days, there was no interference from maternal protection in the suckled piglets. One vaccination only induced a poor antibody response in SPF animals.

Control by vaccination of infections caused by ETEC in neonatal or weaned animals requires constant monitoring as the pressure of vaccination often leads to the emergence of new serotypes, or the same serotypes expressing new virulence attributes. This will be manifested by failure of vaccination.

C. Postweaning Diarrhea (PWD)

PWD is attributed to a complex interaction between changes in the physiology of digestion caused by change of diet at weaning, and the effects of these changes on the proliferation of certain enteropathogens in the small intestine.

In this section the relationship between change of diet and infection with ETEC, rotavirus, or both will be discussed, followed by close examination of the influence of various nutritional factors on the manifestation of the clinical illness.

1. Weaning and Infection

a. The Role of ETEC. Certain ETEC are by far the most important and common infections associated with PWD (Stevens *et al.,* 1972; Svendsen *et al.,* 1974; Tzipori *et al.,* 1980c). A shift in the prevalence of particular serotypes has been observed, serotype O149:(K91):K88ac:-H19 is at present predominant in many countries (Guinée *et al.,* 1980). Serogroups O138, O139, O141, O147, and O157 are known to have been associated with PWD. ETEC serogroup O149, causing PWD, produces LT or LT and ST.

ETEC PWD tends to occur 4 to 7 days after weaning 3- to 4-week-old piglets. This initially coincides with bacterial shedding in the feces by a proportion of pigs, but 7 days after weaning most pigs shed the organism, with or without diarrhea. In herds where the morbidity and mortality are high, shedding of organisms begins earlier and by the fourth day most weaned pigs shed bacteria in their feces (Tzipori *et al.,* 1980c). This relationship between timing of infection with ETEC as it relates to weaning and clinical outcome was examined in gnotobiotic piglets (Tzipori *et al.,* 1980d). Four-week-old gnotobiotic piglets remained clinically susceptible to clinical infection for only 4 days after the change of diet from milk to artificial dry diet. Piglets orally challenged 4 days after the change of diet showed no symptoms of diarrhea at all. Similar results were obtained using SPF piglets (Tzipori *et al.,* 1984b).

A series of experiments designed to examine the effect of change of diet from milk to dry food on gut morphology and physiology with and without infection with ETEC was conducted recently (Tzipori *et al.,* 1984b). Cesarean-derived SPF piglets were maintained on a milk diet until 28 days of age. Two groups were weaned on to a dry diet and one of these was orally challenged with ETEC; one of the remaining two groups on the milk diet was also challenged. Infected piglets on the dry diet developed clinical diarrhea and at necropsy exhibited severe lesions in the small intestine associated with extensive bacterial adherence throughout. Infected piglets on the milk diet had little or no diarrhea, and fecal bacterial counts were lower and adherence in the small intestine was associated with only minor mucosal changes. Control piglets on milk or dry food remained clinically healthy and had normal mucosal morphology. It seems that change of diet from milk to dry food has, in itself, little or no adverse effect on the integrity of the mucosa of the small intestine, which is in contrast to field studies where marked villus atrophy, crypt hyperplasia, and decreased levels of digestive enzyme activity were observed in clinically, apparently healthy, weaned piglets (Gay *et al.*, 1976; Hampson *et al.*, 1982; Kenworthy, 1976). On the other hand, in the absence of sudden change from milk to dry food in similarly infected piglets, there was only limited bacterial colonization of the epithelial cells of the small intestine, with little or no diarrhea. These observations suggest that a sudden dietary change to dry food at weaning creates circumstances which promote proliferation and colonization of the small intestine by K88 *E. coli*, which lead to a more severe clinical and pathological syndrome than either event, weaning or infection, can cause in isolation.

The reason for the severe damage to the mucosal lining observed as a consequence of these events is not clear. However, in addition to the hypersecretion induced by ETEC enterotoxins which is characteristic of infection in neonates, PWD diarrhea is presumably further amplified by brush border malfunction and malabsorption resulting from mucosal damage. It is worth noting that, in another experiment, we had used piglets which had been raised under gnotobiotic conditions and which were shown to be extremely susceptible to infection with ETEC while still on a milk diet at the age of 4 weeks (Tzipori *et al.*, 1980d), whereas in SPF piglets ETEC induced little or no diarrhea (Tzipori *et al.*, 1984b). This suggests that the exposure of gut mucosa to certain microflora, including nonpathogenic *E. coli*, may render the normal gut of a 3- to 4-week-old piglet consuming milk less suitable for extensive colonization by ETEC, even in the absence of maternal antibodies. The next step in this series of studies was to determine whether different levels and sources of dietary energy and protein influence the degree of proliferation and/or colonization of ETEC in the gut.

 b. The Role of Rotavirus. Several investigations have provided evidence which implicates porcine rotavirus in PWD (Bohl *et al.*, 1978; Lecce and King, 1978; Woode *et al.*, 1976).

An investigation designed to determine the relative contribution of ETEC and/or porcine rotavirus to PWD in a major piggery has indicated that ETEC played the major and consistent role while, at best, rotavirus exacerbated the severity of the disease (Tzipori *et al.*, 1980d). This was based on the fact that ETEC was more consistently cultured from affected piglets while rotavirus was present less frequently; rotavirus antibodies were also present in serum collected from the herd before PWD first appeared. There was, however, a decline of circulating antibodies to rotavirus which coincided with the time of weaning, or shortly thereafter. This relationship was further examined under experimental conditions (Tzipori et al., 1980d). Four-week-old gnotobiotic piglets fed milk showed mild symptoms of diarrhea when inoculated with a field strain of porcine rotavirus. Symptoms were more severe when piglets were inoculated after a change of diet from milk to dry food. Piglets infected 4 days after weaning showed little or no symptoms of diarrhea. However, infection among littermates with rotavirus and ETEC given sequentially produced a diarrheal disease that was more severe than that produced by either agent alone. Lecce et al. (1982) inoculated colostrum-deprived piglets of a similar age with porcine rotavirus and observed mild diarrhea, whereas coinfection with ETEC and rotavirus caused prolonged severe diarrhea. In their experiment, however, the ETEC used caused no illness and shedding of bacteria was only for a short duration. In their assessment the rotavirus played the major role. The difference in conclusions between the two studies would seem to be related to the strains of ETEC used.

We have used the O149 serogroup which had the K88ac pilus antigen. Lecce et al. (1982) used O157 serogroup, which also liberates LT and ST, but has no demonstrable colonizing factor. In one piglet infected with both agents there was evidence of colonization in the ileum which the authors presumably interpreted to indicate possession of an as yet unidentified colonizing factor. It has been demonstrated elsewhere that, when the lower small intestine of piglets of similar age is infected with rotavirus, bacteria lacking colonizing factors can often adhere to virus-altered mucosa (Tzipori et al., 1983a). This was observed in piglets which were infected with rotavirus and either *E. coli* J2 (a mutant of O149 which lacks K88) or K12. We attribute the attachment to the lower small intestinal mucosa to the effects of (1) bacterial proliferation resulting from accumulation of undigested and unabsorbed nutrients and a slow moving ingesta in the lower small intestine, and (2) altered mucosa caused by loss of mature enterocytes and loss of protective mucus gel which allows bacteria to gain access to the villous surface. If the O157 strain used by Lecce et al. (1982) lacks a colonizing factor or possesses one which is less efficient than K88, colonization of the anterior small intestine, crucial in terms of clinical outcome, would not occur. Under such circumstances ETEC would play a less dominant role.

These studies reinforce the notion that the stress of weaning, of which the major component is the effect of change of diet on the physiology of digestion, provides an opportunity for infection by a number of different enteric pathogens or combinations thereof. In one nutrition experiment (H. S. Chang and S. Tzipori, unpublished data), several piglets which experienced much more severe PWD than others in the same group, were found to have, in addition to ETEC, extensive infection with *Cryptosporidium* in the large intestine, yet in itself *Cryptosporidium* is not capable of inducing PWD (Tzipori, 1983a).

Using the working hypothesis of Lecce *et al.* (1982, 1983) we can now explain the manner in which the rotavirus in our study was found to prolong the period of postweaning susceptibility to ETEC. ETEC proliferate during the period of physiological adjustment, which in our study was 4 days (Tzipori *et al.*, 1980d), and after which the gut appears to resist proliferation and colonization. Infection with rotavirus after weaning, whether clinical or subclinical, disrupts the mucosa, which in turn may facilitate colonization by ETEC if present, causing PWD beyond 4 days.

2. The Influence of Nutritional Factors

That various dietary factors may predispose newly weaned pigs to PWD, was suspected from the early 1960s. The choice of ingredients and the physical form of diets as well as the level of feeding appear to be associated with physiological disturbances to the mucosa of the pig's small intestine and induce a shift in the gut microflora.

The main energy source of the suckling piglet is fat, with carbohydrate becoming increasingly important as the animal gets older. The nature and physical structure of dietary proteins change as the milk proteins are progressively replaced by proteins of plant origin. In the course of this period, the physiological phenomena of digestion are undergoing significant development, with corresponding changes in the digestive enzymes. A considerable amount of information on digestion and development of digestive enzymes in the young pig has been published. The piglet is not well equipped at weaning with all the necessary enzymes to digest weaner diets. Depending on the composition of the diet, progressive development takes place 1 to 2 weeks after weaning. Therefore, a sudden change of diet at weaning from digestible sow's milk to a less digestible diet will create digestive upsets. Moreover, the earlier weaning takes place the more immature the digestive system and the more time required for adaptation to occur. It has also been shown that levels of digestive enzymes are markedly lowered during the first week after weaning (Gay *et al.*, 1976; Hampson *et al.*, 1982; Hartman *et al.*, 1961) and, therefore, undigested and unabsorbed dietary components that remain in the gut will provide nutrients for selective bacterial proliferation (Kenworthy and Crabb, 1963; Moon, 1974).

a. The Role of Dietary Protein. The data regarding the significance of source and level of dietary proteins are conflicting and they remain inconclusive. The underlying factors thought to contribute to PWD are summarized as follows: the merit of feeding milk-derived versus non-milk protein supplements which include animal and vegetable proteins, and "simple" (a single protein source) versus "complex" (six or more sources) diets containing about 20% crude protein. However, it is established that the apparent digestibility of milk protein is considerably higher than that of soya bean (SB), fish or meat meal, oil meal, or cereal proteins (Grudniewska, 1982; Seve and Aumaitre, 1978) and this may be explained by the progressive development of the digestive function after the suckling period. The implications are that an abrupt change from sow's milk to diets containing a less digestible protein predisposes the small intestine to selective proliferation of bacteria. Other studies have shown that feeding diets based on dried skim milk as the major protein supplement versus diets containing non-milk-protein sources at weaning did not necessarily prevent the occurrence of PWD.

The same applies to feeding of complex versus simple diets. Nielson *et al.* (1980) found that replacing SB meal and barley with increasing levels of skim milk (up to 15%) resulted in corresponding reduction of the incidence of diarrhea. Comparing a complex diet (10% skim milk, 5% fish meal, 5% oat groats, 35% corn, 12% SB meal, and 25% rolled wheat) with a simple diet (containing 65% corn and 25% SB meal), Bayley and Carlson (1970) reported piglets fed the complex diet performed better, but the number of pigs with diarrhea requiring treatment was not significantly different. Others (Okai *et al.,* 1976) found that feeding a complex diet resulted in higher incidence and more severe PWD than piglets fed a simple diet. It appears that, while increasing the level of skim milk powder may reduce the incidence of diarrhea (Nielson *et al,* 1980), the inclusion of other ingredients such as wheat, barley or fish meal in complex diets might account for the greater severity of diarrhea observed. The level of protein fed was also thought to influence the frequency of PWD. Prohazka and Baron (1980) reported PWD in pigs fed 21% crude protein (40% maize, 20% barley, 23% SB meal, and 16% skim milk powder), whereas no diarrhea was observed in pigs fed a 9 or 13% protein diet. Bacteriological examinations showed an increase in the fecal flora of hemolytic *E. coli* in piglets fed 21% crude protein and that this increase coincided with an increase in gastric pH. According to Prohazka and Baron (1980), the cause of diarrhea observed in piglets on high protein diets was the inability of the young pig to produce gastric acid in quantities sufficient for digestion of high protein, resulting in gastric pHs above 5.0, a level which allows multiplication of ETEC strains. The inadequacy of gastric acid secretion in the weaned piglet is due to the fact that the mechanisms controlling acid–base equilibrium take 8–9 weeks to develop, after which the piglet shows greater resistance to the establishment of ETEC. The bactericidal nature of gastric HC1 has been suggested by others (White et al., 1969). High pH also affects protein digestion, undigested protein in the small intestine may provide nutrients for selective bacterial proliferation.

Presentation of dietary proteins which are foreign antigens to the gut immune system results initially in immune recognition. However, with sustained presentation, this is followed by the development of immune tolerance, due to active suppression of any immune response. Before the development of this tolerance the gut immune system of the young pig may experience a period of hypersensitivity. This may be particularly significant in early weaned piglets and is predisposed to by the amount of creep feed eaten before weaning. This transient hypersensitivity to food antigens in the immediate weaning period can cause enteropathy and predispose to ETEC proliferation (Miller et al., 1984). Abrupt weaning, meaning without the introduction of creep feed during the neontal period, was said to have reduced the incidence and severity of PWD in herds where it was practicable (Miller et al., 1984).

b. *The Role of Dietary Carbohydrate.* The newborn piglet is well equipped to digest lactose; however the ability to digest starch at an age less than 5–6 weeks is poor, as the levels of α-amylase and, to a lesser degree, maltase in the mucosa are low. Undigested starch is an excellent substrate for *E. coli* proliferation (Kidder, 1982) but processing of starch in early weaning diets has been shown to improve digestibility by enzymes, cooking in particular can rupture the starch. However, processed starch which reduces polymerization to increase solubility is readily utilized not only by the piglet but by bacteria as well.

c. *The Role of Dietary Fiber.* As young pigs are incapable of utilizing dietary fiber, only approximately 3% of crude fiber is allowed in the weaner diet. However, beneficial effects of fiber at weaning in reducing the incidence of PWD have been suggested by some investigators (Armstrong and Cline, 1976, 1977; Smith and Hall, 1968). Smith and Hall (1968) were able to demonstrate that feeding only barley fiber *ad libitum* to 5-week-old weaned pigs orally challenged with *E. coli* resulted in no diarrhea as compared with those fed either barley meal or a barley/fish meal diet. There was no evidence of bacterial proliferation and adhesion to small intestines of piglets fed fiber.

Studies in ligated gut loops of 3-week-old piglets showed more fluid accumulated in ETEC-inoculated control loops as compared with similar loops in piglets fed crude fiber in the form of 20% ground oats (Armstrong and Cline, 1976). On the other hand, studies by Real *et al.* (1977) and Rivera *et al.* (1978) have shown that the addition of 10 to 30% dietary oats to the diet of weaned pigs had little influence in reducing the severity of PWD.

d. The Role of Dietary Fat. Lipase activity in the newborn pig is high; 40% of total solids in sow's milk consist of fat. Fat is not fermented by bacteria and it is unlikely to contribute to proliferation and diarrhea. Fat composition may affect digestibility, which varies among diets; the indirect effect of fats is not clear.

e. Dietary Energy Level. High dietary energy in weaner diets is said to predispose the intestine to bacterial proliferation (Moon, 1974), presumably because of the readily available nutrients in the small intestine for bacterial proliferation. There was little difference in the manifestation of PWD in 4-week-old gnotobiotic piglets weaned onto high energy diets or low energy diets (Tzipori *et al.*, 1980d). In conventionally reared piglets, weaned at 3–4 weeks of age and fed a high energy diet, the onset of PWD after natural challenge was usually postponed from the fourth day after weaning to the fifth or sixth day, (Tzipori *et al.*, 1980c). The delay in the onset of PWD was associated with reduced mortality and morbidity. Piglets given the high energy diet tended to eat shortly after weaning and ate more often, presumably because of the better palatability of the diet, and appeared to have suffered less severely from diarrhea.

f. Feeding Methods. Undoubtedly the act of weaning imposes stresses on the piglet, whatever the precise etiology of PWD. The disease is a reflection of a range of interrelated management abuses of the pigs' requirements in relation to nutrition, environment, and other factors such as stocking density and peer competition. Measures to reduce the degree of strain on the digestive system and possibly reduce the incidence of PWD include studies on the influence of restricted versus *ad libitum* feeding, and the form, wet or dry, in which it should be fed.

It is generally considered that, when diets are given *ad libitum* at weaning, some pigs may gorge themselves, and such overindulgence often leads to diarrhea caused by an overloading of an as yet unadjusted digestive system. Undigested food may form a substrate for ETEC proliferation. Restricted feeding was shown by a number of investigators to be more beneficial in reducing the incidence and severity of PWD (Ball and Aherne, 1982; English, 1981; Nielson *et al.*, 1980;

Palmer and Hulland, 1965; Smith and Hall, 1968). Smith and Hall (1968) showed that feeding 150 g twice daily of a barley meal/fish meal diet to weaned piglets caused no PWD as compared with *ad libitum* feeding. Feeding simple or semicomplex diets (Ball and Aherne, 1982) at three different levels of feed intake from restricted to unrestricted, revealed that feeding methods had a greater effect on the incidence of PWD than diet complexity. The highest incidence of PWD, however, occurred in piglets that had a time-limited access to feed and this was consequently attributed to their more erratic feed intake and their tendency to overeat when the feeder was first placed in the pen. Intake of large single meals tends to result in temporary stasis of the gastrointestinal tract, followed by fluid accumulation and rapid peristaltic activity, resulting in reduced digestibility, increased rate of passage, and hence reduced absorption (Porter and Rolls, 1971; Ruckabusch and Bueno, 1976). Gut stasis, it is suggested, promotes bacterial proliferation in the lumen leading to PWD.

The relationship between a choice of ingredients with high digestibility fed *ad libitum*, or restricted intake (English, 1981) has shown that, while yet again restricted intake of two commercial diets was superior to *ad libitum* in terms of incidence and severity of PWD, a high digestibility diet (37.5% cooked oat flakes, 10% maize oil, 20% denatured skim milk, 25% milk substitute, and 5% glucose) was superior to commercial diets; *ad libitum* in this instance caused no higher incidence than restricted feeding. The author concluded that restricted feeding of the newly weaned piglet should mainly be applied to diets with low digestibility.

Suckling pigs received their nourishment in liquid milk form, ingested in small quantities at approximately hourly intervals. The sudden shift to dry weaner diet and water is often associated with growth check due to reduced fluid intake. Some investigators have therefore suggested that early weaned pigs should be given a liquid diet, preferably based on skim milk, to encourage food consumption (Hardy, 1978; Kornegay *et al.*, 1979). In experiments designed to determine the role of rotavirus in the pathogenesis of PWD (Lecce *et al.*, 1983), liquid diet (as 19% solid, 30% protein, 40% lactose, and 20% animal fat) given hourly, was found to be superior to feeding three times a day in terms of the incidence and severity of diarrhea. When the same liquid diet was diluted to 6% solid, feeding hourly or three times a day resulted in a low incidence of diarrhea with little difference between the two treatments. Armstrong and Cline (1977) found that piglets weaned on liquid milk replacer diet had faster weight gain and suffered less PWD when challenged with ETEC than piglets fed a dry diet, but of different composition. Generally, wet feeding is thought to keep the pig's stomach more acid and therefore more bacteriocidal (Lawrence, 1972; Thomlinson, 1974). When the stomach is filled with dry matter the centre of the mass has a high pH value (Thorpe and Thomlinson, 1967).

To establish the influence of the consistency of the diet, 35 cesarean-derived SPF piglets were divided into four groups (H. S. Chang and S. Tzipori, unpublished data). They were weaned from liquid cow's milk diet to a basal, milk-based diet, given either wet (two groups) or dry (two groups) at the age of 4 weeks. One group fed liquid and another fed dry were challenged with ETEC O149 serogroup. The remaining two groups were challenged with a laboratory nonpathogenic *E. coli* K12. Piglets infected with ETEC fed dry basal diet became depressed, developed diarrhea followed by dehydration. At necropsy marked mucosal changes in the small intestine were observed. These included villus atrophy, extensive bacterial adherence to the mucosa, and marked reduction in membrane-bound lactase activity. In contrast, piglets fed the same diet in liquid form had milder diarrhea accompanied by limited bacterial adherence and minor mucosal and physiological changes. Piglets fed dry or liquid diets and inoculated with K12 remained clinically healthy and had no mucosal changes. The same experiment was repeated under conventional circumstances where PWD occurred naturally (H. S. Chang and S. Tzipori, unpublished data) using the same diet presented in a liquid form mixed with water or dry. The severity of PWD in 80 piglets was examined clinically and a few were necropsied to assess the extent of mucosal and physiological changes. As with SPF, but to a lesser degree, the incidence of diarrhea and severity among piglets fed a liquid diet was lower, and mucosal changes, including bacterial counts in the lumen and adhesion to the mucosa, were significantly lower. However, feeding diets in a liquid form does not apply to all types of diet: for instance, a SB-based diet fed in a similar set of experiments to SPF and conventionally weaned piglets induced PWD of equal severity and incidence (H. S. Chang and S. Tzipori, unpublished data).

These experiments confirm earlier findings that nutritional factors alone, in the absence of ETEC, had litte or no adverse effect on the integrity of the intestinal mucosa. The performance results obtained for the group fed liquid basal diet indicated a better rate and economy of gain as compared with dry basal diet. The results obtained with SB clearly indicate that the advantage of feeding liquid diet depends on the type of diet used.

Partial replacement of milk protein by SB meal protein adversely affected mucosal morphology and physiology and clinical outcome following challenge with ETEC. This was attributed to the differences in digestibility between the two diets for the newly weaned piglet.

Conclusions that may have emerged from the preceding discussion are that diets for young weaned piglets should be highly digestible, preferably based on milk, with restricted intake, and in liquid form if possible, in order to minimize the level of unabsorbed nutrients which may encourage the rapid proliferation of ETEC while the physiology of digestion is undergoing a period of readjustment. It also seems that transition from a milk-based diet to one containing, for example SBs should be gradual. Weaning in isolation for 1 week has been shown to reduce the level of exposure of the newly weaned pig during the period of 4–6 days of high susceptibility, from piglets weaned the previous week (Tzipori et al., 1980c).

Our studies have shown that, under controlled laboratory experiments, diets vary in their effect on the outcome of infection with ETEC, and diets with low "proliferation indexes" may yet be formulated and these would reduce proliferation of bacteria and intestinal changes to further reduce the incidence and severity of PWD. PWD has no long-term effect on weight gain, and piglets that have recovered from PWD subsequently exhibit compensatory growth (Tzipori et al., 1980c; H. S. Chang and S. Tzipori, unpublished data); this is because the damage inflicted is restricted to the mucosal lining and recovery is rapid and complete.

IV. *Cryptosporidium*

The significance of *Cryptosporidium* as an enteropathogen of veterinary importance was only realized in the past 6–7 years. Since 1980 a considerable amount of information on the infection in a variety of animals, and its significance in calves and in other neonates of small ruminants has become available. The literature regarding the organism and its history, the nature of the infection in various animals, and the disease that it causes under field and experimental conditions has been reviewed (Angus, 1983; Tzipori, 1983a). This information will be covered here very briefly. Emphasis on the other hand will be placed on knowledge that has become available since the publication of these reviews and includes (1) details of the nature and epidemiology of the disease in humans because of the true zoonotic nature of this infection, and in calves (Section VI,A), (2) new methods for diagnosis, (3) new advances in laboratory animals and *in vitro* propagation, and (4) further studies on chemotherapy.

A. Cryptosporidiosis in Animals

Cryptosporidium is a protozoan genus in the subclass Coccidia which completes its life cycle on intestinal and respiratory epithelial cell surfaces of mammals, birds, and reptiles. Cryptosporidiosis is a common infection which, to date, has been described in some 20 different species of animals including man, and in at least 12 of them the infection was associated with some illness (Tzipori, 1983a). The infection was first observed in mice in 1907 (Tyzzer, 1907). The life cycle broadly follows that of other enteric coccidia, with asexual followed by sexual endogenous stages. Distinct features by which cryptosporidiosis achieves greater reproductive potential include cyclic development of the schizogeny and autoinfection, particularly the second feature which allows it to maintain persistent infection in immunologically compromised hosts. Oocysts contain four sporozoites which sporulate endogenously and are therefore infective when discharged in the feces. The oocysts are extremely resistant to the action of disinfectants commonly used in laboratories and hospitals (Campbell *et al.*, 1982).

Detailed morphology of cryptosporidiosis has been described by Vetterling *et al.* (1971) and Bird and Smith (1980), and ultrastructural aspects of the sexual stages of the life cycle were studied by Goebel and Braendler (1982). The organism has so far been observed in the gastrointestinal tracts of clinically healthy mice, rabbits, guinea pigs, raccoons, cats, and birds; clinically ill calves, lambs, goats, piglets, deer, humans, monkeys and snakes, and immunologically deficient foals. The infection was also observed in association with upper respiratory tract infections of birds. Based on recent transmission experiments, *Cryptosporidium* was shown to lack host specificity and, therefore, a potential zoonosis. Organisms from some species can infect a wide variety of other animals, with or without causing illness. Thus, isolates from calves, humans, deer, lambs, and goats readily infect lambs, calves, goats, and piglets causing enterocolitis; and mice, rats, guinea pigs, chickens, dogs, cats, and foals without causing illness.

Cryptosporidiosis has most commonly been studied in calves, and more recently in humans. Studies in animals show that the lower small intestine is the organ most severely affected; in very young animals, however, the entire bowel may be infected. *Cryptosporidium*, unlike other coccidia, does not invade the epithelial cytoplasm, it remains physically outside the cell boundaries firmly embedded in the brush border membrane. The most common mucosal changes observed are stunted, fused, and swollen villi, coated with immature absorptive cells, and the lamina propria is moderately infiltrated with macrophages, neutrophils, and eosinophils. The infection has a marked effect on the level of membrane-bound digestive enzymes, and diarrhea results from brush border maldigestion and malabsorption. Relapses of the disease have been reported several weeks after apparent recovery. The disease has also been described in artificially reared lambs and fawns, and in suckled goat kids and lambs. *Cryptosporidium* was reported to cause moderate to severe upper respiratory tract infection in turkeys and other birds. Some species, although readily infected, appear to possess an innate resistance; in rats, mice and guinea pigs, for example, the infection is asymptomatic with a long incubation period. Ruminants, on the other hand, are susceptible and can become ill if infected at an early age. Whereas the evidence against host specificity is strong, some differences between animal isolates do exist, the extent of which are not fully understood in terms of their behavior in certain hosts and specific organs. These factors, clinical and subclinical infections of various species, with possibly one species genus, would undoubtedly complicate any future attempts to fully understand the epidemiology of this infection in vertebrates.

B. Human Cryptosporidiosis

The history of cryptosporidiosis in humans is short. The first clinical case was reported in 1976 and until 1980 the four or so cases were mostly discovered in individuals with some clinical or congenital immunodeficiency (Lasser *et al.*, 1979; Meisel *et al.*, 1976; Weisburger *et al.*, 1979). However, the occurrence of cryptosporidiosis in immunologically normal persons was also becoming apparent (Nime *et al.*, 1976; Tzipori *et al.*, 1980e). A limited study in 1980 had indicated that cryptosporidiosis may be responsible in an as yet undetermined percentage of cases of diarrhea in immunologically normal humans, particularly in children (S. Tzipori and C. R. Madely, unpublished data). However, it took nearly 3 additional years before this view was accepted (Jokipii *et al.*, 1983; Tzipori *et al.*, 1983b). Simultaneously, the emergence of acquired immunodeficiency syndrome (AIDS) and AIDS-related infection has brought cryptosporidiosis to the forefront. Cryptosporidiosis in humans then manifests as two clinically distinct disease entities: a self-limiting enterocolitis in immunologically normal humans, and a persistent, life-threatening diarrhea in immunologically compromised individuals, particularly those with AIDS.

1. Infection in Immunologically Normal Humans

The infection in immunologically normal humans has so far been reported in detail in more than 30 patients (Anderson *et al.*, 1982;

Current *et al.*, 1983; Fletcher *et al.*, 1982; Nime *et al.*, 1976; Tzipori *et al.*, 1980e). The symptoms of the disease vary from severe diarrhea, vomiting, abdominal pain, fever, nausea, and loss of bodyweight, which require hospitalization and intensive care lasting up to 2 weeks (Current *et al.*, 1983; Fletcher *et al.*, 1982; Tzipori *et al.*, 1980e; Tzipori, 1983b), to transient with mild diarrhea, or asymptomatic (Current *et al.*, 1983; Tzipori, 1983b), recovery being spontaneous. Shedding of oocysts coincides with the clinical diarrhea, as with calves. Rises in antibody following clinical infection can be demonstrated by the indirect IF test using ileal sections of experimentally infected gnotobiotic lambs (Tzipori and Campbell, 1981), piglets (Tzipori, 1983b), or mice (Campbell and Current, 1983). In two infants the IF antibody titers had risen from undetectable levels to above 80 within 7 days; the levels were still the same 3 weeks later (M. Smith and S. Tzipori, unpublished data).

Information relating to the epidemiology of the infection among human patients with clinical diarrhea has begun to appear in the literature. Table VIII provides a record of incidence reported by various investigators. It can be seen that the frequency of detection is well below 10%. The incidence in the general population who require no medical intervention is unknown. The infection is more common in children aged between 6 and 12 months (Hojlyng *et al.*, 1984), or older (Mata *et al.*, 1984; Tzipori *et al.*, 1983b). Studies that were conducted over at least a 12-month period have shown that the frequency of diarrhea attributed to *Cryptosporidium* was higher during the wet summer months (Mata *et al.*, 1984; Tzipori *et al.*, 1983b). However, this pattern of excretion was not repeated the following summer, indicating that while infection may be more common in the summer and autumn months it is not repeated each year (Tzipori *et al.*, 1983b). This period does not coincide with the calving season in Australia, a factor considered significant by some investigators. Symptom-free infections with *Cryptosporidium* are not very common. Our study (Tzipori *et al.*, 1983b) and that of Mata *et al.* (1984) both failed to detect oocysts excretion from patients without diarrhea. There are several instances of individuals that have had contact with animals and humans with cryptosporidiosis and have been shown to excrete oocyst (Current *et al.*, 1983; Nichols and Thom, 1984). Sources of infection are from other humans (Blagburn and Current, 1983; Baxby *et al.*, 1983), possibly contaminated food or water (Holten-Andersen *et al.*, 1983; Jokipii *et al.*, 1983), and domestic animals, particularly calves with diarrhea (Anderson *et al.*, 1982; Current *et al.*, 1983). Upper respiratory tract infection with *Cryptosporidium* has been observed in patients with AIDS (P. Ma, personal communication; Mele *et al.*, 1983). Infection of

TABLE VIII

THE FREQUENCY OF DETECTION OF *Cryptosporidium* OOCYSTS RECENTLY REPORTED IN A NUMBER OF COUNTRIES

Country	Number tested	Percentage with oocysts	Strain used[a]	Comments	Reference
Australia	884	4.1	Giemsa	Children (late summer)	Tzipori et al. (1983b)
Costa Rica	278	4.3	Giemsa	Children (summer)	Mata et al. (1984)
Denmark	800	1.35	MXN	Children and adults	Holten-Anderson et al. (1983)
Finland	154[b]	9.1	MZN	Adults (winter)	Jokipii et al. (1983)
Liberia	278	7.9	MZN	Children	Højlyng et al. (1984)
United Kingdom (Clwyd)	500	1.4	Giemsa	Children (spring)	Casemore and Jackson (1983)
United Kingdom (Clwyd)	1500	1.6	MZN	Children	Casemore et al. (1984)
United Kingdom (Brighton)	800	1	PA	—	Casemore et al. (1984)
United States (N/East)	1290	2.6	MAF	Adult	Wolfson et al. (1984)

[a]MZN, modified Ziehl–Neelsen; MAF, modified acid fat; PA, phenal auramine.
[b]Not clear by which criteria these were short tested from 1422 specimens—could account for high percentage.

the trachea was also demonstrated in gnotobiotic piglets experimentally inoculated with *Cryptosporidium* of human origin (Tzipori, 1983a). The questions are, what is the likelihood of, and how common will be infection of the upper respiratory tract in immunologically normal humans and other mammals; this raises the possibility of aerosol, as well as fecal–oral, transmission.

Cryptosporidiosis, which Mata *et al.*, (1984) place after rotavirus, ETEC, *Campylobacter,* and *Shigella,* may have greater significance in that, on occasions it tends to cause a more severe illness than other enteropathogens. The pathogenic potential of *Cryptosporidium* infection seems high since (1) no infections were found in nondiarrheic individuals (Mata *et al.*, 1984; Tzipori *et al.*, 1983b), and (2) very few cases of mixed infections in children are seen. In older children and adults an association with giardiasis has been observed (Jokipii *et al.*, 1983; Wolfson *et al.*, 1984). The disease in adults has been seen less frequently, presumably for the same reason as other acute enteric infections that are extremely common: continuous exposure to the agent by the majority of individuals through contact with other humans and animal-contaminated environment. In three of the surveys where adults were reported (Holten-Andersen *et al.*, 1983; Jokipii *et al.*, 1983; Tzipori *et al.*, 1983b) the disease was associated with traveling, known otherwise as "Travelers' Diarrhea," and was primarily thought to be due to ETEC infection. The remaining reported adult cases were associated with contact with animals (Anderson *et al.*, 1982; Current *et al.*, 1983). With the exception of the study in Liberia there is little information regarding the infection in developing countries, where there is a greater contact between animals, particularly ruminants, and humans.

2. Infection in Immunologically Compromised Individuals

The infection in immunologically comprised patients takes the form of persistent diarrhea. Cryptosporidiosis has been described in some detail in over 60 patients in whom either humoral or cell-mediated immune defects were present, with protracted diarrhea that was almost invariably unresponsive to therapy and culminated in death (Reviewed by Anon., 1984; Current *et al.*, 1983; Pitlik *et al.*, 1983; Pape *et al.*, 1983; Roberts, 1984; Tzipori, 1983a). Symptoms ranged from persistent watery diarrhea of up to 12 liters/day to periods of constipation, and bowel movements from 25/day to none over periods of months. Associated symptoms included anorexia, nausea, vomiting, and abdominal pain, intermittent fever, headaches, marked lymphadenopathy, and weight loss of 5 to 50% are common. These infections are usually fatal and tend to be complicated by other conditions associated with the immunodeficiencies. Persistent infection and diarrhea resulting in some deaths and loss of bodyweight have been induced in young nude mice which are known to be deficient in regulatory, or effective, or both types of T cells which suggests that these cells are required for the recovery from the infection (Heine et al., 1984). This could help in the future to define the relationship between immunodeficiency and cryptosporidiosis.

C. Diagnosis of *Cryptosporidium* Infection

Diagnosis at present is largely based on identification of *Cryptosporidium* oocysts in feces. A considerable number of techniques have been applied by scientists in order to enhance identification—often to increase the speed of diagnosis and reduce the need for examination with high magnification to allow a quick scan. These methods can broadly be divided into staining techniques of dried fecal smears and examination of wet preparations by phase contrast microscopy.

Among the various staining techniques, the modified Kinyoun acid-fast (cold) method was found by Ma and Soave (1983), who compared six different methods, to be the most sensitive. Garcia et al. (1983b) compared 15 different procedures and recommended the modified Ziehl–Nielsen carbolfuchsin stain, following fixation in 10% formalin. Procedures utilizing wet preparations such as dichromate solution flotation (Willson and Acres, 1982), Sheathers' sugar flotation (Reese et al., 1982), and the formalin–ether sedimentation used by Ma and Soave (1983) have been employed for clarification/concentration of fecal specimens. A three-step procedure which consists of differentiation by iodine wet mount, followed by identification by modified Kinyoun acid-fast staining, and concentration of oocysts by Sheathers' sugar cover-slip flotation method has been suggested for routine examination of human specimens. Unlike differences between serological tests, which often rely on detection of different antigens that may be present in varying quantities, examination of fecal smears, whichever the method of choice, depends on the number of intact oocysts present in the specimen. Sensitivity in itself may not be a problem as, in animals at least, there is a good correlation between shedding of oocysts and infection severe enough to cause clinical illness. By contrast to all the newly described techniques, in terms of rate of detection and morphology, Giemsa stain remains one of the most effective (Garcia et al. 1983b). Demonstration of oocysts in the feces as a method for diagnosis seems to correlate well with intestinal biopsies (Garcia et al., 1983b; Ma and Soave, 1983; Pitlik et al., 1983). Future tests based on antigens from sources other than oocysts discharged in the feces, hemagglutination for instance, may increase the sensitivity and simplify diagnosis.

The most reliable method for diagnosis, however, is identification of the endogenous stages attached to the brush border of epithelial cells by histological examination because it allows an assessment of the extent of the infection. Confirmation of infection of human origin can be verified by inoculation of SPF newborn laboratory animals in which the endogenous stages of the life cycle can be examined histologically, as well as by shedding of oocysts in feces. Oocysts can also be recognized under the EM by negative stain. They have sufficiently characteristic surface markings to be identified when feces are examined for routine enteric viruses (Baxby et al., 1984). Another method which has been suggested recently for diagnosis is the negative staining with migrosins which was said to be as sensitive as the modified Ziehl–Nielsen method (Pohjola, 1984).

D. New Advances in Laboratory Studies

The prospect of detailed studies of the biology, pathogenesis, immunity, and control of cryptosporidiosis has improved greatly. Study of the disease was enhanced with the discovery that *Cryptosporidium* isolated from calves and humans, the most readily available source of organisms, can be propagated in laboratory animals and the disease can be studied in gnotobiotic pigs, lambs, and calves. Initially, the difficulty was to obtain bacteria-free oocysts for experimental studies. This was overcome by treatment of fecal suspensions with ethanol (Tzipori et al., 1982b) or with antibodies (Snodgrass et al., 1984b). The propagation of cryptosporidiosis in 8-day old chicken embryos was a welcome development (Current et al., 1983). Isolates from humans and calves progressed through the same developmental stages as those observed in suckled mice. Oocysts harvested from embryonated eggs 8 days after inoculation infected suckled mice, and no differences were observed between the human and the calf isolates propagated in the chicken embryo. The allantoic route of inoculation was the only one that resulted in complete endogenous development within the microvillous region of endoderm cells of the chorioallantoic membrane. Unfortunately, it was not possible to further passage oocysts derived from chicken embryos.

Cryptosporidium derived from human origins has also been successfully propagated in a number of cell cultures (Current and Haynes, 1984; E. Waldman and S. Tzipori, unpublished data). The parasite completed its life cycle from sporozoites to sporulated oocysts. *Cryptosporidium* propagated more readily in human fetal cell line than in primary chicken kidney or porcine kidney (PK10) cells. Fetal mouse lung cell line was also found to support growth (E. Waldman and S. Tzipori, unpublished data). However, in cell culture there was no evidence of autoinfection, a characteristic of infection in animals and chicken embryos thought to be maintained by generation of "thin-walled" oocysts, in contrast to "thick-walled" oocysts which are discharged in the feces. Seven days after infection of cell cultures, oocysts were the only structures that could be identified. The propagation of *Cryptosporidium* in cell culture, chicken embryo, and gnotobiotic animals should provide means to obtain adequate quantities of uncontaminated purified antigen for development of more sensitive serological tests. Different endogenous stages can be obtained to produce monoclonal antibodies which may provide a method for strain differentiation, and cell culture grown organisms may also be used for "fingerprint" analysis. A more detailed study of the biology of the parasite and its association with cell surfaces can now be examined, so can the action of various chemicals and disinfectants on the survival and viability of oocysts. Finally, it may open up new possibilities for controlling the disease, particularly in calves.

E. Control of Cryptosporidiosis

Prevention or treatment of cryptosporidiosis in calves and humans will undoubtedly be of benefit in some instances. A vaccine prepared from inactivated cell culture-propagated parasites containing mainly endogenous developmental stages seems theoretically feasible. The disease in calves is sufficiently important in some cases to warrant prevention. The antigenicity of such preparations and the immunity that is likely to follow of course require examination. Unlike ETEC and rotavirus which occur shortly after birth, protection against cryptosporidiosis by passive immunization of the pregnant dam seems less likely as the disease most commonly occurs from 1 to 7 weeks after birth. However, vaccination of the newborn calf may be a better option in this case, allowing for active immunity to develop as the calf reaches the susceptible age of 5–7 days.

In humans, unless it will be shown that the incidence of clinical disease in the general population is higher than 2–7% (Table VIII), a vaccine is unlikely to be useful. However, there may be a need for monoclonal antibodies or hyperimmune colostrum raised against sporozoites and/or other endogenous stages which can be used to treat severe cases of cryptosporidiosis in immunologically normal patients, and, more importantly, in immunologically compromised individuals suffering from persistent infection.

Treatment with antimicrobial agents seemed initially a matter of time and, like other infections, a drug would be found to which this parasite will succumb. This, however, has not been the case to date. A list of chemotherapeutic agents that have been used and were found to be ineffective has been published (Tzipori, 1983a). Since then more drugs have been tested in various combinations but were found to be ineffective (Angus et al., 1984).

We have extended our own studies by examining additional drugs in

TABLE IX

CHEMOTHERAPEUTIC AGENTS THAT FAILED TO ARREST *Cryptosporidium* INFECTION IN 5-DAY-OLD GNOTOBIOTIC PIGLETS

Drug	Indication	Dose[a](mg/kg)
Tiamulin hydrogen fumarate (Dynamutalin)	*Mycoplasma* and *Treponema* spp.	40
Tylosin (Tylan)	*Mycoplasma*	40
Amantadine (Antadine)	Antiviral	100
Cyproheptidine (Periactin)	Antihistamine/5-hydroxytramine	4
Avermectin	Antiparasitic	0.02
Pyrimethamine (Daraprim)	Malaria	25
Pyrimethamine and Dapsone (Malaprim)	Malaria	125/100
Pyrazinamide (Zinamide)	Tuberculosis	500
Rifampicin (Rifadine)	Tuberculosis	150
Isoniazid	Tuberculosis	100
Colchicine (Colgout)	Cell division (mitosis)	0.5
Benzimidazole (Thiabenzole)	Anthelmintic	60
Nepthalophos (Rametin)	Anthelmintic	30
Levamisole (Nilvern)	Anthelmintic	12

[a] Dose given twice a day.

gnotobiotic piglets which have the advantage, as compared with mice, of becoming clinically affected. However, we were unsuccessful in any of the drugs tested (Table IX). The procedure we adopted was designed to test the drugs for treatment; therefore, after an incubation of 2–3 days and just before clinical diarrhea was about to begin in control piglets, we commenced treatment which we maintained for 4–6 days. Clinical as well as histological assessment was used.

At present, the testing of chemotherapeutic agents is largely empirical and has proved to be futile. In the future as information on the biology of the parasite becomes available the development of specific drugs directed against specific targets may be more effective.

V. *Clostridium perfringens* Type C

Cl. perfringens, which usually forms a part of the normal intestinal flora of man and animals, has been shown to be associated with a number of disease syndromes. These include gas gangrene, food poisoning in man, and various forms of acute enteritis and fatal enterotoxemia in animals. *Cl. perfringens* is a complex group of organisms which are classified according to the type of any one of four major toxins (Niilo, 1980).

A. Characteristics of the Disease

Cl. perfringens type C causes a range of necrotizing, often hemorrhagic, enteritis in newborn lambs (Griner and Johnson, 1954), adult sheep known as "struck" (McEwan, 1930), calves (Griner and Bracken, 1953), piglets (Barnes and Moon, 1964), foals (Dickie *et al.*, 1978; Niilo and Chalmers, 1982), and young chickens (Nairn and Bamford, 1967). Although the disease has been reported to occur only in several developed countries, the organism probably has a worldwide distribution. It is said that, once the disease is introduced into a herd, it becomes enzootic, causing high morbidity and mortality (Ripley and Gush, 1983).

The infection referred to in the literature as hemorrhagic enterotoxemia, infectious necrotic enteritis, and lamb dysentery, to mention a few, will be referred to here as necrotizing enteritis (NE). The infection affects newborn animals, usually during the first 2 days of life. In some districts of the United States the infection can affect up to 100% of newborn litters of pigs, causing heavy mortality (Bergeland, 1981). In Europe the disease is also associated with mortality (Høgh, 1976). In the United Kingdom, where it was first described by Field and Gibson (1955), it occurs sporadically, affecting up to 10% of pig farms in some districts. The disease tends to be more sporadic and is restricted to newborn calves and lambs in certain areas. The clinical signs and pathology of NE in these species are similar and the reader is referred to Bergeland (1981) for a detailed description of the disease in pigs.

In humans the disease is less frequent; it caused extensive outbreaks at the end of World War II, known as Darmbrand or enteritis necroticans (EN) (Zeissler and Rassfeld-Sternberg, 1949). In the highlands of Papua New Guinea (PNG) it is a persistent cause of disease and death (Murrell et al., 1966; Shepherd, 1979), mostly in children older than 1 year. Cl. perfringens has also been suggested as a possible cause of antibiotic-associated diarrhea (Borriello et al., 1984) and necrotizing enterocolitis in premature babies raised under physical isolation (Blakey et al., 1984), although neither of these studies specified the type of Cl. perfringens thought to be involved. Some strains, particularly those isolated from human cases in PNG, also appear to produce enterotoxin which originally was thought to be characteristic of type A only (Skjelkvale and Duncan, 1975). It is not known how common enterotoxin production is in strains of animal origin. EN due to Cl. perfringens type C has been reported from southeast Asia (Headington et al., 1967), China (Shann et al., 1979), and Africa (Wright, 1966).

B. Characteristics of the Organism

Some 12 antigenic, mostly extracellular, components may be produced by actively dividing organisms. They are designated by letters of the Greek alphabet from α to μ (Niilo, 1980). Type C strains release three extracellular hemolytic toxins along with many other exotoxins and exoenzymes. β-toxin is the principal lethal toxin, and to a lesser extent α-toxin. The β-toxin is temperature and trypsin sensitive and with some strains it is rapidly lost upon laboratory subculture. Various strains produce different quantities of β-toxin, which presumably determine the pathogenicity. The ability of some varieties to produce an enterotoxin antigenically identical to that produced by Cl. perfringens type A, (Skjelkvale and Duncan, 1975), which is a major cause of food poisoning in humans, may also be the cause of strain differences. δ-toxin which is the third extracellular hemolytic toxin released by Cl. perfringens type C is important for diagnosis, particularly in strains that readily lose their ability to produce β-toxin. δ-toxin has been purified (Alouf and Jolivet-Reynaud, 1981) and was found, in adddition to being hemolytic, to be cytotoxic to other mammalian cells including leukocytes, platelets, and peripheral and alveolar macrophages of rabbits (Jolivet-Raynaud et al., 1982).

C. Mechanisms of Diarrhea

Cl. perfringens commonly forms part of the normal intestinal microflora of animals and humans and spores shed in feces can survive in the environment for a considerable length of time. Therefore, the presence of *Cl. perfringens* in the environment or even in the gut, although a prerequisite, is not in itself sufficient to cause illness. Certain conditions are needed to allow the organism (1) to proliferate in the small intestine and produce sufficient β-toxin to act on the mucosa to initiate changes, and (2) to prevent the toxin from being inactivated by proteolytic enzymes to which it is sensitive. It was shown that *Cl. perfringens* was capable of proliferating in the gut only during the first 36 hr of life (Smith and Jones, 1963). Smith and Jones suggested that a low gastric pH limits the growth of ingested bacteria after this time. The presence of trypsin inhibitors in sow's colostrum, and cow's colostrum (Griner, 1963; Pineiro et al., 1975), and presumably in other species of animals, appears to protect the trypsin-sensitive β-toxin. Both gastric pH and trypsin inhibition in the colostrum, ironically, are mechanisms presumably designed to prevent degradation of colostral immunoglobulins, in particular IgG. Bacterial proliferation must, therefore, coincide with these events. Thus, for an infection to cause a disease it needs either to occur shortly after birth, as is the case with NE in newborn piglets, lambs, calves, and foals, or when infection coincides with, for instance, sudden change from prolonged consumption of a protein-deficient diet to a protein-rich diet.

NE in humans, and presumably in older animals, is attributed to dietary factors. Lawrence and Walker (1976) proposed that in "pigbel," an endemic NE in the highlands of PNG, the persistence of the disease has been attributed to reduced protease levels in the intestine caused by a continuous consumption of a low protein diet, and to the presence of protease inhibitors in the dietary staple, sweet potatoes, protecting β-toxin from proteolysis. The sudden consumption of a protein-rich diet at festivals for instance, encourages *Cl. perfringens* to proliferate in the absence of high levels of trypsin in the small intestine. This complex relationship between prolonged consumption of a low protein diet and dietary protease inhibitors, followed by a sudden consumption of a protein-rich diet, allowing proliferation of organisms and toxin production, was subsequently demonstrated in a series of elegant studies in guinea pigs (Lawrence and Cooke, 1980).

Apart from β-toxin, the role of extracellular substances, including the enterotoxin, in the pathogenesis of NE, is not clear.

D. Diagnosis

A presumptive diagnosis can be made on the basis of clinical and pathological findings, particularly when the disease occurs within 48 hr of birth. The observation of diarrhea which can be hemorrhagic, together with necrosis of the mucosa in the small intestine and the characteristic rod-shaped bacteria surrounding ghost-like necrotic villi, are all pathognemonic and suggestive of *Cl. perfringens* type C infection (Bergeland, 1981). However, confirmation, particularly in the nonfatal cases, or in humans, requires identification of the major toxins.

Toxin in intestinal contents or feces may be demonstrated by the mouse inoculation/protection test (Niilo and Chalmers, 1982); alternatively, production of toxin in cultures of organisms in cooked meat medium can be followed by mouse inoculation/protection tests.

In typing *Cl. perfringens* according to their major toxins, some factors need to be considered: (1) toxin production occurs during the growth phase of the organism, therefore 5-hr cultures are the most suitable; (2) toxin production is affected by pH, source, and level of amino acids and carbohydrates in the media; (3) some strains of *Cl. perfringens* may lose the ability to produce one or more of their major toxins in culture. These may require to be identified by detection of the minor toxins which they produce (Buddle, 1954). δ-toxin, for instance, is often used to confirm isolates of *Cl. perfringens* type C that have lost their ability to produce β-toxin. The specificity of production of major toxins is demonstrated by intradermal inoculation of guinea pigs (Carter, 1978). Dermatosis (0.5 to 1.0 cm) is produced if toxin is present in the supernatant of culture fluid. These lesions can be prevented by incubation with a mixture of commercially available antisera raised against types A and C prior to inoculation.

E. Control

Newborn animals can be protected by administration of *Cl. perfringens* antiserum at birth; however, vaccination of pregnant dams with β-toxin is a much more practical and cheaper method. Adequate protection was achieved by inoculation of pregnant sows at mid gestation and 2 weeks before farrowing (Høgh, 1976), or at service and 3 weeks before farrowing (Ripley and Gush, 1983).

The terms hemorrhagic and enterotoxemia should be avoided in relation to type C as diarrhea may or may not be hemorrhagic and, while toxins produced by the organisms in the gut may reach the systemic circulation, enterotoxemia is not known to play a clear role in the pathogenesis of NE.

VI. Calf Diarrhea

A. Epidemiology

Enteric infections of newborn and young calves were shown in one study in the United States to constitute approximately 40% of all infections affecting calves aged up to 60 days (Bulgin *et al.*, 1982). Tables X and XI indicate that rotavirus, *Cryptosporidium*, bovine coronavirus, and ETEC are the four major causes of diarrhea in calves and that they are responsible for 75 to 95% of infections worldwide. The relative frequency of each of the four differ between locations and must indeed vary between seasons and years. Therefore, the data presented in Tables X and XI are the frequency taken from a small sample at a time stated. Nevertheless, trends can be recognized, for instance, with few exceptions, rotavirus is the most prominent cause of diarrhea in calves; bovine coronavirus appears to be the most prominent in North America and France, less so in the United Kingdom. It has been detected serologically in Northern Ireland but appears to cause little or no diarrhea (M. S. McNulty, personal communication). In Australia, coronavirus has been observed on several occasions, but appears to be of low virulence as experimental inoculation of gnotobiotic calves failed to cause diarrhea (S. Tzipori, unpublished data). *Cryptosporidium* has gained prominence in recent times and is second to rotavirus in most studies.

Table X shows the prevalence of one or two pathogens reported for several countries. The data indicate that between 25 and 40% of infections are attributed to *Cryptosporidium* alone, or in combination with others. Infection with more than one pathogen is found in from 20 to 50% of calves. Table XI further indicates that ETEC is detected in 30 to 40% of cases of diarrhea in North America, and up to 58% in France as compared with 4 and 6% in the United Kingdom and Australia respectively. Generally, the higher frequency of isolation of rotavirus from cases with diarrhea compared with other agents may also be due to the physical resistance of these viruses as compared with coronavirus and

TABLE X

FIELD SURVEYS REPORTED FOR A NUMBER OF COUNTRIES OF THE PREVALENCE OF ONE OR MORE ENTEROPATHOGENS IN DIARRHEIC CALVES

Country	Number examined		Enteropathogen(s)[a] (percentage)	Years monitored	Reference
	Herds	Calves			
United States (Idaho)	73	284	CR (38.7)	1981	Anderson and Hall (1982)
Canada	26	161	CR (26)	1974–1981	Sanford and Josephson (1982)
Federal Republic of Germany	125	254	CR (37.6)	1979–1981	Fiedler et al. (1982)
Hungary	110	497	CR (27)	1978–1979	Nagy and Pohlenz (1982)
Switzerland	NP[b]	132	CR (28)	1978–1979	Nagy and Pohlenz (1982)
Czechoslovakia	2	75	CR (40)	1980–1981	Pavlasek (1982)
United States	NP[b]	279	RV (54), CV (46)	1978–1979	Benfield and Francis (1981)
Canada	59	222	RV (31), ETEC (37)	1973	Acres et al. (1977)
German Democratic Republic	81	202	RV (39), CV (32)	1978–1979	Schulz (1982)
France	20	21	RV (43)	1978–1979	de Rycke et al. (1981)
Mexico	4	140	RV (14)	1974–1980	Trejo Medina et al. (1982)

[a] CR, *Cryptosporidium*; RV, rotavirus; CV, coronavirus; ETEC, enterotoxigenic *E. coli*.
[b] Not provided.

TABLE XI
The Relative Frequency of Enteric Pathogens in Diarrheic Calves Reported for Different Countries

Country	Number examined		Percentage of calves infected with[a]				Mixed infection	Unknown	Monitored during	Reference
	Herds	Calves	RV	CV	CR	ETEC				
Canada	47	51	72	47	33	29	50	6	1977?	Morin et al. (1978)
United States (Dakotas)	NP[b]	147	19	22	3	39	22	24	1978–1979	Benfield and Francis (1981)
United States	12	32	34	22	19	28	34[c]	25	1977?	Moon et al. (1978)
The Netherlands	11	325	46	16	39	6	23	17	1981	de Leeuw et al. (1983)
France	38	50	30	52	NP[b]	59	36	12	1981?	Renault et al. (1982)
United Kingdom	34	286	54	9	22	4	21	27	1981	Snodgrass and Sherwood (1984)
Australia	9	91	49	0	36	6	19	15	1982	Jerrett (1982)

[a] RV, rotavirus; CV, coronavirus; CR, *Cryptosporidium*; ETEC, enterotoxigenic *E. coli*.
[b] Not provided.
[c] Approximate estimate (the author).

Cryptosporidium, which are not present in large numbers in the feces. Although demonstration of ETEC may be difficult because neither the ST_a or the K99 are easily detected, it can be readily diagnosed as it tends to affect calves aged less than 2 days. In contrast, rotavirus and coronavirus affect calves from 3 days up to 4 weeks, while *Cryptosporidium* affects calves from at least 5 days up to 4–6 weeks. Differences in the frequency of isolation of pathogens were detected between beef and dairy calves suffering from diarrhea. Bulgin *et al.* (1982) found that coronavirus and ETEC were much more common in beef calves (42 and 17%, respectively), than in dairy calves (13 and 7.6%), while Snodgrass and Sherwood (1984) showed that rotavirus (68%) was much higher in dairy calves. House (1978) has estimated the average annual loss of calves for the 7-year period 1970–1976 to be $95,000,000/year. Based on data obtained from two separate studies it was concluded that, in terms of mortality, rotavirus was the least important (5%) as compared with coronavirus which, although of lower incidence than rotavirus, is more important ($\approx$ 30%) in terms of mortality and hence economic loss; ETEC was the most impoartant (50%). *Cryptosporidium* and rotavirus are similar in this respect. On the basis of age, the younger the calf affected the higher the mortality rate, hence ETEC would be responsible for higher economic losses when it occurs in a herd. Infections that occur later, such as rotavirus and *Cryptosporidium*, although they may have a higher incidence, have a lower mortality rate. Coronavirus is an exception because it is a more virulent pathogen in North America than *Cryptosporidium* and rotavirus, and hence, while its incidence may be lower, its economic impact is greater.

Table XI further indicates that of between 6 and 27% of cases of diarrhea in calves, the etiology remains unknown. Diagnosis on a herd basis would tend to reduce this figure; however, Snodgrass and Sherwood (1984) failed to establish a firm diagnosis in 8 of 34 farms experiencing outbreaks of diarrhea, although 1 or more enteric pathogens were detected in each of the 8 farms.

B. Infections Specific to Calves

In addition to the four enteropathogens listed above there are others which ought to be considered. Some have been known for a long time but their role has been ill defined, e.g., *Salmonella* and *Campylobacter* spp. and bovine viral diarrhea virus; others have been identified but their role is not as yet clear. These include the Breda/Berne family of viruses and bovine calicivirus.

1. Salmonella and Other Enteric Bacteria

Salmonellosis in young calves has been reported by several investigators. It is not often included in routine diagnosis of calf diarrhea, presumably because (1) traditionally it is not thought to cause illness in very young calves, and (2) salmonellosis, unlike other enteric infections which are restricted to the gut, can be systemic and therefore, often manifests a recognizable clinical syndrome. Bulgin et al. (1982) have attributed 31.9% of infections affecting diarrheic calves aged up to 60 days in the United States to salmonellosis, more than half of the incidences occurring in the first 4 weeks of life. In Australia, *Salmonella* spp. were isolated from 12% of diarrheic calves (Jerrett, 1982) with an age range of 8 to 18 days. They were observed, however, on only two of nine dairy farms examined. Snodgrass and Sherwood (1984), on the other hand, failed to detect *Salmonella* in their study of dairy or beef herds.

Cl. perfringens type C causes acute bloody diarrhea within the first few days of life. The disease tends to be fatal, and is restricted to certain geographical areas. In the study by Bolgin et al. (1982), approximately 2% of symptomatic infections of calves were attributed to *Cl. perfringens*. Recently, calf dysentery was reported in young calves which was attributed to a non-ETEC strain. The disease was reproduced experimentally in gnotobiotic calves (Chanter et al., 1984).

2. Campylobacter Species

The case for *Campylobacter* spp. as a cause of enteritis leading to diarrhea in calves is not very convincing. *Campylobacter fetus* subsp. *intestinalis* has long been recognized as a causative agent of infertility and abortion in cattle and sheep, while *Campylobacter jejuni* and *Campylobacter coli* are incriminated in intestinal disorders, dysentery, and diarrhea in various animals. Their role as a primary cause of diarrhea in calves is probably insignificant; neither field observations nor experimental data provide evidence to suggest otherwise.

C. fetus and *C. jejuni* have both been isolated from enteric lesions of cattle (Al-Mashat and Taylor, 1980a). Similar lesions were induced experimentally in calves with both agents (Al-Mashat and Taylor, 1980b, 1983). Experiments in young calves and lambs revealed that, in some instances, infections can cause intestinal irritation (Firehammer and Myers, 1981; F. Krautil and S. Tzipori, unpublished data) with little or no diarrhea (F. Krautil and S. Tzipori, unpublished data). *C. jejuni* also failed to induce diarrhea in five gnotobiotic calves (Morgan et al., 1983). In our laboratory we orally inoculated six colostrum-fed calves aged up to 6 days of age with 10^9–10^{11} of *C. jejuni;* two calves passed mucoid and bloody feces for 1 day with no other symptoms. After an incubation period of 6 days one 6-day-old calf given 8×10^{11} bacteria developed mucoid bloody diarrhea lasting almost 10 days. Throughout the illness the calf remained alert and continued to drink milk with no apparent loss of body condition (F. Krautil and S. Tzipori, unpublished data). The prevalence of the organism in bovines is high. Firehammer and Myers (1981) isolated *C. jejuni* from 40% of 127 diarrheic calves in the United States and 3 from each of 3 normal calves, while Garcia et al. (1983a) recovered the organism from 50 of 100 slaughtered beef. Eighty-one of 103 cultures which were typed belonged to 14 serotypes, with serotype 7 being the most frequent (35% of isolates). These serotypes are also commonly isolated from humans. In the United Kingdom, *C. jejuni* and *E. coli* were recovered from 25% of healthy calves and 34% of diarrheic calves. *C. jejuni* was not shown to be a sole agent in any outbreak of diarrhea (Morgan et al., 1983). While there is no supportive evidence that *Campylobacter* spp. are a primary cause of diarrhea, one suspects that under some yet undefined conditions their ability to cause intestinal lesions may result in illness.

The significance of *Campylobacter* spp. lies, however, in their emergence from obscurity as a veterinary pathogen to a cause of enteritis in humans. However, their involvement in human disease is largely based on epidemiological observations and on other circumstantial evidence; they are isolated more frequently from patients with diarrhea—simultaneous isolations may be obtained from stools and blood—respond to treatment with erythromycin, and have studied in volunteers (Blaser and Reller, 1981). The infection in humans has an incubation period of 2 to 7 days and the disease tends to occur either sporadically or in outbreaks, and it affects all ages. Clinical signs consist of fever, vomiting, diarrhea, often with blood and colicky periumbilical pain (Kirubakaran et al., 1981). The incidence in humans varies from 5% (Kirubakaran et al., 1981; Young et al., 1980) up to 10% or higher (Bruce et al., 1977; Georges et al., 1984). Asymptomatic infection of up to 25% among humans is also common (Blaser and Reller, 1981).

Like *Salmonella*, *Campylobacter* is sensitive to gastric acid. The sites of tissue injury include the jejunum, ileum, and colon. The lesions include diffuse, bloody, edematous, and exudative enteritis. The mechanism of diarrhea is not clear; bacteremia and cellular infiltration suggest tissue invasiveness; cellular invasiveness may also occur, although it has only been demonstrated *in vitro*. It now appears that many strains of *C. jejuni* and *C. coli* produce a cholerae-like, heat-labile enterotoxin (Klipstein and Engert, 1984; McCardell et al., 1984;

Ruiz-Palacios et al., 1983) which produces a cytotonic response in Y-1 and CHO cells, increases permeability in the rabbit skin test, and evokes fluid secretion in ligated ileal loops. This enterotoxin is immunologically related to E. coli LT and its B subunit. It remains to be established whether the enterotoxin production will prove to be a contributory factor in the pathogenesis of secretory-type diarrhea caused by C. jejuni that is common in children from developing countries.

3. The Breda/Berne and Other Enteric Viruses

A new virus of calves was reported in 1982 by Woode et al. (1982) and was named the Bredavirus after the town in the United States in which the calf was found. Bredavirus was shown to be antigenically different from coronaviruses, which it resembles morphologically. This virus caused diarrhea when fed to gnotobiotic calves. A second, serologically related by IF, and morphologically similar virus, Bredavirus 2, was isolated in Ohio and showed enough serological differences to be regarded as a distinct serotype. Another similar virus was isolated in tissue culture from a horse in Berne in 1972, and is known as the Berne virus (Weiss et al., 1983). It was found to be antigenically related to the two Bredavirus strains (Weiss et al., 1983). A virus morphologically similar and serologically related to the two Bredaviruses (but more distinctly to the Bredavirus 2 by immunoelectron microscopy) was observed in the stools of 20 patients with gastroenteritis, most of whom were children (Beards et al., 1984). These isolations suggested the existence of yet another previously unknown and therefore taxonomically unclassified family of viruses. These corona-like particles are pleomorphic, measuring 100 (Beards et al., 1984) to 120–140nm (Weiss et al., 1983) with a fringe of closely applied peplomers (7–9 nm in length), with occasional large ones (20 nm) (Weiss et al., 1983). The Berne virus, as seen in cell culture, is enveloped with an elongated core structure, budding at the plasma membrane, its growth is unaffected by iododeoxyuridine and it is inactivated by organic solvents. This family of viruses appears to be widespread in animals including horses, cattle, sheep, goats, and pigs. Antibodies were not detected in sera from dogs, cats and, surprisingly, humans (Weiss et al., 1983). It is not clear whether "fringed particles," a name which has been applied to a 100-nm corona-like virus by Mebus et al. (1978), observed by electron microscopy in calf feces during an outbreak of diarrhea in a beef herd in the United States, is related or identical to the Bredavirus. Another virus described as a "mini-coronavirus" was recently detected in gut contents of calves with diarrhea in Quebec dairy herds. It measures only 45–65 nm, is antigenically unrelated to bovine coronavirus, and seems too small to be a member of this family (Dea *et al.,* 1983).

When fed to gnotobiotic calves aged 3 to 40 days, Bredavirus induced mild diarrhea 3 to 5 days later; virus shedding in the feces lasted 4 to 6 days. There was evidence of villus atrophy and infection was confined to the epithelial lining cells. Inoculation of five older colostrum-fed calves, resulted in mild diarrhea in two of them (Saif *et al.,* 1981). While these viruses appear to be widespread, the frequency of their detection in calves with diarrhea is low, presumably due either to failure by electron microscopists to identify them or, like bovine calcivirus which is also able to induce diarrhea in gnotobiotic calves, are seldom detected by routine fecal examination.

Several other infections of the intestine leading to diarrhea in calves have been reported once or twice and include hemorrhagic and necrotizing gastroenteritis associated with viral damage to epithelial cells caused by an enteric bovine adenovirus (Bulmer *et al.,* 1975; Thompson *et al.,* 1981). Other pathogens such as parvovirus have previously been reviewed (Tzipori, 1981) and no additional incriminating field evidence has since come forward.

Astroviruses, another group of small viruses occasionally seen in the feces of pigs, calves, and other species, have been shown to be nonpathogenic, causing only transient diarrhea in gnotobiotic pigs (Saif *et al.,* 1980) or in calves (Woode *et al.,* 1984), but they may exacerbate infections caused by another diarrheagenic virus in gnotobiotic calves (Woode *et al.,* 1984). Bovine viral diarrhea virus, which is not normally considered in the differential diagnosis of calf diarrhea, may need to be reappraised. Bulgin *et al.* (1982) identified the infection in 8% of cases of diarrhea, particularly among dairy calves aged less than 30 days.

VII. Piglet Enteritis

A. Epidemiology

Piglet enteritis is a syndrome which the author has divided for the sake of convenience into three distinct entities: postnatal, neonatal, and postweaning diarrhea (Tzipori *et al.,* 1980b). The first and third are caused almost exclusively by ETEC. Postnatal diarrhea occurs within the first 2 days of life and is invariably associated with ST_a-producing ETEC. *Cl. perfringens* type C, which also occurs immediately after birth, is readily distinguished because it causes mostly hemorrhagic diarrhea and is restricted to certain geographical locations. The third entity, PWD, occurs 4 to 7 days after weaning, is caused largely by ETEC and is discussed elsewhere (Section III,C). Neonatal diarrhea occurs from the fourth day after birth and up to weaning and it may be attributed to one or more of the following enteropathogens according to location: TGE, rotavirus, ETEC, coccidia, adenovirus, and porcine epidemic diarrhea (PED) virus. Some of the pathogens mentioned above occur only in some areas.

Enteric colibacillosis in piglets is characterized by profuse watery diarrhea, rapid dehydration, and no vomiting. Morbidity and mortality can be up to 100% in litters born to gilts (Morin et al., 1983). Colibacillosis and transmissible gastroenteritis, two diseases of young piglets which have been known for many years, have been extensively studied and reported by many investigators.

The data on rotavirus infection under field conditions are conflicting and the economic significance of the disease is, therefore, not entirely clear. The following are observations made by the author over a number of years with regard to field and experimental infections.

Porcine rotavirus causes occasional diarrhea in 2- to 3-week-old piglets. The disease tends to be sporadic, although some outbreaks may be seen from time to time which can occur at any time of the year. The morbidity is mostly low (Table XII) and so is the mortality rate. The low incidence and late onset of rotavirus diarrhea in piglets is due neither to lack of sufficient virus in the environment to cause disease, nor is it due to its low pathogenicity for piglets. The reason is that the suckled piglet is, mostly, well protected by passive immunity. Rotavirus is widespread worldwide, and unlike other potential pathogens, e.g., TGE and coccidia, is certain to be present in almost every herd. Virus particles are extremely resistant and are shed into the environment in large quantity. This must provide continuous, strong antigenic stimulation to the population, much more effectively, it seems, than other enteropathogens. Sublinical infection of suckled piglets also probably takes place during this time, allowing the neonate to develop its own active immunity. Development of active immunity while consuming specific antibodies against the virus has been demonstrated experimentally (Bridger et al., 1982).

Porcine rotavirus infection in piglets, devoid of maternal protection, is devastating, causing severe diarrhea, dehydration, vomiting, and death (Tzipori and Williams, 1978). In this regard rotavirus to piglets is no less a pathogen than TGE or ETEC. Rotavirus infection exerts its most severe effect in piglets that are artificially weaned at a young age (Coalson and Lecce, 1973; Lecce et al., 1976). Indeed, in Australia

TABLE XII

THE RELATIVE FREQUENCY OF ENTERIC PATHOGENS IN DIARRHEIC PIGLETS REPORTED FOR SEVERAL COUNTRIES

Country	Number examined		Percentage of piglets infected with[a]				Mixed infection	Unknown	Monitored during	Reference
	Outbreaks	Piglets	TGE	RV	ETEC	Cocc.				
Canada	182	749	52	9	22	15	12	9	1977–1981	Morin et al. (1983)
United States (midwest)	NP[b]	1975	16	14	31	18	14	16	1981?	Bergeland and Henry (1982)
Australia (Victoria)	23	388	0	4	82	1	3	7	1978–1983	Tzipori (unpublished data)
Austria	NP	2009	NP	NP	74	NP	NP	26	1969–1978	Awad-Masalmeh (1982)

[a]TGE, transmissible gastroenteritis; RV, rotavirus; ETEC, enterotoxigenic *E. coli*; Cocc., coccidiosis.
[b]NP, not provided.

rotavirus infection was first discovered in piglets during an attempt to wean piglets aged 36 to 48 hr onto artificial diets (Rodger et al., 1975). The role of maternal protection provided by milk to the suckled piglet, in contrast to their littermates, which were being artificially reared (after consumption of colostrum), was demonstrated when both groups were challenged with rotavirus; the suckled piglets had mild or no diarrhea, while their artificially reared littermates suffered severe illness and most of them died (Tzipori and Williams, 1978). Rotavirus diarrhea is unquestionably a more serious and economically more important disease of calves than of pigs. Curiously, piglets devoid of colostrum are more susceptible to rotavirus infection than colostrum-deprived calves (Tzipori et al., 1981). The significance of the disease in both species, calves and piglets, is directly related to the degree of maternal protection provided by the dam. It is less important in pigs because of good lactogenic protection; conversely, it is important in calves because of poor lactogenic protection.

It has been stated in a report by the Meat and Livestock Commission of 1983 that in the United Kingdom the average annual loss of live piglets before weaning is approximately 12% and that a large number of these deaths are attributed to infection with ETEC, up to half of which are caused by K88 serotypes (Walters and Sellwood, 1984).

Table XII provides the relative frequency of isolation of four major enteropathogens involved in the etiology of outbreaks of piglet enteritis in various locations. They were extracted from investigations published; it is surprising how few there are. Table XII points out the diverse frequencies encountered in different places and, presumably, at different times. By far the most comprehensive study is that by Morin et al. (1983). It is clear from their report that ETEC and TGE are the two most important pathogens. The emergence of coccidiosis in recent years places it as the third most important enteropathogen. However, coccidiosis, as with TGE, appears to occur only in some locations. In Australia, in the absence of TGE and with coccidia having only been sighted (R. S. Cutter and R. T. Jones, unpublished data; S. Tzipori, unpublished data), ETEC becomes the single most important pathogen. In some outbreaks of postnatal diarrhea in Australia up to 26% of piglets may be lost less than 48 hr after birth (Tzipori et al., 1980b). PWD has been estimated to cause an average of 4% mortality in herds that experience the disease.

Rotavirus, according to the table, is the fourth commonest pathogen encountered. Mixed infection does not seem to be as common as other reports suggest (Sanford and Josephson, 1981). The portion of cases without positive diagnosis is relatively low, and presumably is much lower when taken on an outbreak basis. The indicence of *Cl. perfringens* is low, apparently because where the disease is enzootic it is readily controlled by vaccination. These studies highlight the complexity of the etiology of diarrhea in piglets and may indicate in part the reason why this disease can be difficult to control.

B. INFECTIONS SPECIFIC TO PIGLETS

1. Coccidiosis

The first report dealing with coccidiosis as a possible cause of diarrhea in suckled piglets was that by Sangster et al. (1976). The disease was later reported in the United States (Bergeland, 1977; Stuart and Lindsay, 1979), Canada (Morin et al., 1980; Sanford and Josephson, 1981), and Scotland (Roberts et al., 1980). There are nine known species of coccidia in pigs (Vetterling, 1965) and, until recently, they were thought to be innocuous. However, the pathogenicity to piglets of *Isopora suis* was suspected earlier by Biester and Murray (1934). The toxonomy and life cycle of *Isopora suis* have been reviewed (Harleman and Meyer, 1983).

The disease is characterized by a yellow to gray, foul-smelling diarrhea, which could lead to dehydration, and occasional vomiting. Necropsy reveals multifocal villus atrophy, often with a marked necrotizing enteritis of the small intestine, especially in the middle and distal jejunum and ileum. Morbidity is variable but can be high; mortality, however, is low. Simultaneous infection with other enteric pathogens results in more severe lesions and clinical disease.

Experiments with SPF piglets showed that the disease is dose and age related; young piglets given high doses developed more severe clinical illness, as compared with mild lesions in piglets aged between 2 and 6 weeks given a similar dose. Lower doses tended to increase the incubation period from 4 days and result in milder illness. The severity of the illness is related to the extent of villus atrophy which results in maldigestion and malabsorption (Robinson et al., 1983). Multifocal, rather than diffuse lesions seen in the infected mucosa, may be the reason for low mortality rates caused by coccidiosis.

Examination of feces for the presence of oocysts by the flotation technique is not very reliable. Oocysts measure between 18–20 and 20–23 μm and contain two ellipsoidal sporocysts, each containing four sporozoites. Detection of shedding by piglets infected with coccidia in the feces can be as low as 7% (Sanford, 1983) or up to 50% (Robinson and Morin, 1982). Diagnosis, therefore, is more reliably based on demonstration of endogenous coccidia, i.e., by histopathological examination of the small intestine of live piglets necropsied soon after the beginning of diarrhea. Multifocal lesions of villus atrophy in the mid and lower jejunum and ileum, with epithelial cells containing largely asexual stages of the life cycle of the parasite, can readily be recognized. Extensive lesions of necrotic enteritis may also be present in severe cases (Bergeland, 1977; Robinson and Morin, 1982).

The disease occurs all year round with higher incidence during the summer and fall months (Sanford and Josephson, 1981; Robinson and Morin, 1982). The incidence of intestinal coccidiosis has increased steadily in recent years in parts of North America (Robinson and Morin, 1982; Sanford and Josephson, 1981; Stevenson and Andrews, 1982), and is thought to relate to rapid expansion of operations committed to total confinement and continuous farrowing.

Coccidiosis can be suspected in herds with diarrhea occurring between 5 and 15 days of age, which tends to eliminate ETEC but not TGE. However, the age span of piglets affected by TGE is wider. In Ontario, Canada, Sanford and Josephson (1981), who had identified coccidiosis in 82 scouring piglets from 34 herds, observed that ETEC and TGE are the agents most commonly identified, whereas rotavirus, *Cl. perfringens,* and other miscellaneous agents are seen only occasionally. Coccidia, it seems, are the next most important enteropathogens that cause diarrhea in suckling piglets; 79% had ETEC and/or TGE in addition to coccidia, while 29% had coccidia only.

More recently, coccidiosis was detected in feces from 298 of 1453 (20.5%) diarrheic piglets submitted to a veterinary diagnostic laboratory in Ontario, Canada, which indicates a substantial increase in incidence from earlier reports (Sanford, 1983).

Solid immunity develops after infection. The infection causes diarrhea in suckled piglets and is rarely seen in weaned piglets (Harleman and Meyer, 1983). However, it is most commonly seen in piglets aged between 5 and 15 days of age, which suggests that secretory antibodies present in the milk at this time are not adequate for protection. In herds where the infection is enzootic oocysts have also been detected in the feces of pregnant gilts or sows.

Treatment of sows with amprolium hydrochloride or decoquinate shortly before and after farrowing produced variable results according to some (Robinson and Morin, 1982). Others have reported success in reducing oocyst output with the above drugs plus a host of others including sulfaquinidine, nitrofurazone, and monensin (Harleman and Meyer, 1983; Roberts and Walker, 1981; Sanford and Josephson, 1981).

2. Porcine Epidemic Diarrhea (PED) Virus

PED virus was first isolated in the late 1970s in Europe (Pensaert and Debouck, 1978; Wood, 1979). This virus, a coronavirus which is antigenically distinct from TGE virus, was associated with epidemics of diarrhea in piglets in England and Belgium. Experimental infection of colostrum-deprived piglets with the Belgium isolate caused severe watery diarrhea and death. Pathogenesis studies have shown that the virus replicates in epithelial cells lining the small intestine and the colon (Debouck *et al.*, 1981), showing many similarities to other existing coronavirus infections in animals. Further, outbreaks with PED virus were also reported in Germany (R. G. Hess, personal communication).

Epidemiological studies in herds affected by this virus indicate that it does not become enzootic on a farm after an outbreak and may, therefore, explain why PED outbreaks are rather explosive in nature (Pensaert *et al.*, 1982). Serological studies indicate that the distribution of antibodies to PED virus is widespread in Europe with the exception of Scandinavia and Northern Ireland. No antibodies were detected in porcine sera from the United States or Australia (Debouck *et al.*, 1982).

3. Adenovirus Enteritis

Porcine adenovirus was first isolated in 1964 from a pig with diarrhea (Haig *et al.*, 1964). Although adenovirus intranuclear inclusion bodies have been seen in enterocytes of the small intestine of piglets (Fujiwara *et al.*, 1968), their role remains obscure. Experimental transmission with one porcine adenovirus in hysterectomy-derived piglets resulted in diarrhea (Coussement *et al.*, 1981; Ducatelle *et al.*, 1981, 1982). One comprehensive study from Ontario, Canada has shown that of 979 live pigs autopsied and examined for various causes, 43 (4.4%) derived from 38 different farms had evidence of adenovirus intranuclear inclusions in the intestinal epithelium. Affected piglets ranged in age from 5 days to 24 weeks; 23 had diarrhea, only 4 of which had no other known enteropathogens (Sanford and Hoover, 1983). These authors concluded from their study that the limited histological changes, and in most cases the lack of enteric disease, suggested that enteric adenovirus infection in conventional pigs is incidental and largely asymptomatic. The study by Morin *et al.* (1983) has attributed only 0.3% of 749 cases of piglet enteritis examined to adenovirus infection; these were among 1- to 2-week-old animals.

VIII. Diarrhea in Foals

Diarrhea is said to be the most common clinical disease of young foals and during the first 6 weeks of life some 50% of all foals may be expected to have one or more diarrheic episodes. With the exception of diarrhea that occurs within the first 5 days of life, the disease tends to be transient and the overall mortality is low. In terms of overall numbers, diarrhea in foals may seem to be less significant than that in other domestic species. However, on some horse studs, which is where outbreaks normally occur, a loss of 1 foal may be equal in economic terms to 50 or more calves.

Despite the relatively high incidence of diarrhea in foals, the etiology of the majority of outbreaks remains unresolved. Textbooks and general articles concerned with clinical aspects of diarrhea have a tendency to list enteropathogens that are traditionally associated with enteric infection in calves, lambs, and piglets. Thus, the role of ETEC, although suspected for many years as a major cause, is not clear. Of the enteric viruses, only rotavirus has so far been shown to be associated with some cases of diarrhea in foals.

A. Rotavirus Diarrhea

From a limited number of field studies (Strickland et al., 1982; Tzipori and Walker, 1978) and experimental inoculation of foals with foal rotavirus (Conner and Darlington, 1980; Kanitz, 1977; Tzipori et al., 1982c), the clinical picture which emerges is characterized by depression and anorexia, followed by profuse watery diarrhea and elevated rectal temperature. Dehydration and loss of body condition may follow in a disease course lasting from 1 to 12 days. Outbreaks tend to occur in well-managed studs where mares and their newborn foals are brought together for breeding (Strickland et al., 1982; Tzipori and Walker, 1978). The proportion of affected foals under such conditions is normally high. Foals with confirmed rotavirus diarrhea are affected between the ages of 5 days to 7 weeks; the older they are, the milder the illness. The age span is presumably the main reason for low mortalities attributed to this infection. Experimentally infected foals develop similar signs after an incubation period of 2 to 4 days, depending on the age of the foal. Kanitz (1977) described a fairly severe clinical disease in some of the foals, particularly those fed gut contents. On the other hand, in our experience diarrhea failed to develop in colostrum-deprived or colostrum-fed newborn foals with one of our strains of rotavirus without coinfection with ETEC derived from calves (Tzipori

TABLE XIII

FREQUENCY OF ROTAVIRUS ISOLATIONS FROM FOALS WITH DIARRHEA

Country	Number of samples	Samples containing rotavirus Percentage	Reference
United States (New York)	105	61.9	Gillespie et al. (1984)
Australia (Victoria)	52 (30)[a]	23 (40)	Tzipori (unpublished data)
United States (Kentucky)	86	30	Conner and Darlington (1980)
Ireland (South)	35	34	Strickland et al. (1982)
Japan (Hokkaido)	40 (14)[b]	12 (35)	Imagawa et al. (1984)

[a] When foals older than 4 days are considered.
[b] When only foals with acute diarrhea are considered.

et al., 1982c). The foals did become depressed and anorexic and two of the three had marked constipation. Constipation following rotavirus infection was also observed by Kanitz (1977). There are at least two known distinct serotypes of equine rotavirus (Section II,E,3.) whose pathogenicity in foals was not reported. We have since, however, isolated another strain of foal rotavirus which causes moderate diarrhea in foals of a few days old (S. Tzipori, unpublished data). It is, therefore, likely that rotavirus of different serotypes may induce varying degrees of clinical illness in foals.

Data on the epidemiology of diarrhea in foals are scarce, and the portion attributed to rotavirus infection can, therefore, only be presumed (Table XIII). The majority of these investigators did not account for other enteropathogens; even so, one point is clear from this table, that at most rotavirus may be responsible for one-third of the cases of diarrhea occurring in foals. The majority of serious field cases we encountered in recent years have been in foals younger than 5 days, an age where mortality and/or intensive treatment have a serious economic consequences for the industry. It is, therefore, obvious that there must be other as yet unidentified infections in this species.

In our laboratory, research efforts to determine the cause of diarrhea in foals were conducted along two lines: (1) examination under experimental conditions of suspected, or potential, pathogens isolated from field cases of diarrhea by inoculation of foals and/or other species of animals, and (2) determination of the pathogenicity in foals of agents known to cause diarrhea in other mammalian species. These included

ETEC of calf and pig origin, *C. jejuni* and *Cryptosporidium* derived from calves, and the role of mixed infection.

In addition to rotavirus which was reported earlier, we examined the role of a number of bacteria which we had encountered in field cases of diarrhea. These include *Cl. perfringens* type C, *Streptococcus durans*, and several *E. coli* strains.

B. *Streptococcus durans*

In an outbreak of diarrhea in foals less than 4 days old, fecal examination and culture yielded no recognizable enteropathogens. A fecal suspension from these foals induced diarrhea in 7-day-old foals 2 days after inoculation. Bacterial counts at necropsy revealed high counts (10^7 to 10^8) for *E. coli* and an α-hemolytic *Streptococcus* throughout the small intestine. Histological examination of the small intestine revealed an extensive colonization of the entire mucosal surface by Gram-positive cocci which were subsequently identified by PAP-staining to be *S. durans*, a most unlikely enteropathogen. Gram-positive cocci are rarely implicated as a cause of enteritis and diarrhea in mammals, least of all enterococci, which are commonly found in feces of animals and humans. Enterococci are Group D streptococci, a group which includes *S. fecalis*, *S. faecium*, and *S. durans*. *S. faecium*, to which *S. durans* is very closely related, has been extensively studied and well characterized. *S. faecium* has been suggested as a means to control colibacillosis in piglets (Section III,B,2,b) (Underdahl *et al.*, 1982). Other strains of *S. faecium* have been shown to adhere to the duodenal epithelium of chickens, causing growth retardation (Fuller *et al.*, 1981; Houghton *et al.*, 1981).

This initial observation led to a further isolation of *S. durans* from foals with diarrhea and it was used for experimental inoculation of foals, piglets, and calves (Tzipori *et al.*, 1984c). Oral inoculation of five suckled foals aged 1–4 days with *S. durans* and a sixth which became infected by contact, caused profuse diarrhea mostly within 24 hr. The most consistent and predominant histological feature of all these foals was the extensive colonization of the mucosal surface of the small intestine by cocci identified as *S. durans* by PAP staining. Three of these foals also had high counts of *E. coli*, which proved subsequently to be nonpathogenic to foals. Colonization of the small intestine by *S. durans* appears to promote proliferation of other bacteria, particularly *E. coli* in the lumen. Over recent years we have examined the small and large intestines of a considerable number of foals inoculated with various serotypes of *E. coli* including those isolated from foals with diarrhea; seldom had we encountered *E. coli* counts as high as those seen in foals infected with *S. durans*. The author believes that the small intestine of newborn foals is normally not very suitable for *E. coli* proliferation because of alkaline pH (B. Smyth, personal communication). Proliferation of *S. durans*, a lactic acid-producing bacterium, may induce more favorable conditions, and reduced pH may be one of them.

S. durans has also induced diarrhea in gnotobiotic piglets similar to that observed in foals with extensive colonization of the epithelial surface of the small intestine. Calves, however, remained healthy after oral inoculation. The mechanism by which *S. durans* causes diarrhea in foals is not clear. The bacteria failed to cause dilatation of pig gut loop, and did not attach in the *in vitro* adherence test to equine brush borders. Changes to mucosal architecture were not severe, although the activity of brush border digestive enzymes was markedly depressed, suggesting a direct mechanical interference with brush border digestion and absorption. The prevalence of this infection in the equine population is unknown, nor is the incidence of diarrhea attributed to infection with *S. durans*. The organism is usually described together with other Group D streptococci and only very recently were *S. durans* and *S. faecium* shown unequivocally to be two separate species (Farrow *et al.*, 1983). They are often isolated together with *S. faecium* and *S. fecalis* from cases of pneumonia, arthritis, endocarditis, and various other infections in domestic animals and from cystitis and endocarditis in humans. The clinical signs, the occurrence of the disease shortly after birth, and the high *E. coli* counts which *S. durans* seems to promote may have for years caused this disease to be confused with colibacillosis.

C. *Cl. perfringens* Type C

Necrotic entertis attributed to *Cl. perfringens* type C has been described in two foals from Colorado (Dickie *et al.*, 1978) and one from Canada (Niilo and Chalmers, 1982). A similar condition, not previously recognized in Australia, was noted over two consecutive foaling seasons of 1981 and 1982 (Sims *et al.*, 1984) and involved several fatal cases. The affected foals developed severe diarrhea in the first 48 hr of life and displayed signs of severe abdominal pain and profuse yellow–brown watery diarrhea which became bloody. In one outbreak, 6 of 29 newborn thoroughbred foals were affected and in a second stud,

5 of 17 foals. Three of these foals died within hours of the beginning of clinical illness, despite intensive treatment which included, in addition to fluid, electrolyte, and antibiotic therapy, administration of one liter of pooled horse serum. The remaining affected foals recovered after similar treatment. Affected foals, which subsequently recovered, passed yellow–brown, fetid diarrheic feces, and rapidly became dehydrated. It seems that once diarrheic feces became bloody, foals had little chance of recovery. Necropsies carried out on dead foals revealed large volumes of bloody fluid of up to 4 liters in the small and mostly in the large, intestine. Significant changes were restricted to the gastrointestinal tract which included vascular congestion of the serosal surface of the distal two-thirds of the small intestine. The mucosal surface of the small intestine from the anterior jejunum to the ileocecal junction was deeply congested. The stomach, which was partly filled, and the large intestine which contained the bulk of the fluid, appeared normal.

Histological examination revealed severe necrotizing enteritis extending from the jejunum to the terminal ileum. The villi in affected areas were necrotic and surrounded by massive numbers of Gram-positive rods. The villi were devoid of internal structure, and a large number of neutrophils and macrophages were seen within the villi and outside in the lumen. Inflammatory changes were seen in some areas of the muscularis layer. The mucosa of the stomach and large intestine appeared to be unaffected (Sims *et al.*, 1984).

Studies in piglets show that the organisms invade the epithelial lining of the jejunum and multiply along the basement membrane (Arbuckle, 1972). This occurs along the tips of the villi, and is followed by desquamation and necrosis of the lamina propria. Necrotic villi surrounded by masses of bacteria are then released into the lumen; bacteria may also invade deeper tissue involving the crypts, submucosa, and the muscularis layer (Arbuckle, 1972).

NE was successfuly induced in newborn foals after oral inoculation with either gut contents (two foals) or *Cl. perfringens* type C cultivated from foals with NE (two foals). The disease was also reproduced using a laboratory strain CN3714 (three foals). Clinical signs of illness began within 12 hr, mostly 4–6 hr after inoculation. The foals displayed signs of severe abdominal pain, manifested by straining, flank watching, and arching of the back. They became further depressed and anorectic, and those most severely affected began to pass dark brown feces which subsequently became bloody. Foals that were less severely affected were depressed, anorectic, and passed yellow–brown feces (L. D. Sims and S. Tzipori, unpublished data).

D. OTHER ENTEROPATHOGENS

1. Bacteria Isolated from Foals with Diarrhea

A number of strains of *E. coli* (O2:HNM, O16:H48, O22:H7, O77:H28, O23:H16, and O88:H21), which were isolated from foals with diarrhea, lacked virulence attributes such as a colonizing factor, as tested in the *in vitro* adhesion test of porcine and equine brush borders, and liberated no recognizable enterotoxins. A number of them (O23:H16, O88:H21, and O133:H29) were fed to colostrum-deprived (CD) newborn foals, and others were fed to gnotobiotic piglets. None caused illness or colonization of the small intestine in these animals. *Salmonella* has also been observed in one outbreak of diarrhea in foals involving eight animals less than 1 week of age. *Salmonella* was detected in the feces of three, and from the tissue and intestine of one dead foal aged 6 days.

2. Enteropathogens from Other Species Studied in Foals

Experimental inoculations of 3–4 foals aged from 1–5 days with *Cryptosporidium* or *C. jejuni*, both derived from calves with diarrhea, failed to cause illness. *C. jejuni* was shed in the feces from 2–5 days after inoculation. Of four foals inoculated with *Cryptosporidium*, two of which were CD, only one shed the organism in the feces 7 days after inoculation. Necropsy on this foal revealed small numbers of organisms attached to the jejunum.

Inoculation of five CD, or suckled, foals with calf ETEC (two with O20:KX106, K99:HNM, and three with strain B44) resulted in mild watery diarrhea in one CD foal in less than 24 hr, and lasted 8 hr. None of these foals, which were necropsied between 2 and 4 days after oral inoculation, showed any evidence of extensive proliferation in the lumen or colonization of intestinal mucosa. Exhaustive *in vitro* adhesion tests on equine *E. coli* recovered from diarrheic foals, or ETEC from other animals, showed that *E. coli* with K88ab or K88ac were the only types to attach convincingly to small intestinal brush border membranes of young and adult horses (Tzipori *et al.*, 1984a). Inoculation of foals with ETEC-bearing K88 was generally without effect. Two foals were inoculated with a LT-ST_b producer (O149 serogroup) and a ST_a producer (O20 serogroup). Only a foal inoculated with a high oral dose of O149 developed watery diarrhea in less than 24 hr.

There was evidence of some proliferation in the upper ileum with focal bacterial attachment to surface epithelium, identified as an organism with K88 by PAP-staining (Tzipori *et al.*, 1984a).

There has been a suggestion, which will need further confirmation, that *Aeromonas* spp. may also be involved in diarrhea of young foals. In particular, *Aeromonas hydrophila* has been observed in two cases of acute diarrhea in 3-day-old foals (D. A. Pass, personal communication). *Aeromonas* spp. isolated from human patients with gastroenteritis have been shown to produce ST-like enterotoxin and to cause watery diarrhea in gnotobiotic piglets (S. Tzipori, unpublished data).

IX. Concluding Remarks

Rotavirus research at present is progressing along two major themes: development of rotavirus vaccines which, in human medicine, has only begun; and definition of the extent of antigenic diversity, which also includes the assessment of the significance of atypical rotaviruses. A unifying system for rotavirus serotyping which will extend across species barriers should eventually emerge. ETEC, although known to cause diarrhea in animals long before any of the newer pathogens had emerged, were a difficult group to sort out. Sensitive and rapid methods for diagnosis are now available, the relationship between various virulence characteristics are now better understood and vaccines, some of which are effective, have been developed. Research on ETEC owes many of its advances to the application of new technology. Vaccines incorporating several antigenic determinants should prove more efficient. PWD may take longer to control. Research on *Cryptosporidium* is in its infancy. While the infection in various hosts has been examined and the disease in susceptible species has been characterized, the protozoology requires further studies and, with *in vitro* cultivation, this should be possible. Means to treat or control this disease are not yet available; there is no question that in some cases of human infections treatment will be of great value.

Some enteropathogens appear to be universal; they are found throughout the world and infect most vertebrates. These include rotavirus, *E. coli, Cryptosporidium,* and *Campylobacter* spp. Others are more prominent in certain geographical locations and have a restricted host range; bovine coronavirus of calves, and TGE and coccidiosis of pigs are examples.

In calves, rotaviruses, followed by *Cryptosporidium,* are the most common causes of diarrhea. Where bovine coronavirus occurs it tends to cause a more severe disease than the previous two, even if fewer calves are involved. ETEC can vary from being insignificant to being a major cause of economic loss. In piglets ETEC are by far the most important cause of diarrhea. However, where TGE occurs it is the leading cause of devastating infection in young piglets. Coccidiosis has emerged in recent times and ranks as the third most important cause. Rotavirus and other infections are *mostly* less significant.

Infection with more than one enteropathogen, whether they are acting synergistically or their combined effect is additive, irrespective of species, tends to lead to a more severe clinical outcome. The literature regarding mixed infections with ETEC and rotavirus in domestic animals has been reviewed elsewhere (Tzipori *et al.*, 1983a).

Vaccines of varying efficiency are either being developed or already being used against diarrhea in calves caused by rotavirus and ETEC. No efficient vaccine is available as yet against bovine coronavirus, nor is there a treatment against cryptosporidiosis. Undoubtedly, future research is required to improve the quality of vaccines that are already in existence for rotavirus and ETEC, and develop one for bovine coronavirus, as well as search for control of *Cryptosporidium*. Similarly, better vaccines are expected to emerge in the near future against ETEC diarrhea in piglets. Vaccines against TGE, although available, can be improved. Long-term control of coccidiosis, on the other hand, may require approaches other than treatment with chemicals.

The etiology of diarrhea in foals is far from being resolved. It is clear that the range of enteric pathogens in horses is somewhat different from those observed in other domestic animals. In this regard, studies on enteritis in foals are lagging behind, as knowledge acquired from studies of other animals can be only partially applied. Control will only be possible with further research on etiology.

Understanding the nature of virulence by which organisms mediate their effect and the host response, both of which can often be clearly demonstrated by *in vitro* techniques, or in gnotobiotic animals, explains only in part the disease process. The underlying difficulties, a common denominator to enteric infections in all species, are related to defining the intervening factors which may promote or inhibit any one, or all, of the sequence of events leading to infection of the gastrointestinal tract and diarrhea. This process, which on balance determines whether an infection takes place, remains subclinical, or induces illness, remains largely a gray area and will need to be addressed in the future.

References

Acres, S. D., and Babiuk, L. A. (1978). *J. Am. Vet. Med. Assoc.* **173**, 555–559.
Acres, S. D., Saunders, J. R., and Radostits, O. M. (1977). *Can. Vet. J.* **18**, 113–121.
Acres, S. D., Isaacson, R. E., Babiuk, L. A., and Kapitany, R. A. (1979). *Infect. Immun.* **25**, 121–126.

Acres, S. D., Forman, A. J., and Kapitany, R. A. (1982). *Am. J. Vet. Res.* **43,** 569–575.
Al-Mashat, R. R., and Taylor, D. J. (1980a). *Vet. Rec.* **107,** 31–34.
Al-Mashat, R. R., and Taylor, D. J. (1980b). *Vet. Rec.* **107,** 459–464.
Al-Mashat, R. R., and Taylor, D. J. (1983). *Vet. Rec.* **112,** 54–58.
Alouf, J. E., and Jolivet-Reynaud, C. (1981). *Infect. Immun.* **31,** 536–546.
Altmann, K., and Mukkur, T. K. S. (1983). *Res. Vet. Sci.* **35,** 234–239.
Anderson, B. C., and Hall, R. F. (1982). *J. Am. Vet. Med. Assoc.* **181,** 484–485.
Anderson, B. C., Donndelinger, T., Wilkins, R. M., and Smith, J. (1982). *J. Am. Vet. Med. Assoc.* **180,** 408–409.
Angus, K. W. (1983). *J. R. Soc. Med.* **76,** 62–70.
Angus, K. W., Hutchinson, G., Campbell, I., and Snodgrass, D. R. (1984). *Vet. Rec.* **114,** 166–168.
Aning, K. G., Thomlinson, J. R., Wray, C., Sojka, W. J., and Coulter, J. (1983). *Vet. Rec.* **112,** 251.
Anonymous. (1982). *New Sci.* **94,** 22.
Anonymous. (1984). *Lancet* **1,** 492–493.
Arbuckle, J. B. R. (1972). *J. Pathol.* **106,** 65–72.
Arias, C. F., Lopez, S., and Espejo, R. T. (1982). *J. Virol.* **41,** 42–50.
Armstrong, W. D., and Cline, T. R. (1976). *J. Anim. Sci.* **42,** 592–598.
Armstrong, W. D., and Cline, T. R. (1977). *J. Anim. Sci.* **45,** 1042–1050.
Askaa, J., and Bloch, B. (1984). *Arch. Virol.* **80,** 291–303.
Atroshi, F., Alaviuhkola, T., Schildt, R.. and Sandholm, M. (1983). *Comp. Immun. Microbiol. Infect. Dis.* **6,** 235–245.
Awad-Masalmeh, M. (1982). *Wien. Tieraerztl. Monatsschr.* **69,** 358–364.
Babiuk, L. A., Mohammed, K., Spence, L., Fauvel, M., and Petro, R. (1977). *J. Clin. Microbiol.* **6,** 610–617.
Bachmann, P. A., Hess, R. G., Dirksen, G., and Schmid, G. (1984). *Proc. Int. Symp. Neonatal Diarrhea 4th.*
Back, E., Svennerholm, A. M., Holmgren, J., and Mollby, R. (1979). *J. Clin. Microbiol.* **10,** 791–795.
Ball, R. O., and Aherne, F. X. (1982). *Can. J. Anim. Sci.* **62,** 907–913.
Barnes, D. M., and Moon, H. W. (1964). *J. Am. Vet. Med. Assoc.* **144,** 1391–1394.
Barnett, B. B., Spendlove, R. S., and Clark, M. L. (1979). *J. Clin. Micriobiol.* **10,** 111–113.
Bastardo, J. W., McKimm-Breschkin, J. L., Sonza, S., Mercer, L. D., and Holmes, I. H. (1981). *Infect. Immun.* **34,** 641–647.
Bayley, H. S., and Carlson, J. A. (1970). *J. Anim. Sci.* **30,** 394–401.
Baxby, D., Hart, C. A., and Taylor, C. (1983). *Br. Med. J.* **287,** 1760–1761.
Baxby, D., Getty, B., Blundell, N., and Ratcliffe, S. (1984). *J. Clin. Microbiol.* **19,** 566–567.
Beards, G. M., Hall, C., Green, J., Flewett, T. H., Lamouliatte, F., and Du Pasquier, P. (1984). *Lancet* **1,** 1050–1052.
Benfield, D. A., and Francis, D. H. (1981). *Proc. Int. Symp. Neonatal Diarrhea 3rd,* 361–372.
Bergeland, M. E. (1977). *Proc. Annu. Meet. Am. Assoc. Vet. Lab. Diagnost. 20th,* 151–158.
Bergeland, M. E. (1981). *In* "Diseases of Swine" (H. W. Leman, R. D. Glock, W. L. Mengeling, R. H. C. Penny, E. Scholl, and B. Straw, eds.), 5th ed., pp. 418–431. Iowa State Univ. Press, Ames.
Bergeland, M. E., and Henry, S. C. (1982). *In* "The Veterinary Clinics of North America: Swine Diseases" (L. G. Biehl, ed.), pp 389–399. Saunders, Philadelphia.

Bertschinger, H. U., Moon, H. W., and Whipp, S. C. (1972). *Infect. Immun.* **5**, 595–605.
Biester, H. E., and Murray, C. (1934). *J. Am. Vet. Med. Assoc.* **85**, 207–219.
Bijlsma, I. G. W., de Nijs, A., van der Meer, C., and Frik, J. F. (1982). *Infect. Immun.* **37**, 891–894.
Bird, R. G., and Smith, M. D. (1980). *J. Pathol.* **132**, 217–233.
Bishop, R. F., Davidson, G. P., Holmes, I. H., and Ruck, B. J. (1973). *Lancet* **2**, 1281–1283.
Blagburn, B. L., and Current, W. L. (1983). *J. Infect. Dis.* **148**, 772–773.
Blakey, J. L., Lubitz, L., Campbell, N. T., Gillman, G. L., Bishop, R. F., and Barnes, G. L. (1984). (In press).
Blaser, M. J., and Reller, L. B. (1981). *New Engl. J. Med.* **305**, 1444–1452.
Bohl, E. H., Kohler, E. M., Saif, L. J., Cross, R. F., Agnes, A. G., and Theil, K. W. (1978). *J. Am. Vet. Med. Assoc.* **172**, 458–463.
Bohl, E. H., Saif, L. J., Theil, K. W., Agnes, A. G., and Cross, R. F. (1982). *J. Clin. Microbiol.* **15**, 312–319.
Bohl, E. H., Theil, K. W., and Saif, L. J. (1984). *J. Clin. Microbiol.* **19**, 105–111.
Borriello, S. P., Larson, H. E., Welch, A. R., Barclay, F., Stringer, M. F., and Bartholomew, B. A. (1984). *Lancet* **1**, 305–307.
Bridger, J. C. (1980). *Vet. Rec.* **107**, 532–533.
Bridger, J. C., and Brown, J. F. (1981). *Infect. Immun.* **31**, 906–910.
Bridger, J. C., and Woode, G. N. (1976). *J. Gen. Virol.* **31**, 245–250.
Bridger, J. C., Clarke, I. N., and McCrae, M. A. (1982). *Infect. Immun.* **35**, 1058–1062.
Brill, B. M., Wasilauskas, B. L., and Richardson, S. H. (1979). *J. Clin. Microbiol.* **9**, 49–55.
Brock, J. H., Arzabe, F. R., Ortega, F., and Pineiro, A. (1977). *Immunology* **32**, 215–219.
Bruce, D., Zochowski, W., and Ferguson, I. R. (1977). *Br. Med. J.* **2**, 1219.
Buddle, M. B. (1954). *J. Comp. Pathol. Ther.* **64**, 217–224.
Bulgin, M. S., Anderson, B. C., Ward, A. C. S., and Evermann, J. F. (1982). *J. Am. Vet. Med. Assoc.* **180**, 1222–1226.
Bulmer, W. S., Tsai, K. S., and Little, P. B. (1975). *J. Am. Vet. Med. Assoc.* **166**, 233–238.
Burgess, M. N., Bywater, R. J., Cowley, C. M., Mullan, N. A., and Newsome, P. M. (1978). *Infect. Immun.* **21**, 526–531.
Burki, F., Schusser, G., and Szekely, H. (1983). *Zentralbl. Veterinaer med.* **30**, 237–250.
Campbell, I., Tzipori, S., Hutchison, G., and Angus, K. W. (1982). *Vet. Rec.* **111**, 414–415.
Campbell, P. N., and Current, W. L. (1983). *J. Clin. Microbiol.* **18**, 165–169.
Carter, G. R. (1978). *In* "Diagnostic Procedures in Veterinary Microbiology," 3rd ed. Thomas, Springfield, Illinois.
Casemore, D. P., and Jackson, B. (1983). *Lancet* **2**, 679.
Casemore, D. P., Armstrong, M., and Jackson, B. (1984). *Lancet* **1**, 734–735.
Chandler, D. S., Chandler, H. M., Luke, R. J. K., Tzipori, S. R., and Craven, J. A. (1985). *Vet. Microbiol.* (in press).
Chanock, R. M. (1982). *In* "Viral Diseases in South-East Asia and the Western Pacific" (J. S. Mackenzie, ed.), pp. 139–155. Academic Press, Australia.
Chanter, N., Morgan, J. H., Bridger, J. C., Hall, G. A., and Reynolds, D. J. (1984). *Vet. Rec.* **114**, 71.
Chasey, D., and Davies, P. (1984). *Vet. Rec.* **114**, 16–17.
Ciosek, D., Truszczynski, M., and Jagodzinski, M. (1983). *Comp. Immun. Microbiol. Infect. Dis.* **6**, 313–319.
Clark, S. M., Roth, J. R., Clark, M. L., Barnett, B. B., and Spendlove, R. S. (1981). *J. Virol.* **39**, 816–822.

Clarke, I. N., and McCrae, M. A. (1981). *J. Virol. Methods* **3**, 261–269.
Clarke, I. N., and McCrae, M. A. (1983). *J. Virol. Methods* **64**, 1877–1884.
Coalson, J. A., and Lecce, J. G. (1973). *J. Anim. Sci.* **36**, 1114–1121.
Conner, M. E., and Darlington, R. W. (1980). *Am. J. Vet. Res.* **41**, 1699–1703.
Contrepois, M. Girardeau, J. P., Dubourguier, H. C., Gouet, P., and Levieux, D. (1978). *Ann. Rech. Vet.* **9**, 385–388.
Coussement, W., Ducatelle, R., Charlier, G., and Hoorens, J. (1981). *Am. J. Vet. Res.* **42**, 1905–1911.
Cranwell, P. D., Noakes, D. E., and Hill, K. J. (1976). *Br. J. Nutr.* **36**, 71–86.
Current, W. L., and Haynes, T. B. (1984). *Science* **224**, 603–605.
Current, W. L., and Long, P. L. (1983). *J. Infect. Dis.* **148**, 1108–1113.
Current, W. L., Reese, N. C., Ernst, J. V., Bailey, W. S., Heyman, M. B., and Weinstein, W. M. (1983). *New Engl. J. Med.* **308**, 1252–1257.
Daerr, H. C., Jaeger, O., Smith, S. E. G., and Becker, W. (1980). *Blauen Hefte Tierarzt* **61**, 26–31.
Darfeuille A., LaFeuille, B., Joly, B., and Cluzel, R. (1983). *Ann. Microbiol. (Paris)* **134A**, 53–64.
Dauvergne, M., Brun, A., and Soulebot, J. P. (1983). *Dev. Biol. Stand.* **53**, 245–255.
Dea, S., Roy, R. S., and Elazhary, M. A. S. Y. (1983). *Can. J. Comp. Med.* **47**, 88–91.
Dean, A. G., Ching, Y., Williams, R. G., and Harden, L. B. (1972). *J. Infect. Dis.* **125**, 407–411.
Debouck, P., Pensaert, M., and Coussement, W. (1981). *Vet. Microbiol.* **6**, 157–165.
Debouck, P., Callebaut, P., and Pensaert, M. (1982). *Proc. Congr. Int. Pig Vet. Soc. 7th, Mexico City.*
de Leeuw, P. W., Ellens, D. J., Talmon, F. P., Zimmer, G. N., and Kommerij, R. (1980). *Res. Vet. Sci.* **29**, 142–147.
de Leeuw, P. W., Moerman, A., Pol, J. M. A., Tiessink, J. W. A., and van Zijderveld, F. G. (1983). *Proc. Int. Symp. World Assoc. Vet. Microbiol. Immun. 8th, Perth.*
de Rycke, J., Le Roux, P., Melik, N., and Raimbault, P. (1981). *Ann. Rech. Vet.* **12**, 403–411.
Dickie, C. W., Klinkerman, D. L., and Petrie, R. J. (1978). *J. Am. Vet. Med. Assoc.* **173**, 306–307.
Dimitrov, D. H., Estes, M. K., Rangelova, S. M., Shindarov, L. M., Melnick, J. L., and Graham, D. Y. (1983). *Infect. Immun.* **41**, 523–526.
Dobrescu, L., and Huygelen, C. (1976). *Zentralbl. Veterinaermed.* **23**, 79–88.
Donta, S. T., Moon, H. W., and Whipp, S. C. (1974). *Science* **183**, 334–336.
Dorner, F., Mayer, P., and Leskova, R. (1980). *Zentralbl. Veterinaermed.* **27**, 207–221.
Ducatelle, R., Coussement, W., and Hoorens, J. (1981). *Arch. Virol.* **69**, 219–228.
Ducatelle, R., Coussement, W., and Hoorens, J. (1982). *Vet. Pathol.* **19**, 179–189.
Dyall-Smith, M. L., and Holmes, I. H. (1981). *J. Virol.* **38**, 1099–1103.
Dyall-Smith, M. L., and Holmes, I. H. (1982). *J. Virol.* **40**, 720–728.
Dyall-Smith, M. L., Elleman, T. C., Hoyne, P. A., Holmes, I. H., and Azad, A. A. (1983). *Nucleic Acids Res.* **11**, 3351–3362.
Ebina, T., Sato, A., Umezu, K., Ishida, N., Ohyama, S., Ohizumi, A., Aikawi, K., Katagiri, S., Katsushima, N., Imai, A., Kitaoka, S., Suzuki, H., and Konno, T. (1983). *Lancet* **2**, 1029–1030.
Echeverria, P., Seriwatana, J., Patamaroj, U., Moseley, S. L., McFarland, A., Chityothin, O., and Chaicumpa, W. (1984). *J. Clin. Microbiol.* **19**, 489–491.
Edman, J. C., Hallewell, R. A., Valenzuela, P., Goodman, H. M., and Rutter, W. J. (1981). *Nature (London)* **291**, 503–506.

Eichhorn, W., Bachmann, P. A., Baljer, G., Plank, P., Schneider, P. (1983). *Dev. Biol. Stand.* **53**, 237–243.
Eidels, L., Proia, R. L., and Hart, D. A. (1983). *Microbiol. Rev.* **47**, 596–620.
Elias, M. M. (1977). *J. Gen. Virol.* **37**, 191–194.
Elleman, T. C., Hoyne, P. A., Dyall-Smith, M. L., Holmes, I. H., and Azad, A. A. (1984). *Nucleic Acids Res.* **11**, 4689–4701.
English, P. R. (1981). *Proc. Pig Vet. Soc.* **7**, 29–37.
Escherich, T. (1885). *Fortschr. Med.* **3**, 515.
Espejo, R. T., Lopez, S., and Arias, C. (1981). *J. Virol.* **37**, 156–160.
Farrow, J. A. E., Jones, D., Phillips, B. A., and Collins, M.D. (1983). *J. Gen. Microbiol.* **129**, 1423–1432.
Fiedler, H. H., Bahr, K. H., and Hirchert, R. (1982). *Tieraerztl. Umsch.* **37**, 497–500.
Field, H. I., and Gibson, E. A. (1955). *Vet. Rec.* **67**, 31–35.
Finkelstein, R. A., and Yang, Z. (1983). *J. Clin. Microbiol.* **18**, 23–28.
Finkelstein, R. A., Yang, Z., Moseley, S. L., and Moon, H. W. (1983). *J. Clin. Microbiol.* **18**, 1417–1418.
Firehammer, B. D., and Myers, L. L. (1981). *Am. J. Vet. Res.* **42**, 918–922.
Fletcher, A., Sims, T. A., and Talbot, I. C. (1982). *Br. Med. J.* **285**, 22–23.
Flewett, T. H., and Woode, G. N. (1978). *Arch. Virol.* **57**, 1–23.
Flewett, T. H., Bryden, A. S., and Davies, H. (1973). *Lancet* **2**, 1497.
Fonteyne, J., Zissis, C., and Lambert, J. P. (1978). *Lancet* **1**, 983.
Francis, D. H. (1983). *Am J. Vet. Res.* **44**, 1884–1888.
Frantz, J. C., and Robertson, D. C. (1981). *Infect. Immun.* **33**, 193–198.
Freter, R. (1969). *Tex. Rep. Biol. Med.* **27**, 299–316.
Freter, R. (1981). *In* "Adhesion and Microorganism Pathogenicity" (K. Elliott, M. O'Connor, and J. Whelan, eds.), pp. 36–47. Pitman, London.
Freter, R., Smith, Jr., H. L., and Sweeney, F. J. (1961). *J. Infect. Dis.* **109**, 35–42.
Fujiwara, H., Minamimoto, S., and Namioka, S. (1968). *Natl. Inst. Anim. Health Q.* **8**, 53–54.
Fuller, R., Houghton, S. B., and Brooker, B. E. (1981). *Appl. Environ. Microbiol.* **41**, 1433–1441.
Furer, E., Cryz, Jr., S. J., Dorner, F., Nicolet, J., Wanner, M., and Germanier, R. (1982). *Infect. Immun.* **35**, 887–894.
Garcia, M. M., Lior, H., Stewart, R. B., Ruckerbauer, G. M., and Skljarevski, A. (1983a). *Campylobacter II. Proc. Int. Workshop Campylobacter Infect. 2nd*, Brussels.
Garcia, L. S., Bruckner, D. A., Brewer, T. C., and Shimizu, R. Y. (1983b). *J. Clin. Microbiol.* **18**, 185–190.
Gaul, S. K., Simpson, T. F., Woode, G. N., and Fulton, R. W. (1982). *J. Clin. Microbiol.* **16**, 495–503.
Gay, C. C., Barker, I. K., and Moore, P. (1976). *Proc. Congr. Int. Pig Vet. Soc. 4th, Ames*, 11.
Georges, M. C., Wachsmuth, I. K., Meunier, D.M.V., Nebout, N., Didier, F., Siopathis, M. R., and Georges, A. J. (1984). *J. Clin. Microbiol.* **19**, 571–575.
Giannella, R. A., Drake, K. W., and Luttrell, M. (1981). *Infect. Immun.* **33**, 186–192.
Gillespie, J., Kalica, A., Connor, M., Schiff, E., Barr, M., Holmes, D., and Frey, M. (1984). *Vet. Microbiol.* **9**, 1–14.
Goebel, E., and Braendler, U. (1982). *Protistologica* **18**, 331–344.
Greenberg, H. B., Sack, D. A., Rodriguez, W., Sack, R. B., Wyatt, R. G., Kalica, A. R., Horswood, R. L., Chanock, R. M., and Kapikian, A. Z. (1977). *Infect. Immun.* **17**, 541–545.

Greenberg, H. B., Kalica, A. R., Wyatt, R. G., Jones, R. W., Kapikian A. Z., and Chanock, R. M. (1981). *Proc. Natl. Acad. Sci. U.S.A.* **78,** 420–424.
Greenberg, H. B., Wyatt, R. G., Kapikian, A. Z., Kalica, A. R., Flores, J., and Jones, R. (1982). *Infect. Immun.* **37,** 104–109.
Greenberg, H. B., Valdesuso, J., van Wyke, K., Midthun, K., Walsh, M., McAuliffe, V., Wyatt, R. G., Kalica, A. R., Flores, J., and Hoshino, Y. (1983). *J. Virol.* **47,** 267–275.
Gregory, D. W., Cardella, M. A., and Myers, L. L. (1983). *Am. J. Vet. Res.* **44,** 2073–2077.
Griner, L. A. (1963). *Bull. Off. Int. Epizoot.* **59,** 1443–1452.
Griner, L. A., and Bracken, F. K. (1953). *J. Am. Vet. Med. Assoc.* **122,** 99–102.
Griner, L. A., and Johnson, H. W. (1954). *J. Am. Vet. Med. Assoc.* **125,** 125–127.
Gross, R. J. (1983). *J. Infect.* **7,** 177–192.
Grudniewska, B. (1982). *Pig News Infor.* **3,** 401–408.
Guerrant, R. L., Brunton, L. L., Schnaitman, T. C., Rebhun, L. I., and Gilman, A. G. (1974). *Infect. Immun.* **10,** 320–327.
Guinée, P. A. M., and Jansen, W. H. (1979). *Infect. Immun.* **23,** 700–705.
Guinée, P. A. M., Jansen, W. H., Wadstrom, T., and Sellwood, R. (1980). *In* "Laboratory Diagnosis in Neonatal Calf and Pig Diarrhea" (P. W. de Leeuw, P. A. M. Guinee, eds.), pp. 126–160. Martinus Nijhoff, The Hague.
Gyles, C. L., Stevens, J. B., and Craven, J. A. (1971). *Can J. Comp. Med.* **35,** 258–266.
Hadad, J. J., and Gyles, C. L. (1982). *Can. J. Comp. Med.* **46,** 21–26.
Haig, D. A., Clarke, M. C., and Pereira, M. S. (1964). *J. Comp. Pathol.* **74,** 81–84.
Hampson, D. J., Kidder, D. E., and Hampson, E. M. (1982). *Proc. Congr. Int. Pig Vet. Soc. 7th, Mexico City*, p. 256.
Hardy, B. (1978). *Pig Farming Dec,* 24.
Harleman, J. H., and Meyer, R. C. (1983). *Vet. Q.* **5,** 178–185.
Harnett, N. M., and Gyles, C. L. (1983). *Am. J. Vet. Res.* **44,** 1210–1214.
Hartman, D. A., Hays, V. W., Baker, R. O., Neagle, L. H., and Catron, D. V. (1961). *J. Anim. Sci.* **20,** 114–123.
Hartmann, H., Bechtel, D., Otto, P., and Schonhev, W. (1982). *Arch. Exp. Veterinaermed.* **36,** 611–621.
Headington, J. T., Sathornsumathi, S., Simark, S., and Sujatanond, W. (1967). *Lancet* **1,** 802–806.
Heine, J., Moon, H. W., and Woodmansee, D. B. (1984). *Infect. Immun.* **43,** 856–859.
Hess, R. G., Bachmann, P. A., Eichhorn, W., Frahm, K., and Plank P. (1982). *Fortschr. Veterinaermed.* **35,** 103–108.
Høgh, P. (1976). *Dev. Biol. Stand* **32,** 69–76.
Hojlyng, N., Molbak, K., Jepsen, S., and Hansson, A. P. (1984). *Lancet* **1,** 734.
Holmes, I. H. (1979). *Prog. Med. Virol.* **25,** 1–36.
Holmes, I. H. (1983). *In* "The Reoviridae" (W. K. Joklik, ed.), pp. 359–423. Plenum, New York.
Holten-Andersen, W., Gerstoft, J., and Henriksen, S. A. (1983). *New Engl. J. Med.* **309,** 1325–1326.
Honda, T., Arita, M., Takeda, Y., and Miwatani, T. (1982). *J. Clin. Microbiol.* **16,** 60–62.
Honda, T., Samakoses, R., Sornchai, C., Takedo, Y., and Miwatani, T. (1983). *J. Clin. Microbiol.* **17,** 592–595.
Hoshino, Y., Wyatt, R. G., Greenberg, H. B., Kalica, A. R., Flores, J., and Kapikian, A. Z. (1983a). *Infect. Immun.* **41,** 169–173.
Hoshino, Y., Wyatt, A. G., Greenberg, H. B., Kalica, A. R., Flores, J., and Kapikian, A. Z. (1983b). *J. Clin. Microbiol.* **18,** 585–591.

Hoshino, Y., Wyatt, R. G., Greenberg, H. B., Flores, J., and Kapikian, A. Z. (1984). *J. Infect. Dis.* **149,** 694–702.
Houghton, S. B., Fuller, R., Coats, M. E. (1981). *J. Appl. Bacteriol.* **51,** 113–120.
House, J. A. (1978). *J. Am. Vet. Med. Assoc.* **173,** 573–576.
Imagawa, H., Wada R., Hirasawa, K., Akiyama, Y., and Oda, T. (1984). *Jpn. J. Vet. Sci.* **46,** 1–9.
Isaacson, R. E. (1981). *Proc. Int. Symp. Neonatal Diarrhea 3rd,* 213–236.
Isaacson, R. E., Dean, E. A., Morgan, R. L., and Moon, H. W. (1980). *Infect. Immun.* **29,** 824–826.
Jerrett, I. V. (1982). *Aust. Adv. Vet. Sci. Proc. Aust. Vet. Assoc.,* pp. 163–165.
Jokipii, L., Pohjola, S., and Jokipii, A. M. M. (1983). *Lancet* **2,** 358–361.
Jolivet-Reynaud, C., Cavaillon, J., and Alouf, J. E. (1982). *Infect. Immun.* **38,** 860–864.
Jones, G. W., and Rutter, J. M. (1972). *Infect. Immun.* **6,** 918–927.
Jones, G. W., and Rutter, J. M. (1974). *J. Gen. Microbiol.* **84,** 135–144.
Kalica, A. R., Sereno, M. M., Wyatt, R. G., Mebus, C. A., Chanock, R. M.,and Kapikian, A. Z. (1978). *Virology* **87,** 247–255.
Kalica, A. R., Greenberg, H. B., Wyatt, R. G., Flores, J., Sereno, M. M., Kapikian, A. Z., and Chanock R. M. (1981). *Virology* **112,** 385–390.
Kanitz, C. L. (1977). *Proc. Annu. Conf. Am. Assoc. Equine Practice 22nd,* pp. 155–165.
Kantharidis, P., Dyall-Smith, M. L., and Holmes, I. H. (1983). *J. Virol.* **48,** 330–334.
Kapikian, A. Z., Kim, H. W., Wyatt, R. G., Rodriguez, W. J., Ross, S., Cline, W. L., Parrott, R. H., and Chanock, R. M. (1974). *Science* **185,** 1049–1053.
Kapikian, A. Z., Cline, W. L., Greenberg, H. B., Wyatt, R. G., Kalica, A. R., Banks, C. E., James, H. D., Jr., Flores, J., and Chanock, R. M. (1981). *Infect. Immun.* **33,** 415–425.
Kauffman, F. (1947). *J. Immunol.* **57,** 71–100.
Kenworthy, R. (1976). *Res. Vet. Sci.* **21,** 69–75.
Kenworthy, R., and Crabb, W. E. (1963). *J. Comp. Pathol.* **73,** 215–228.
Kidder, D. E. (1982). *Pig News Info.* **3,** 25–28.
Kirubakaran, C., Davidson, G. P., Darby, H., Hansman, D., McKay, G., Moore, B., and Lee, P. (1981). *Med. J. Aust.* **2,** 333–335.
Kleid, D., Yansura, D., Small, B., Dowbenko, D., Moore, D., Grubman, M., McKercher P., Morgan, D., Robertson, B., and Bachrach, H. (1981). *Science* **214,** 1125–1129.
Klipstein, F. A., and Engert, R. F. (1984). *Lancet* **1,** 1123–1124.
Klipstein, F. A., Engert, R. F., Houghten, R. A., and Rowe, B. (1984). *J. Clin. Microbiol.* **19,** 798–803.
Kohler, E. M. (1974). *Am. J. Vet. Res.* **35,** 331–338.
Kohler, E. M., Cross, R. F., and Bohl, E. H. (1975). *Am. J. Vet. Res.* **36,** 757–764.
Kornegay, E. T., Tinsley, S. E., and Bryant, K. L. (1979). *J. Anim. Sci.* **48,** 999–1006.
Kudoh, Y., Zen-Yoji, H., Matsushita, S., Sakai, S., and Maruyama, T. (1977). *Microbiol. Immunol.* **21,** 175–178.
Lambert, J. P., Marissens, D., Marbehant, P., and Zissis, G. (1983). *J. Med. Virol.* **11,** 31–38.
Lasser, K. H., Lewin, K. L., and Ryning, F. W. (1979). *Hum. Pathol.* **10,** 234–240.
Lawrence, G. W., and Cooke, R. A. (1980). *Br. J. Exp. Pathol.* **61,** 261–271.
Lawrence, G. W., and Walker, P. D. (1976). *Lancet* **1,** 125–126.
Lawrence, T. L. J. (1972). *Vet. Rec.* **91,** 84–88.
Lecce, J. G., and King, M. W. (1978). *J. Clin. Microbiol* **8,** 454–458.
Lecce, J. G., King, M. W., and Mock, R. (1976). *Infect. Immun.* **14,** 816–825.
Lecce, J. G., Balsbaugh, R. K., Clare, D. A., and King, M. W. (1982). *J. Clin. Microbiol.* **16,** 715–723.

Lecce, J. G., Clare, D. A., Balsbaugh, R. K., and Collier, D. N. (1983). *J. Clin. Microbiol.* **17,** 689–695.
Lee, C. H., Moseley, S. L., Moon, H. W., Whipp, S. C., Gyles, C. L., and So, M. (1983). *Infect. Immun.* **42,** 264–268.
Levine, M. M. (1983). *Scand. J. Gastroenterol.* **18,** 121–134.
Levine, M. M., Kaper, J. B., Black, R. E., and Clements, M. L. (1983). *Microbiol. Rev.* **47,** 510–550.
Logan, E. F., and Meneely, J. D. (1981). *Vet. Rec.* **109,** 513–514.
Lourenco, M. H., Nicolas, J. C., Cohen, J., Scherrer, R., and Bricout, F. (1981). *Ann. Virol. (Paris)* **132E,** 161–173.
Ma, P., and Soave, R. (1983). *J. Infect. Dis.* **147,** 824–828.
McCardell, B. A., Madden, J. M., and Lee, E. C. (1984). *Lancet* **2,** 448–449.
McCrae, M. A., and Faulkner-Valle, G. P. (1981). *J. Virol.* **39,** 490–496.
McCrae, M. A., and McCorquodale, J. A. (1982). *Virology* **117,** 435–443.
McEwan, A. D. (1930). *J. Comp. Pathol.* **43,** 1–21.
McNulty, M. S. (1978). *J. Gen. Virol.* **40,** 1–18.
McNulty, M. S., Allan, G. M., Todd, D., and McFerran, J. B. (1979). *Arch. Virol.* **61,** 13–21.
McNulty, M. S., Allan, G. M., Todd, D., McFerran, J. B., McKillop, E. R., Collins, D. S., and McCracken, R. M. (1980). *Avian Pathol.* **9,** 363–375.
McNulty, M. S., Allan, G. M., Todd, D., McFerran, J. B., and McCracken, R. M. (1981). *J. Gen. Virol.* **55,** 405–413.
Mann, G. (1983). *Arch. Exp. Veterinaermed.* **37,** 323–326.
Mata, L., Bolarios, H., Pizarro, D., and Vives, M. (1984). *Am. J. Trop. Med. Hyg.* **33,** 24–29.
Matsuno, S., Inouye, S., and Kono, R. (1977). *J. Clin. Microbiol.* **5,** 1–4.
Matsuno, S., Hasegawa, A., Kalica, A. R., and Kono, R. (1980). *J. Gen. Virol.* **48,** 253–256.
Matthews, R. E. F. (1979). *Intervirology* **11,** 133–135.
Mebus, C. A., Underdahl, N. R., Rhodes, M. B., and Twiehaus, M. J. (1969). *Univ. Nebr. Agric. Exp. Stn. Res. Bull.* **233,** 1–16.
Mebus, C. A., White, R. G., Bass, E. P., and Twiehaus, M. J. (1973). *J. Am. Vet. Med. Assoc.* **163,** 880.
Mebus, C. A., Rhodes, M. B., and Underdahl, N. R. (1978). *Am. J. Vet. Res.* **39,** 1223–1228.
Meisel, J. L., Perera, D. R., Meligro, C., and Rubin, C. E. (1976). *Gastroenterology* **70,** 1156–1160.
Mele, L., Nadler, H., Pappalardo, S., Forgacs, P., Shea, J., Kurtz, S., and Ma, P. (1983). *Proc. 83rd Annu. Meet. Am. Soc. Microbiol.,* Abstr. C96.
Middleton, P. J., Szymanski, M. T., Abbott, G. D., Bortolussi, R., and Hamilton, J. R. (1974). *Lancet* **1,** 1241–1244.
Miller, B. G., Newby, T. J., Stokes, C. R., and Bourne, F. J. (1984). *Vet. Rec.* **114,** 296–297.
Mills, K. W., Tietze, K. L., and Phillips, R. M. (1983). *Am J. Vet. Res.* **44,** 2188–2189.
Mooi, F. R., de Graaf, F. K., and van Embden, J. D. A. (1979). *Nucleic Acids Res.* **6,** 849–865.
Moon, H. W. (1974). *Adv. Vet. Sci. Comp. Med.* **18,** 179–211.
Moon, H. W., and Runnels, P. L. (1984). *Proc. Int. Symp. Neonatal Diarrhea 4th,* 558–569.
Moon, H. W., and Whipp, S. C. (1970). *J. Infect. Dis.* **122,** 220–223.

Moon, H. W., McClurkin, A. W., Isaacson, R. E., Pohlenz, J., Skartvedt, S. M., Gillette, K. G., and Baetz, A. L. (1978). *J. Am. Vet. Med. Assoc.* **173**, 577–583.
Moon, H. W., Isaacson, R. E., and Pohlenz, J. (1979). *Am. J. Clin. Nutr.* **32**, 119–127.
Moon, H. W., Kohler, E. M., Schneider, R. A., and Whipp, S. C. (1980). *Infect. Immun.* **27**, 222–230.
Moon, H. W., Baetz, A. L., and Giannella, R. A. (1983). *Infect. Immun.* **39**, 990–992.
Morgan, J. H., Hall, G. A., Reynolds, D. J., and Parsons, K. (1983). *Campylobacter* II. *Proc. Int. Workshop Campylobacter Infect. 2nd,* Brussels.
Morgan, R. L., Isaacson, R. E., Moon, H. W., Brinton, C. C., and To, C. C. (1978). *Infect. Immun.* **22**, 771–777.
Morin, M., Lariviere, S., Lallier, R., Begin, M., Roy, R., and Ethier, R. (1978). *Proc. Int. Symp. Neonatal Diarrhea 2nd,* pp. 347–367.
Morin, M., Robinson, Y., and Turgeon, D. (1980). *Can. Vet. J.* **21**, 65.
Morin, M., Turgeon, D., Jolette, J., Robinson, Y., Phaneuf, J. B., Sauvageau, R., Beauregard, M., Teuscher, E., Higgins, R., and Lariviere, S. (1983). *Can. J. Comp. Med.* **47**, 11–17.
Morris, J. A., Thorns, C. J., and Sojka, W. J. (1980). *J. Gen. Microbiol.* **118**, 107–113.
Morris, J. A., Thorns, C. J., Scott, A. C., Sojka, W. J., and Wells, G. A. H. (1982). *Infect. Immun.* **36**, 1146–1153.
Morris, J. A., Thorns, C. J., Wells, G. A. H., Scott, A. C., and Sojka, W. J. (1983). *J. Gen. Microbiol.* **129**, 2753–2759.
Moseley, S. L., Echeverria, P., Seriwatana, J., Tirapat, C., Chaicumpa, W., Sakuldaipeara, T., and Falkow, S. (1982). *J. Infect. Dis.* **145**, 863–869.
Moseley, S. L., Hardy, J. W., Huq, M. I., Echeverria, P., and Falkow, S. (1983). *Infect. Immun.* **39**, 1167–1174.
Murakami, Y., Nishioka, N., Hashiguchi, Y., and Kuniyasu, C. (1981). *Microbiol. Immunol.* **25**, 1097–1100.
Murakami, Y., Nishioka, N., Hashiguchi, Y., and Kuniyasu, C. (1983). *Infect. Immun.* **40**, 851–855.
Murrell, T. G. C., Roth, L., Egerton, J., Samels, J., and Walker, P. D. (1966). *Lancet* **1**, 217–222.
Myers, L. L. (1978). *Am. J. Vet. Res.* **39**, 761–765.
Myers, L. L. (1980). *Am. J. Vet. Res.* **41**, 1952–1956.
Myers, L. L., and Snodgrass, D. R. (1982). *J. Am. Vet. Med. Assoc.* **181**, 486–488.
Nagy, B. (1980). *Infect. Immun.* **27**, 21–24.
Nagy, B., and Pohlenz, J. (1982). *Tieraerztl. Prax.* **10**, 163–172.
Nagy, B., Moon, H. W., and Isaacson, R. E. (1976). *Infect. Immun.* **13**, 1214–1220.
Nagy, B., Moon, H. W., and Isaacson, R. E. (1977). *Infect. Immun.* **16**, 344–352.
Nagy, B., Moon, H. W., Isaacson, R. E. To, C. C., and Brinton, C. C. (1978). *Infect. Immun.* **21**, 269–274.
Nagy, L. K., Bhogal, B. S., Walker, P. D., and MacKenzie, T. (1979). *Proc. Int. Symp. Neonatal Diarrhea 2nd,* pp. 411–424.
Nairn, M. E., and Bamford, V. W. (1967). *Aust. Vet. J.* **43**, 49–54.
Newsome, P. M., Burgess, M. N., and Mullan, N. A. (1978). *Infect. Immun.* **22**, 290–291.
Nichols, G., and Thom, B. T. (1984). *Lancet* **1**, 735.
Nicolas, J. C., Cohen, J., Fortier, B., Lourenco, M. H., and Bricout, F. (1983). *Virology* **124**, 181–184.
Nielson, H. E., Danielsen, V., Aherne, F. X., and Young, L. G. (1980). *Proc. Congr. Int. Pig Vet. Soc. 6th, Copenhagen,* p. 295.
Niilo, L. (1980). *Can. Vet. J.* **21**, 141–148.

Niilo, L., and Chalmers, G. A. (1982). *Can. Vet. J.* **23**, 299–301.
Nime, F. A., Burek, J. D., Page, D. L., Holscher, M. A., and Yardley, J. H. (1976). *Gastroenterology* **70**, 592–598.
Norrby, E. (1983). *Arch. Virol.* **76**, 163–177.
Ojeh, C. K., Snodgrass, D. R., and Herring, A. J. (1984). *Arch. Virol.* **79**, 161–171.
Okai, D. B., Aherne, F. X., and Hardin, T. R. (1976). *Can. J. Anim. Sci.* **56**, 573–586.
Ørskov, I., Ørskov, F., Smith, H. W., and Sojka, W. J. (1975). *Acta Pathol. Microbiol. Scand. Sect. B:Microbiol* **83**, 31–36.
Palmer, N. C., and Hulland, T. J. (1965). *Can Vet. J.* **6**, 310–316.
Pape, J. W., Liautaud, B., Thomas, F., Mathurin, J. R., St. Amand, M. M.-A., Boncy, M., Pean, V., Pamphile, M., Laroche, A. C., and Johnston, W. D., Jr. (1983). *New Engl. J. Med.* **309**, 945–950.
Patamaroj, U., Seriwatana, J., and Echeverria, P. (1983). *J. Clin. Microbiol.* **18**, 1429–1431.
Pavlasek, I. (1982). *Vet. Med. (Prague)* **27**, 729–740.
Pedley, S., Bridger, J. C., Brown, J. F., and McCrae, M. A. (1983). *J. Gen. Virol.* **64**, 2093–2101.
Pensaert, M. B., and Debouck, P. (1978). *Arch. Virol.* **58**, 243–247.
Pensaert, M. B., Callebaut, P., and Debouck, P. (1982). *Proc. Congr. Int. Pig Vet. Soc. 7th, Mexico City*.
Pineiro, A., Ortega, F., and Uriel, J. (1975). *Biochim. Biophys Acta* **379**, 201–206.
Pitlik, S. D., Fainstein, V., Garza, D., Guarda, L., Bolivar, R., Rios, A., Hopfer, R. L., and Mansell, P. A. (1983). *Arch. Intern. Med.* **143**, 2269–2275.
Pohjola, S. (1984). *Res. Vet. Sci.* **36**, 217–219.
Porter, J. W. G., and Rolls, B. A. (1971). *Proc. Nutr. Soc.* **30**, 17–25.
Porter, P., and Linggood, M. A. (1983). *J. Infect.* **6**, 111–121.
Porter, P., Kenworthy, R., Noakes, D. E., and Allen, W. D. (1974). *Immunology* **27**, 841–853.
Porter, P., Parry, S. H., and Allen, W. D. (1977). *Ciba Found. Symp.* **46**, 55–75.
Prohazka, L., and Baron, F. (1980). *Zentralbl. Veterinaermed. Reihe B* **27**, 222–232.
Real, C. E., Tanksley, T. D., Jr., and Purser, K. W. (1977). *Am. Soc. Anim. Sci. 68th Annu. Meet.* p. 105 (Abstr.).
Reese, N. C., Current, W. L., Ernst, J. V., and Bailey, W. S. (1982). *Am. J. Trop. Med. Hyg.* **31**, 226–229.
Renault, L., Laporte, J., and Alamagny, A. (1982). *Bull. Mens. Soc. Vet. Pratique Fr.* **66**, 701–710.
Rijke, E. O., Webster, J., and Baars, J. C. (1983). *Dev. Biol. Stand.* **53**, 155–160.
Ripley, P. H., and Gush, A. F. (1983). *Vet. Rec.* **112**, 201–202.
Ritchey, M. B., Palese, P., and Kilbourne, E. D. (1976). *J. Virol.* **18**, 738–744.
Rivera, E. R., Armstrong, W. D., Clawson, A. J., and Linnerud, A. C. (1978). *J. Anim. Sci.* **46**, 1685–1693.
Roberts, L., and Walker, E. J. (1981). *Vet. Rec.* **108**, 62.
Roberts, L., Walker, E. J., Snodgrass, D. R., and Angus, K. W. (1980). *Vet. Rec.* **107**, 156–157.
Roberts, R. B. (1984). In "The Acquired Immune Deficiency Syndrome and Infections of Homosexual Men" (P. Ma and D. Armstrong, eds.), pp. 302–316. Yorke Medical Books, Technical Publishing, U.S.A.
Robins-Browne, R. M. (1980). *South Afr. J. Sci.* **76**, 352–359.
Robins-Browne, R. M., Still, C. S., Miliotis, M.D., and Koornhof, H. J. (1979). *Infect. Immun.* **25**, 680–684.

Robinson, Y., and Morin, M. (1982). *Can. Vet. J.* **23**, 212–216.
Robinson, Y., Morin, M., Girard, G., and Higgins, R. (1983). *Can. J. Comp. Med.* **47**, 401–407.
Rodger, S. M., and Holmes, I. H. (1979). *J. Virol.* **30**, 839–846.
Rodger, S. M., Craven, J. A., and Williams, I. (1975). *Aust. Vet. J.* **51**, 536.
Rodger, S. M., Bishop, R. F., Birch, C., McLean, B., and Holmes, I. H. (1981). *J. Clin. Microbiol.* **13**, 272–278.
Rodger, S. M., Bishop, R. F., and Holmes, I. H. (1982). *J. Clin. Microbiol.* **16**, 724–726.
Rodriguez, W. J., Kim, H. W., Brandt, C. D., Yolken, R. H., Arrobio, J. O., Kapikian, A. Z., Chanock, R. M., and Parrott, R. H. (1978). *Lancet* **2**, 37.
Ronnberg, B., and Wadstrom, T. (1983). J. Clin. Microbiol **17**, 1021–1025.
Rosenberg, M. L., Koplan, J. P., Wachsmuth, I. K., Wells, J. G., Gangarosa, E. J., Guerrant, R. L., and Sack, D. A. (1977). *Ann. Intern. Med.* **86**, 714–718.
Ruckabusch, Y., and Bueno, L. (1976). *Br. J. Nutr.* **35**, 397–405.
Ruiz-Palacios, G. M., Torres, J., Torres, N. I., Escamilla, E., and Ruiz-Palacios, B. R. (1983). *Lancet* **2**, 250–252.
Runnels, P. L., Moon, H. W., and Schneider, R. A., (1980). *Infect. Immun.* **28**, 298–300.
Russell, S. M., and Liew, F. Y. (1979). *Nature (London)* **280**, 147–148.
Rutter, J. M., Burrows, M. R., Sellwood, R, and Gibbons, R. A. (1975). *Nature (London)* **257**, 135–136.
Sack, D. A., Huda, S., Neogi, P. K. B., Daniel, R. R., Spira, W. M. (1980). *J. Clin. Microbiol.* **11**, 35–40.
Saif, L. J., and Smith, K. L. (1984). *Proc. Int. Symp. Neonatal Diarrhea 4th*, pp. 394–423.
Saif, L. J., Bohl, E. H., Theil, K. W., Kohler, E. M., and Cross, R. F. (1980). *Annu. Conf. Res. Work. Anim. Dis. 61st,* Abst. no. **149**, Chicago.
Saif, L. J., Redman, D. R., Theil, K. W., Moorhead, P. D., and Smith, C. K. (1981). *Annu. Conf. Res. Work. Anim. Dis. 62nd*, abst. no. **236**, Chicago.
Saif, L. J., Redman, D. R., Smith, K. L., and Theil, K. W. (1983). *Infect. Immun.* **41**, 1118–1131.
Saif, L. J., Smith, K. L., Landmeier, B. J., Bohl, E. H., Theil, K. W., and Todhunter, D. A. (1984). *Am. J. Vet. Res.* **45**, 49–58.
Sanford, S. E. (1983). *Calif. Vet.* **37**, 26.
Sanford, S. E., and Hoover, D. M. (1983). *Can. J. Comp. Med.* **47**, 396–400.
Sanford, S. E., and Josephson, G. K. A. (1981). *Can. Vet. J.* **22**, 282–285.
Sanford, S. E., and Josephson, G. K. A. (1982). *Can. Vet. J.* **23**, 343–347.
Sangster, L. T., Seibold, H. R., and Mitchell, F. E. (1976). *Am. Assoc. Vet. Lab. Diagnost.* **19**, 51–55.
Sanyal, S. C., Singh, S. J., and Sen, P. C. (1975). *J. Med. Microbiol.* **47**, 195–198.
Sato, K., Inaba, V., Shinozaki, T., Fujii, R., and Matumoto, M. (1981). *Arch. Virol.* **69**, 155–160.
Schnagl, R. D., Rodger, S. M., and Holmes, I. H. (1981). *Infect. Immun.* **33**, 17–21.
Schulz, W. (1982). *Monatsh. Veterinaermed.* **37**, 849–851.
Sellwood, R., Gibbons, R. A., Jones, G. W., and Rutter, J. M. (1975). *J. Med. Microbiol.* **8**, 405–411.
Seve, B., and Aumaitre, A. (1978). *World Rev. Anim. Prod.* **14**, 25–32.
Shann, F., Lawrence, G., and Pan Jun-Di. (1979). *Lancet* **1**, 1083–1084.
Shepherd, A. (1979). *Papua New Guinea Med. J.* **22**, 18–23.
Sherman, D. M., Acres, S. D., Sadowski, P. L., Springer, J. A., Bray, B., Raybould, T. J. G., and Muscoplat, C. C. (1983). *Infect. Immun.* **42**, 653–658.
Shipley, P. L., Dougan, G., and Falkow, S. (1981). *J. Bacteriol* **145**, 920–925.

Simmon, A., Chrystie, I. L., Tottderdell, B. M., Banatvala, J. E., Rice, S. J., and Walker-Smith, J. A. (1981). *Lancet* **2,** 1174.
Simonson, R. R., Isaacson, R. E., Jacob, C. R., and Newman, K. Z. (1984). *Proc.* 4th *Int. Symp. Neonatal Diarrhea 4th,* pp. 548–557.
Sims, L. D., Tzipori, S., Hazard, G., and Carroll, C. L. (1984). *Aust. Vet. J.* **62,** 194–196.
Skjelkvale, R., and Duncan, C. L. (1975). *Infect. Immun.* **11,** 563–575.
Smith, H. W. (1980). *In* "Recent Advances in Gastrointestinal Pathology" (R. Wright, ed.), pp. 135–150. Saunders, Philadelphia.
Smith, H. W., and Gyles, C. L. (1970). *J. Med. Microbiol.* **3,** 387–401.
Smith, H. W., and Hall, S. (1967). *J. Pathol. Bacteriol.* **93,** 499–529.
Smith, H. W., and Hall, S. (1968). *J. Med. Microbiol.* **1,** 45–59.
Smith, H. W., and Huggins, M. B. (1978). *J. Med. Microbiol.* **11,** 471–492.
Smith, H. W., and Huggins, M. B. (1982). *J. Gen. Microbiol.* **128,** 307–318.
Smith, H. W., and Huggins, M. B. (1983). *J. Gen. Microbiol.* **129,** 2659–2675.
Smith, H. W., and Jones, J. E. T. (1963). *J. Pathol. Bacteriol.* **86,** 387–412.
Smith, H. W., and Linggood, M. A. (1971). *J. Med. Microbiol.* **4,** 467–485.
Smith, M. L., Lazdins, I., and Holmes, I. H. (1980). *J. Virol.* **33,** 976–982.
Snodgrass, D. R., and Sherwood, D. (1984). *Proc. Int. Symp. Neonatal Diarrhea 4th,* pp. 162–170.
Snodgrass, D. R., and Wells, P. W. (1976). *Arch. Virol.* **52,** 201–205.
Snodgrass, D. R., Fahey, K. J., Wells, P. W., Campbell, I., and Whitelaw, A. (1980). *Infect. Immun.* **28,** 344–349.
Snodgrass, D. R., Nagy, L. K., Sherwood, D., and Campbell, I. (1982). *Infect. Immun.* **37,** 586–591.
Snodgrass, D. R., Herring, A. J., Campbell, I., Inglis, J. M., and Hargreaves, F. D. (1984a). *J. Gen. Virol.* **65,** 909–914.
Snodgrass, D. R., Angus, K. W., and Gray, E. W. (1984b). *J. Comp. Pathol.* **94,** 141–152.
Snodgrass, D. R., Ojeh, C. K., Campbell, I., and Herring, A. J. (1984c). *J. Clin. Microbiol.* **20,** 342–346.
Soderlind, O., Olsson, E., Smyth, C. J., and Mollby, R. (1982). *Infect. Immun.* **36,** 900–906.
Sojka, W. J., Wray, C., and Morris, J. A. (1978). *J. Med. Microbiol.* **11,** 493–499.
Stevens, A. J., and Blackburn, P. W. (1967). *Vet. Rec.* **80,** 637–638.
Stevens, J. B., Gyles, C. L., and Barnum, D. A. (1972). *Am. J. Vet. Res.* **33,** 2511–2526.
Stevenson, G. W., and Andrews, J. J. (1982). *Vet. Med. Small Anim. Clin.* **77,** 111–112.
Strickland, K. L., Lenihan, P., O'Connor, M. G., and Condon, J. C. (1982). *Vet. Rec.* **111,** 421.
Stuart, B. P., and Lindsay, D. (1979). *J. Am. Vet. Med. Assoc.* **175,** 328–329.
Svendsen, J. (1979). Ph.D. thesis: Swedish University of Agricultural Sciences, Uppsala, Sweden.
Svendsen, J., Larsen, J. L., and Bille, N. (1974). *Nord. Veterinaermed.* **26,** 314–322.
Svennerholm, A.-M., and Ahren, C. (1982). *Acta Pathol. Microbiol. Immunol. Scand. Sect.* **C90,** 1–6.
Svennerholm, A.-M., and Holmgren, J. (1978). *Curr. Microbiol.* **1,** 19–23.
Takeuchi, A., Inman, L. R., O'Hanley, P. D., Cantey, J. R., and Lushbaugh, W. B. (1978). *Infect. Immun.* **19,** 686–694.
Tao, H., Guangmu, C., Changan, W., Henli, Y., Zhaoying, F., Tungxin, C., Zinyi, C., Weiwe, Y., Xuejian, C., Shuasen, D., Xiaoquang, L., and Weicheng, C. (1984). *Lancet* **1,** 1139–1142.
Theil, K. W., Bohl, E. H., and Agnes, A. G. (1977). *Am. J. Vet. Res.* **38,** 1765–1768.
Thomlinson, J. R. (1974). *Proc. Int. Pig. Vet. Sci. Congr. 3rd., Lyon,* pp. 1–4.

Thompson, K. G., Thomson, G. W., and Henry, J. N. (1981). *Can. Vet. J.* **22**, 68–71.
Thorpe, E., and Thomlinson, J. R. (1967). *J. Pathol. Bacteriol.* **93**, 601–610.
Thouless, M. E. (1979). *J. Gen. Virol.* **44**, 187–197.
Thouless, M. E., Bryden, A. S., Flewett, T. H., Woode, G. N., Bridger, J. C., Snodgrass, D. R., and Herring, J. A. (1977). *Arch. Virol.* **53**, 287–294.
To, S. C. (1984). *Mod. Vet. Pract.* **65**, 39–41.
Trejo Medina, A., Espejo Torres, R., and Romero, P. (1982). *Veterinaria Mexico City* **13**, 79–83.
Tyzzer, E. E. (1907). *Proc. Soc. Exp. Biol. Med.* **5**, 12–13.
Tzipori, S. (1981). *Vet. Rec.* **108**, 510–514.
Tzipori, S. (1983a). *Microbiol. Rev.* **47**, 84–96.
Tzipori, S. (1983b). *Communicable Diseases Intelligence Bull.* No. 83/24, pp. 3–5. (Publ: Dept. of Health, Canberra).
Tzipori, S., and Campbell, I. (1981). *J. Clin. Microbiol.* **14**, 455–456.
Tzipori, S., and Spradbrow, P. B. (1978). *Aust. Vet. J.* **54**, 323–328.
Tzipori, S., and Walker, M. (1978). *Aust. J. Exp. Biol. Med. Sci.* **56**, 453–457.
Tzipori, S. and Williams, R. W. (1978). *Aust. Vet. J.* **54**, 188–192.
Tzipori, S., Makin, T. J., and Smith, M. L. (1980a). *Aust. J. Exp. Biol. Med. Sci.* **58**, 309–318.
Tzipori, S., Jones, R. T., and Fahy, V. A. (1980b). *Aust. Vet. J.* **56**, 154–155.
Tzipori, S., Chandler, D., Smith, M., Makin, T., and Hennessy, D. (1980c). *Aust. Vet. J.* **56**, 274–278.
Tzipori, S., Chandler, D., Makin, T., and Smith, M. (1980d). *Aust. Vet. J.* **56**, 279–284.
Tzipori, S., Angus, K. W., Gray, E. W., and Campbell, I. (1980e). *New Engl. J. Med.* **303**, 818.
Tzipori, S., Makin, T., Smith, M., and Chandler, D. (1980f). *Proc. Congr. Int. Pig Vet. Soc. 6th,* Copenhagen, p. 128.
Tzipori, S., Makin, T., Smith, M., and Krautil, F. (1981). *J. Clin. Microbiol.* **13**, 1011–1016.
Tzipori, S., Chandler, D., Smith, M., Makin, T., and Halpin, C. (1982a). *Aust. Vet. J.* **59**, 93–95.
Tzipori, S., Smith, M. L., Makin, T. J., and Halpin, C. L. (1982b). *Vet. Parasitol.* **11**, 121–126.
Tzipori, S., Makin, T., Smith, M., and Krautil, F. (1982c). *Aust. Vet. J.* **58**, 20–23.
Tzipori, S., Chandler, D., and Smith, M. (1983a). *Prog. Food Nutr. Sci.* **7**, 193–205.
Tzipori, S., Smith, M., Birch, D., Barnes, G., and Bishop, R. (1983b). *Am. J. Trop. Med. Hyg.* **32**, 931–934.
Tzipori, S., Smith, M., Halpin, C., Makin, T., and Krautil, F. (1983c). *Vet. Microbiol.* **8**, 35–43.
Tzipori, S., Withers, M., Robins-Browne, R., Ward, K. L., and Hayes, J. (1984a). *Vet. Microbiol.* **9**, 561–570.
Tzipori, S., McCartney, E., Chang, H. S., and Dunkin, A. (1984b). *FEMS Microbiol. Lett.* **24**, 313–317.
Tzipori, S., Hayes, J., Sims, L., and Withers, M. (1984c). *J. Inf. Dis.* **150**, 589–593.
Underdahl, N. R., Torres-Medina, A., and Doster, A. R. (1982). *Am. J. Vet. Res.* **43**, 2227–2232.
Urasawa, T., Urasawa, S., and Taniguchi, K. (1981). *Microbiol. Immunol.* **25**, 1025–1035.
van Opdenbosch, E., Wellemans, G., Strobbe, R., de Brabander, D. L., and Boucque, Ch. V. (1981). *Comp. Immun. Microbiol. Infect. Dis.* **4**, 293–300.
Verly, E., and Cohen, J. (1977). *J. Gen. Virol.* **35**, 583–586.

Vesikari, T., Isolauri, E., D'Hondt, E., Delem, A., Andre, F. E., and Zissis, G. (1984). *Lancet* **1**, 977–981.
Vetterling, J. M. (1965). *J. Parasitol.* **51**, 897–912.
Vetterling, J. M., Takeuchi, A., and Madden, P. A. (1971). *J. Protozool.* **18**, 248–260.
Vonderfecht, S. L., and Osburn, B. I. (1982). *J. Clin. Microbiol.* **16**, 935–942.
Waldman, S. A., O'Hanley, P., Falkow, S., Schoolnik, G., and Murad, F. (1984). *J. Infect. Dis.* **149**, 83–89.
Walters, J. R., and Sellwood, R. (1984). *Proc. Br. Soc. Anim. Protection Winter Meet. Scarborough.*
Watson, D. L., and Lascelles, A. K. (1975). *Res. Vet. Sci.* **18**, 182–185.
Weisburger, W. R., Hutcheon, D. F., Yardley, J. H., Roche, J. C., Hillis, W. D., and Charache, P. (1979). *Am. J. Clin. Pathol.* **72**, 473–478.
Weiss, M., Steck, F., and Horzinek, M. C. (1983). *J. Gen. Virol.* **64**, 1849–1858.
White, F. G., Wenham, G., Sharman, G. A. M., Jones, A. S., Rattrag, E. E. S., and McDonald, J. (1969). *Br. J. Nutr.* **23**, 847–858.
Willson, P. J., and Acres, S. D. (1982). *Can. Vet. J.* **23**, 240–246.
Wolfson, J. S., Hopkins, C. C., Weber, D. J., Richter, J. M., Waldron, M. A., and McCarthy, D. M. (1984). *New Engl. J. Med.* **310**, 788.
Wood, E. N. (1979). *Br. Vet. J.* **135**, 305–314.
Woode, G. N., Bridger, J. C., Hall, G. A., Jones, J. M., and Jackson, G. (1976). *J. Med. Microbiol.* **9**, 203–209.
Woode, G. N., Bew, M. E., and Dennis, M. J. (1978). *Vet. Rec.* **103**, 32–34.
Woode, G. N., Reed, D. E., Runnels, P. L., Herrig, M. A., and Hill, H. T. (1982). *Vet. Microbiol.* **7**, 221–240.
Woode, G. N., Kelso, N. E., Simpson, T. F., Gaul, S. K., Evans, L. E., and Babiuk, L. (1983). *J. Clin. Microbiol.* **18**, 358–364.
Woode, G. N., Pohlenz, J. F., Kelso Gourley, N. E., and Fagerland, J. A. (1984). *J. Clin. Microbiol.* **19**, 623–630.
Wright, D. H. (1966). *East Afr. Med. J.* **43**, 544–549.
Wyatt, R. G., Mebus, C. A., Yolken, R. H., Kalica, A. R., James, H. D., Jr., Kapikian, A. Z., and Chanock, R. M. (1979). *Science* **203**, 548–550.
Wyatt, R. G., Greenberg, H. B., James, W. D., Pittman, A. L., Kalica, A. R., Flores, J., Chanock, R. M., and Kapikian, A. Z. (1982). *Infect. Immun.* **37**, 110–115.
Wyatt, R. G., James, H. D., Jr., Pittman, A. L., Hoshino, Y., Greenberg, H. B., Kalica, A. R., Flores, J., and Kapikian, A. Z. (1983). *J. Clin. Microbiol.* **18**, 310–317.
Yaguchi, H., Murata, H., Kagota, K., and Namioka, S. (1980). *Br. Vet. J.* **136**, 63–70.
Yolken, R. H., Greenberg, H. B., Merson, M. H., Sack, R. B., and Kapikian, A. Z. (1977). *J. Clin. Microbiol.* **6**, 439–444.
Young, J. R., Callahan, P., Drew, W. L., and Hadley, W. K. (1980). *Curr. Chemother. Infect. Dis. Proc. Interscience Conf. Antimicrobial Agents Chemother., 19th*, pp. 939–940.
Zeissler, J., and Rassfeld-Sternberg, L. (1949). *Br. Med. J.* **1**, 267.
Zissis, G., Lambert, J. P., Marbehant, P., Marissens, D., Lobmann, M., Charlier, P., Delem, A., and Zygraich, N. (1983). *J. Infect. Dis.* **148**, 1061–1068.

Fimbriae: Relation of Intestinal Bacteria and Virulence in Animals

DWIGHT C. HIRSH

School of Veterinary Medicine
University of California
Davis, California

I.	Introduction	207
II.	The Bacterial Cell Surface	210
	A. Capsule	210
	B. Lipopolysaccharide	211
	C. Fimbriae	212
III.	The Epithelial Cell Surface	226
IV.	Fimbriae in the Clinical Setting (A Summary Statement)	228
	References	231

I. Introduction

The gastrointestinal tract is an ecosystem. The microbial flora that comprise the major part of this system do not appear to be randomly associated with the tract. Rather, the flora are associated in a unique fashion, each species or strain of microbe inhabiting that part of the tract for which it is best suited (Savage, 1970, 1972). This association is regulated by the host as well as by the microorganisms inhabiting the tract.

Microorganisms produce substances that result in a relatively stable association within an ecological niche or site in the tract. Microbial products that are important in this regard are those excreted by the microorganism as well as those expressed on its surface. Products excreted by microorganisms regulate not only the numbers of that particular species, but those of competitors as well (Impey *et al.*, 1982). Metabolic by-products, such as the short-chained fatty acids and antibiotic-like substances, the bacteriocins, are two of the most well-known substances.

Short-chained fatty acids are a metabolic by-product of the obligatory anaerobic bacteria, the major species of microbes inhabiting the gastrointestinal tract. The obligate anaerobes secrete acetic, butyric, and lactic acids which, under the conditions of the large bowel, are very toxic to other taxa of microorganisms, especially members of the family Enterobacteriaceae (Meynell, 1963; Hentges and Maier, 1970; Hentges, 1969; Bergeim *et al.*, 1941; Bergeim, 1940). The bacteriocins, on the other hand, are secreted by virtually every species of microorganism. The colicins are examples of bacteriocins secreted by members of the family Enterobacteriaceae (Nomura, 1967). Colicins inhibit microorganisms belonging to the family Enterobacteriaceae, but those species with the genetic capability to secrete a particular colicin will be immune to that particular colicin. Colicins, though active *in vitro*, have not been shown to have a demonstrable influence *in vivo* (Ikari *et al.*, 1969; Craven *et al.*, 1971).

There are structures on the surface of microorganisms that enable a microbe to become established in a particular site or niche. These substances, termed adhesins, anchor the microbe to epithelial cells that comprise or line the niche (Duguid, 1959). Many different genera have been shown to produce adhesins. Examples include *Salmonella, Escherichia, Shigella, Enterobacter, Klebsiella, Proteus, Pseudomonas,* and *Bacteroides* (Constable, 1956; Duguid, 1959; Duguid and Gillies, 1957, 1958; Duguid *et al.*, 1955, 1966, 1975, 1976, 1979; Fader *et al.*, 1982; Korhonen *et al.*, 1980; Paranchych *et al.*, 1978; Schreil and Schleich, 1955; Thornley and Horne, 1962; Watts *et al.*, 1983; Adegbola and Old, 1983; Pruzzo *et al.*, 1984). Some adhesins are involved with the initiation of disease. Adhesins are particularly important to those bacteria that are destined to inhabit, or produce disease of the small intestine. Because of the strong peristaltic movements present in the small intestine, bacteria not adhering to the epithelial surface are swept away (Abrams and Bishop, 1966; Dixon, 1960).

The epithelial cells comprising the niche also play a role in the establishment and maintainence of the ecosystem. Substances on the surface of the epithelial cell serve as receptors for bacterial adhesins. These receptors are somewhat specific in that some epithelial cells have receptors only for certain microbes, whereas other epithelial cells situated at a different location might have other receptors.

To cause disease in the gastrointestinal tract, bacterial pathogens must adhere to, and induce an abnormal behavior of, a target cell. The first step is crucial. This so-called "selective adsorption" must occur for disease to result (Savage, 1970, 1972, 1980). Selective adsorption can be prevented either by antibodies specific for antigenic determinants on the surface of the adhesin, or by other bacteria already living on the target cell (Impey et al., 1982).

Adhesins on the surface of certain strains of bacteria play a well defined, central role in the pathogenesis of the noninvasive diarrheal diseases of newborn animals. This disease is produced by strains of *Escherichia coli* possessing genes encoding information for the production of protein adhesins that have an affinity for certain target epithelial cells of the small intestine. In addition, these strains possess the genetic information to produce an exotoxin, called enterotoxin, that affects the target epithelial cells. Such strains are called enterotoxigenic *E. coli*. If a strain of *E. coli* is without either trait, disease will not be produced by that particular strain.

Enterotoxin, a plasmid-encoded protein, comes in two forms (Smith and Gyles, 1970; Smith and Linggood, 1971, 1972; Smith and Orcult, 1925). One form, labile toxin or LT, so named because of its lability to heat, is a large protein (91,000 MW and immunogenic (Clements et al., 1980). The other, stable toxin or ST, is a small protein (2000 MW and nonimmunogenic (Burgess et al., 1978, 1980). The enterotoxins affect the regulation of cyclic nucleotide activity within the cell. LT affects the adenylate cyclase system, and ST the guanylate cyclase. The mechanism of action of LT is best known. LT is composed of two subunits, A and B. The B subunit is a multimer that binds to receptors on the surface of the cell (GM_1 ganglioside), followed by the translocation of the A subunit across the cell membrane (Holmgren et al., 1982; Middlebrook and Dorland, 1984). The A subunit, after activation, cleaves nicotinamide from NAD and then couples the remaining ribosyl adenine diphosphate onto a regulatory protein of the adenylate cyclase enzyme system. This results in the deregulation of the adenylate cyclase enzyme, causing the overproduction of cyclic AMP (Gill and Richardson, 1980). The result is an active secretion of chloride ions by the epithelial cell, followed by water, sodium, and bicarbonate ions. This produces hypovolemia, metabolic acidosis, and, if the acidosis is severe, hyperkalemia (Merrit, 1980).

The objective of this article is to discuss the information known about structures on the surface of pathogenic Gram-negative microorganisms that interact with receptors on the surface of epithelial cells lining the gastrointestinal tract. Particular emphasis will be given to those strains of *E. coli* that cause disease of the gastrointestinal tract of domestic animals.

II. The Bacterial Cell Surface

The surface of a bacterial cell includes substances that govern the manner in which it interacts with the outside world. Some of these substances are those that will interact with the cells of the host.

A. CAPSULE

The capsule of a Gram-negative bacterium lies outside the cell wall. Most capsules are composed of acidic polysaccharides. The constituents are organized into different configurations, resulting in numerous antigenic determinants. As might be expected, there are a great many immunologically different types of capsules (Orskov et al., 1977; Orskov and Orskov, 1983). *Escherichia coli*, for example, produces at least 70 antigenically different types of capsule. The composite of antigenic determinants defines a particular capsular type, termed the K antigen (for the German word for capsule, Kapsule). Thus, all of the members of the family Enterobacteriaceae have K antigens if they are encapsulated. Most members of the genus *Salmonella* are unencapsulated. Those that are encapsulated express one type of capsule, termed the Vi antigen (Vi for virulence).

The polysaccharides that make up the capsule impart a hydrophilic character to the bacterial cell (Van Oss and Gillman, 1972; Stendahl et al., 1979). Since the membranes of eukaryotic cells are relatively hydrophobic, the capsular polysaccharide acts as a repelling substance (Perers et al., 1977; Weir and Ogmundsdottir, 1977). This is an advantage to extracellular pathogenic microorganisms since they would be destroyed if ingested by phagocytic cells. Encapsulated microorganisms, on the other hand, suffer no such fate because of the repulsive forces that occur between the hydrophilic capsular substance and the hydrophobic membrane of the phagocytic cell. Antibodies binding to the antigenic determinants on the surface of the capsule increase the hydrophobicity of the bacterial particle (Magnusson et al., 1978, 1979; Magnusson and Stjernstrom, 1981; Stjernstrom et al., 1977; Stendahl et al., 1974; Edebo et al., 1980). Likewise, complement components enhance the hydrophobicity of the cell surface (Horwitz and Silverstein, 1980; Stjernstrom et al., 1977). In addition, there are receptors on the surface of phagocytic cells for antibodies and the complement components. Thus, the increase in hydrophobicity together with antibody and complement-binding receptors on the surface of the phagocytic cell serve to bring about close apposition of the two surfaces, bacterial and phagocytic. Such apposition is necessary if phagocytosis is to occur.

Other nonimmune mechanisms may bring encapsulated bacteria in contact with the surface of a host cell. Certain proteins (lectins) on the surface of host cells have an affinity for carbohydrates, and the carbohydrates in the capsule of certain strains of bacteria are attracted to these lectins. Clearance of certain Gram-negative organisms, *E. coli,* for example, has been shown to occur by this mechanism (Tavendale *et al.,* 1983; Perry and Ofek, 1984).

B. LIPOPOLYSACCHARIDE

Lipopolysaccharide lies just beneath the capsule. This substance is part of, and extrudes from, the outer membrane of the Gram-negative cell wall. The lipid portion of this substance is embedded in the outer membrane and has the toxic properties associated with endotoxin. The polysaccharide portion protrudes to the exterior of the bacterial cell and may be covered by the capsule, if one is present. The carbohydrate portion of the lipopolysaccharide is made up of hexoses, including the unusual dideoxyhexoses. The type of linkage between the various sugars, as well as the kinds and number of sugars, present different spatial configurations and, therefore, different antigenic determinants. As with capsules, different antigenic determinants generate many different types. These antigens describe the O or somatic antigens of the Gram-negative bactrium. For members of the family Enterobacteriaceae, O-antigens form the basis for serological typing schemes. For *E. coli,* for example, there are 164 different O-antigens (Orskov *et al.,* 1977).

Lipopolysaccharide, when attached to the bacterial cell, imparts a hydrophilic nature to the particle. This property is due to carbohydrate protruding from the lipid backbone. As with the capsule, this characteristic decreases the potential for association with cell membranes of the host (Van Oss and Gillman, 1972). The role that lipopolysaccharide plays as an adhesin is not known. Without other adhesive structures, however, bacteria expressing only lipopolysaccharide on their surfaces will not adhere to eukaryotic cell membranes (Magnusson *et al.,* 1980; Stendahl *et al.,* 1973, 1979). Deletions of portions of the polysaccharide side chain will result in an increase in hydrophobicity, and, in turn, an increase in association with the eukaryotic cell membrane (Magnusson *et al.*, 1980). Rough mutants of Gram-negative bacteria are less virulent than smooth ones. An increase in relative hydrophobicity may, in large part, account for this observation. Likewise, IgG on the surface of smooth *Salmonella* will result in an increase in the hydrophobicity of the particles which then become more associated with neutrophils (Stendahl *et al.*, 1974; Stjernstrom *et al.*, 1977).

Aside from contributing to our ability to serologically define strains of bacteria, the role of the lipopolysaccharide in the life style of the bacterium is unclear. Certainly, lipopolysaccharide possesses toxic activities and it may be a true virulence determinant. This notion is strengthened by the fact that antibodies to lipopolysaccharide will protect the host from septic shock (Johns *et al.*, 1983; Konstantinov *et al.*, 1982; Morrison, 1983).

C. Fimbriae

The most important adhesins appear to be the whiskerlike protrusions from the bacterial cell wall. These structures have been called various names, two of the more common being fimbriae or pili (Brinton, 1959; Duguid *et al.*, 1955, 1966). The term fimbriae will be used herein because of historical precedence (Duguid *et al.*, 1955).

Evidence that fimbriae existed was first reported in 1908, following the observation that certain strains of bacteria agglutinated red blood cells (Guyot, 1908). Proof that fimbriae were responsible for hemagglutination included the finding that only those strains that produce fimbriae (as demonstrated by electron microscopy) hemagglutinate, and antibodies against the fimbriae inhibit hemagglutination (Anderson, 1949; Duguid *et al.*, 1955; Houwink and Van Iterson, 1950; Salit and Gotschlich, 1977a,b; Schreil and Schleich, 1955).

Studies of the interaction between erythrocytes and bacteria expressing fimbriae resulted in the discovery that certain substances, in particular mannose-containing carbohydrates, affected the hemagglutinating reaction (Collier and De Miranda, 1955; Collier and Jacoeb, 1955). Hemagglutinating microorganisms were subdivided into two groups, those whose hemagglutination reaction was inhibited by mannose (mannose-sensitive hemagglutination), and those not inhibited (mannose-resistant hemagglutination). Microorganisms, especially *E. coli*, expressing mannose-resistant adhesins (hemagglutinins) are intimately involved with diarrheal diseases of the neonatal farm animal.

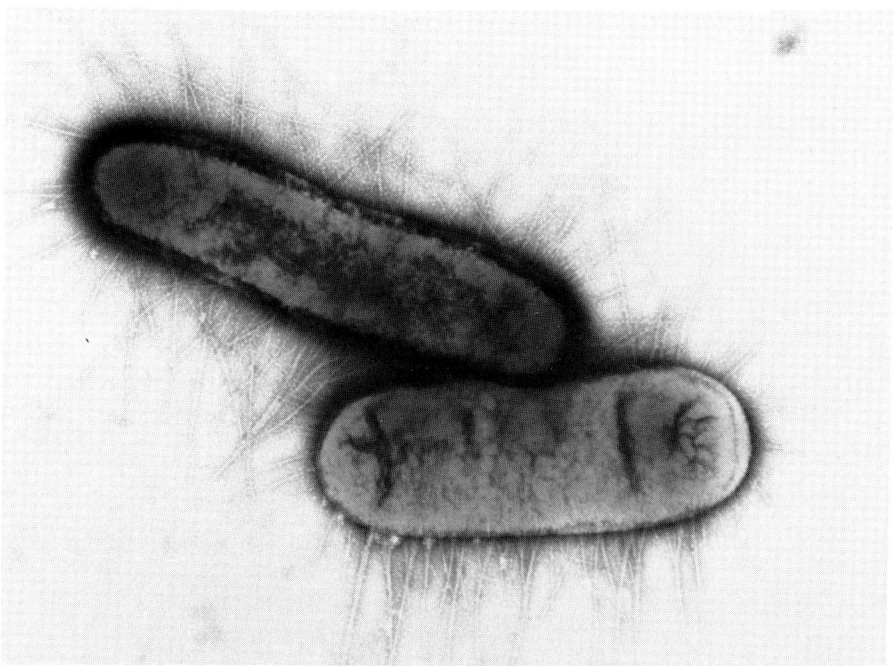

FIG. 1. Transmission electron micrograph demonstrating the expression of type 1 fimbriae on the surface of a wild strain of *Escherichia coli*. (Photograph kindly provided by J. S. Ikeda, University of California, Davis.)

1. *Type 1 or Common Fimbriae*

Type 1 fimbriae are rigid structures, 7 nm in diameter and up to 100 nm in length, with approximately 300–400 per cell (Fig. 1) (Abraham *et al.*, 1983; Anderson, 1949; Brinton, 1959; Brinton *et al.*, 1964; Duguid *et al.*, 1955; Isaacson and Richter, 1981). In three dimensions, they appear as coiled springs complete with hollow centers (Abraham *et al.*, 1983; Brinton, 1965). Fimbriae are made of identical protein subunits hooked together noncovalently, $3\frac{1}{8}$ subunits per turn (Abraham *et al.*, 1983; Brinton, 1965). The molecular weight of the subunit varies with the species and strain of bacteria. The molecular weight of the subunit of type 1 fimbriae from *E. coli* strain K-12 (a laboratory strain) is 17,000 (Abraham *et al.*, 1983; Dodd and Eisenstein, 1982; Eshdat *et al.*, 1981; Salit and Gotschlich 1977b; Brinton, 1965), whereas the molecular weight of the subunit of a fimbria from a clinical isolate of *E. coli* is 19,000 (Dodd and Eiserstein, 1982), for *Salmonella* it is 21,000 (Korhonen et al., 1980), and for *Klebsiella*, 21,500 (Fader et al., 1982).

The structure responsible for mannose-sensitive hemagglutination is found on more than half of the members of the family Enterobacteriaceae (Duguid and Gillies, 1957; Duguid et al., 1955, 1975, 1979). This chromosomally encoded structure has been termed type 1 or common fimbria (Brinton and Baron, 1960; Brinton et al., 1961; Hull et al., 1981). Bacteria expressing this type of fimbria agglutinate erythrocytes from a variety of species of animal, but erythrocytes of the guinea pig are most commonly used (Constable, 1956; Duguid, 1959; Duguid and Gillies, 1957, 1958; Duguid et al., 1966; Fader et al., 1982; Kauffmann, 1948). Other, less commonly considered items agglutinated by bacteria expressing this fimbria are molds (*Aspergillus* and *Penicillium*), *Trichomonas vaginalis*, baker's yeast, and pollen granules (Duguid, 1959; Duguid et al., 1966; Korhonen, 1979; Rosenthal, 1943). In addition to mannose, the hemagglutination reaction is inhibited by strucures or compounds containing this sugar, such as yeast mannan (Bar-Shavit et al., 1977).

Expression of type 1 fimbriae *in vitro* depends upon the conditons of culture. Type 1 fimbriae, as with all the fimbriae studied, are not expressed if bacteria are grown at 15–20°C or over 44°C (Duguid et al., 1955, 1966). Nutritionally rich media tend to suppress expression, as does glucose, whereas minimal media promote expression (Collier and Jacoeb, 1955; Salit and Gotschlich, 1977b). Static culture conditions, resulting in poor oxygen diffusion (but not anaerobic conditions), promote expression of type 1 fimbriae (Brinton, 1965; Duguid et al., 1955, 1966; Ofek et al., 1977). In liquid media, fimbrianated bacteria form a pellicle (Duguid et al., 1966), and on agar surfaces (e.g., nutrient agar) such strains form smaller, more dense colonies than nonfimbrianated (Salit and Gotschlich, 1977b; Brinton, 1959).

Amino acid analysis of the type 1 fimbria reveals the presence of a disproportionately large amount of hydrophobic amino acids, explaining the increased relative hydrophobicity of fimbrianated strains (Salit and Gotschlich, 1977b; Lindahl et al., 1981; Brinton, 1965; Van Oss and Gillman, 1972). Though this finding is significant, the relative hydrophobicity of strains of *E. coli* bearing type 1 fimbriae is less than strains bearing other known fimbrial adhesins (Faris et al., 1981; Lindahl et al., 1981).

The relationship between the various type 1 fimbriae, as judged by amino acid sequence homology, is somewhat confused. The N-terminus of the type 1 fimbria of *Klebsiella pneumoniae*, for example, is 79% homologous with the type 1 fimbria of *Salmonella typhimurium*, but dissimiliar to the common fimbria of *Pseudomonas aeruginosa* (Fader et al., 1982). Yet, strains expressing these fimbriae hemagglutinate erythrocytes; a hemagglutination inhibited by D-mannose.

Gram-negative bacteria expressing type 1 fimbriae adhere to epithelial cells of various animal species (Firon et al., 1984; Isaacson et al., 1978a; Ofek and Beachey, 1978; Runnels et al., 1980; Salit and Gotschlich, 1977a; Duguid et al., 1966; Fader et al., 1979). This adherence is reversibly inhibited by D-mannose and substances containing this carbohydrate (Fader et al., 1979; Ofek et al., 1977). Although this adhesion may be useful for habitation of the surface of an epithelial cell that comprises an ecological niche, it does have liabilities for the microbe. Bacteria expressing type 1 fimbriae associate with the cell membrane of phagocytic cells as well (Bar-Shavit et al., 1977, 1980; Rottini et al., 1979; Silverblatt et al., 1979; Bjorksten and Wadstrom, 1982; Leunk and Moon, 1982). In fact, this adhesion is probably a major means by which bacteria that are not opsonized by antibodies and/or complement become associated with phagocytic cells. Antibodies to fimbriae do not enhance opsonization nor complement-mediated bacteriolysis, but instead reduce phagocytosis of bacteria, presumably by decreasing the hydrophobicity imparted by the presence of the fimbriae (Weinstein and Silverblatt, 1983). Binding to phagocytic cells usually brings about ingestion, but not necessarily so (Ohmann et al., 1982; Silverblatt et al., 1979; Rottini et al., 1979; Bar-Shavit et al., 1980). The receptor for fimbriae on the phagocytic cell is thought to be a major outermembrane, mannose-containing glycoprotein of 140,000 MW. Binding to this receptor may be the crucial event in phagocytosis of bacteria expressing type 1 fimbriae (Perry et al., 1983; Williams and Becker, 1984). The adhesion is not dependent upon any enzymatic process or temperature conditions (Fader et al., 1979; Bar-Shavit et al., 1977; Salit and Gotschlich, 1977a). In addition to having an affinity for cell membranes, type 1 fimbriae bind to lysozyme (McMichael and Ou, 1979). This may be another host-defence mechanism aimed at fimbrianated bacteria that gain entrance into the host.

There is a suggestion that capsule, a mannose-resistant hemagglutinin (e.g., K88), and type 1 fimbriae act together to enhance adherence of pathogenic strains of *E. coli* to target epithelial cells, i.e., that type 1 fimbriae might be a virulence determinant (Knutton et al., 1983). Vaccination of dams with type 1 fimbriae, however, does not result in protection of offspring from enteric disease following challenge with enterotoxigenic *E. coli* expressing both type 1 fimbriae and a mannose-resistant hemagglutinin virulence determinant. This was so even though antibodies against type 1 fimbriae were present in colostrum, serum, or milk (Levine et al., 1982; To et al., 1984). The results of these trials also confirm that the receptors on the target intestinal epithelial cells are specific for each of the different types of fimbria, i.e., *E. coli* expressing type 1 fimbriae will not prevent binding to an epithelial cell by *E. coli* expressing another fimbria, such as K88 (Isaacson et al., 1978a).

The function of the type 1 fimbria is unknown. Evidence gathered to date indicates that this type of fimbria is not involved in the pathogenesis of disease, even when carried or expressed by a pathogenic strain of a bacterium, though such strains will be found in the feces following oral challenge for longer periods of time (Duguid et al., 1976). It has been suggested that type 1 fimbriae are involved with the adherence of bacteria to epithelial cells that comprise the ecological niche for those particular microorganisms (Duguid and Gillies, 1957).

2. K88 Fimbriae

The small intestine of the normal neonatal animal contains very few bacteria (Smith and Jones, 1963). A major reason for this is thought to be the strong propulsive forces exerted on the lumenal contents by peristalsis (Dixon, 1960). Animals with diarrheal disease, on the other hand, have large numbers of bacteria, mainly *E. coli,* in the lumen of the small intestine (Bertschinger et al., 1971; Carpenter and Woods, 1924; Saunders et al., 1963; Smith and Jones, 1963; Smith and Orcutt, 1925; Lariviere et al., 1975). This important observation was the first clue that certain strains of *E. coli* may be the cause of the diarrheal syndrome observed in the neonatal animal. A major obstacle to this hypothesis was that an explanation was needed to account for the multiplication of such strains in such an active environment. Thus, proposals were made that, if *E. coli* was to cause disease in the small intestine, the organism had to adhere to the epithelial cells (Arbuckle, 1970; Drucker et al., 1967; Smith and Halls, 1968).

Studies of the surface structures of *E. coli* strain E68 revealed that this strain had a surface component in addition to, and different from, the carbohydrate capsule (Kelen et al., 1959; Orskov et al., 1961). At this time, it was believed that strain E68 had two different types of capsule. Basic to this difference was that one of the capsule types was heat labile (then designated as an L-type capsule) (Kauffman, 1943; Orskov et al., 1961). This heat-labile surface structure of strain E68 was given the designation K88 because it was serologically distinct from other K antigens so far described.

In time, the K88 antigen was found to be different in a number of ways from the classic K antigens, the most significant difference being that it was protein rather than polysaccharide (Mooi and de Graaf, 1979; Stirm et al., 1967b).

The K88 antigen is a fimbrial structure, seen as fine filaments under the electron microscope (Stirm et al., 1967a). The fimbriae are composed of subunits, 23,000 MW, that are linked together noncovalently to make a structure 4.8 nm in diameter and approximately 100–500 nm long (Pearce et al., 1980).

The genes responsible for the production of K88 are plasmid encoded (Orskov et al., 1964; Stirm et al., 1967a,b; Bak et al., 1972; Orskov and Orskov, 1966; Orskov et al., 1961). Most isolates possess these genes on nonconjugal plasmids of approximately 50 MDa in size (Shipley et al., 1978; Bak et al., 1972; Orskov and Orskov, 1966). Occasionally, conjugal plasmids containing the K88 genes are found, apparently the result of the insertion of a fertility factor (transfer factor) onto a nonconjugal K88 fimbria-encoding plasmid (Bak et al., 1972). In addition, the ability to use raffinose as a carbon source is linked to the genes encoding the K88 fimbria, a useful phenotypic trait when studying transfer of the plasmid (Shipley et al., 1978).

The genes involved with the synthesis of the K88 fimbria are on a 4.3-MDa fragment of DNA, upon which four cistrons responsible for the synthesis of six polypeptides involved in the production of the K88 fimbria are found (Kehoe et al., 1981; Mooi et al., 1981). These genes encode information not only for the subunit, but also for the proteins responsible for translocation of the subunit from the periplasmic space, where it is extruded following translation, to the exterior of the bacterial cell (Mooi et al., 1983).

The K88 fimbria is expressed when bacteria possessing the appropriate plasmid grow at 37°C, but not at 18°C (Isaacson et al., 1977; Jones and Rutter, 1972, 1974; Sellwood et al., 1975). The attachment phase is not temperature dependent, occurring at 4 or 37°C (Sellwood et al., 1975). Expression of the fimbrial protein *in vitro* is dependent upon the medium employed. A medium containing essential salts, citric acid, and glucose (E medium) seems to be the best, although Minca medium may be equally satisfactory (Francis et al., 1982).

There are three serologically detectable variations of the K88 fimbria: K88ab, K88ac, and K88ad (Guinee et al., 1977; Orskov et al., 1964). The "a" portion of each of the variants is conserved and is thought to be the portion responsible for the adherence of the fimbria to the receptor on the epithelial cell (Mooi and de Graaf, 1979).

Expression of the K88 fimbria increases the relative hydrophobicity of the bacterial cell (Lindahl et al., 1981; Smyth et al., 1978). The degree of hydrophobicity is more than that endowed by the type 1 fimbria, but less than that contributed by other fimbrial proteins, such as colonization factor antigens (Lindahl et al., 1981). This increase in hydrophobicity is directly related to the fimbrial protein, which is composed of a large number of hydrophobic amino acids, especially at the C-terminus (Klemm, 1981; Gaastra et al., 1979). Expression of such proteins, when in the lumen of the bowel, enhances adhesion to the epithelial cell surface. Adhesion is strongest if the receptor for the K88 fimbria is also present on the host epithelial cell. Perhaps the hydrophobic interaction helps to stabilize the fimbriae–epithelial cell union in a manner similar to that proposed for the capsule (Chan et al., 1982). Bacteria expressing K88 fimbriae adhere to phagocytic cells as well. Indeed, salmonellae, into which the plasmid encoding K88 fimbria has been placed, are less virulent than K88-negative strains following parenteral injection (Smith and Linggood, 1971).

Escherichia coli strains expressing K88 fimbriae agglutinate guinea pig erythrocytes (Jones and Rutter, 1974; Stirm et al., 1967a; Gibbons et al., 1975). Mannose or mannose-containing substances do not interfere with this reaction, which is a mannose-resistant hemagglutination (Jones and Rutter, 1974). The substances that are most inhibitory to hemagglutination are the β-D-galactosides (Gibbons et al., 1975).

The K88 fimbria plays a central role in the pathogenesis of the diarrheal disease of the newborn pig. This disease is not the result of invasion by the enteropathogen. The strains of *E. coli* that produce this disease, enterotoxigenic *E. coli*, adhere to the target cell, in this case the epithelial cells of the small intestine, and produce enterotoxin (Anderson et al., 1980; Hohmann and Wilson, 1975; Isaacson et al., 1977; Jones and Rutter, 1972; Runnels et al., 1980; Sellwood et al., 1975; Smith and Linggood, 1971; Wilson and Hohmann, 1974; Deneke et al., 1984). The key to the initiation or production of this disease is the ability of the enterotoxigenic *E. coli* to adhere to the target epithelial cell. The target epithelial cell is sensitive to the action of the toxin, whereas other cells of the tract are not as sensitive (Smith and Halls, 1967). If the bacteria do not adhere, disease will not occur (Smith and Linggood, 1971). A major strategy in the prevention of this disease is to elicit the production of antibodies specific for the adhesins. Such antibodies adhere to the fimbriae and prohibit the adherence of the fimbriae and, therefore, the bacteria to the epithelial cell surface (Jones and Rutter, 1972; Sellwood et al., 1975; Wilson et al., 1974). Inhibition of adhesion is due in part to steric hindrance, and in part to the hydrophilic character of the secretory immunoglobulins found in intestinal secretions, colostrum, or milk (Magnusson et al., 1978, 1979, 1981). There is also evidence that antibodies to surface constitutents other than K88 fimbriae will induce the loss of the plasmid and, thus, the ability to express the fimbria in vivo (Porter and Linggood, 1983).

Most enterotoxigenic E. coli isolated from the small intestine of newborn pigs suffering from enterotoxigenic diarrhea express the K88 fimbria (Gyles et al., 1974; Moon et al., 1980; Wittig, 1965). Strains expressing this fimbria are rarely found in the intestinal tract of normal pigs (Gyles et al., 1974). Aside from 987P, another fimbria discussed below, strains expressing the other adhesins related to virulence, such as K99 and F41, are not commonly found on enterotoxigenic E. coli isolated from pigs (Guinee and Jansen, 1979). Thus, preparations containing K88 fimbriae have been used to immunize sows in order that antibodies to antigenic determinants on the K88 fimbria would be passed to their offspring. The rationale for this approach stems from the finding that antibodies specific for the K88 fimbria block adhesion of bacteria expressing this fimbria to intestinal epithelial cells (Jones and Rutter, 1972; Sellwood et al., 1975; Wilson and Hohmann, 1974). Sows immunized with products containing K88 fimbriae produce colostrum that contains antibodies to the K88 antigen (Svendsen and Wilson, 1971). Piglets ingesting this colostrum, or given colostral whey, show a significant reduction in mortality when challenged with K88-expressing strains of enterotoxigenic E. coli, even though they develop diarrhea (Svendsen and Wilson, 1971; Smith, 1972; Rutter and Jones, 1972; Rutter et al., 1976). The small intestine and feces of baby pigs suckling sows that were not given K88 protein contain large numbers of the K88-positive challenge strain (Moon et al., 1968; Smith and Halls, 1968; Rutter et al., 1976). Antibodies to the b or c variant will only bind to those strains carrying that particular determinant. For example, antibodies to K88ab will not block strains with K88ac from binding to their target cell (Wilson et al., 1974). An interesting, and as yet unexplainable, finding is that even though the K88 antigen is the most important, capsules and somatic antigens play some role since the best protection is seen when the vaccine and the challenge strain are the same (Smith, 1972). The role played by these other surface structures in the elicitation of antibodies which will induce the loss of the plasmid encoding K88 fimbriae has been eluded to above (Porter and Linggood, 1983). Such loss might help explain the added protection observed with homologous vaccination and challenge. Colostrum from the sow also contains glycoproteins that are similiar to the receptors for the K88 fimbria (Gibbons et al., 1975). Conceivably, these colostral glycoproteins compete with the target epithelial cell for enterotoxigenic E. coli expressing K88 fimbriae.

3. K99 Fimbriae

Enterotoxigenic E. coli, producing disease in calves and lambs, most often possess the adhesin, K99 (Orskov et al., 1975). This adhesin is 5–8 nm in diameter, approximately 50–300 nm in length, and helical in shape (Isaacson et al., 1977; de Graaf et al., 1981). Morphologically, the fimbriae appear as hairlike protrusions from the surface of the bacterial cell (de Graaf et al., 1980b). As in the case of the other adhesins so far discussed, the K99 fimbria is a protein composed of subunits 18,500 MW (de Graaf and Roorda, 1982). Earlier studies had found that the molecular weight of the subunit of the K99 fimbria was larger than this value (22,500–29,500), and preparations of fimbrial protein seemed to be composed of two chemically different subunits (Isaacson, 1977; Morris et al., 1978; Isaacson et al., 1981). These studies describe anionic and cationic components in preparations of fimbrial proteins (Morris et al., 1978). These two components were later found to be two different fimbriae, K99 and one subsequently named F41, so named because it was isolated from the E. coli strain B41 (Morris et al., 1980a, 1982). The K99 fimbria was the cationic component, with an isoelectric point of 9–10 (de Graaf et al., 1981; Isaacson, 1977; Morris et al., 1980a, 1982).

The genes encoding the K99 fimbria are most often found on conjugal plasmids (Orskov et al., 1975; de Graaf et al., 1980b). There are seven genes responsible for the production of the K99 fimbria (de Graaf et al., 1984). One gene encodes information for a protein of 18.2 kDa in size that is responsible for adherence and is the subunit for the K99 fimbria (de Graaf et al., 1984). The size of the segment of DNA responsible for the production of the K99 fimbria is about 4.4–4.6 MDa (de Graaf et al., 1984; Van Embden et al., 1980). A deletion in any of the genes results in K99 fimbria not being expressed. Although there is little homology between DNA encoding the K88 fimbria and that encoding the K99 fimbria, there are enough data to prompt the suggestion that they have a common ancestor (Kehoe et al., 1982).

Expression of the K99 adhesin *in vitro* is important from a diagnostic standpoint. As with other adhesins, expression of K99 is dependent upon the temperature of growth, 18 up to 30°C inhibiting expression, and 37°C promoting it (Burrows et al., 1976; de Graaf et al., 1980b). A medium that is too rich is inhibitory, especially one containing the amino acid alanine (de Graaf et al., 1980a,b; Orskov et al., 1975).

Glucose, pyruvate, arabinose, and lactose have been shown to be repressive as well (Guinee et al., 1977; Isaacson, 1980). Cyclic AMP and glycerol are stimulatory (Isaacson, 1980). The best medium is reported to be E agar, though Minca plus 1% isovitelex, without glucose, is satisfactory (Guinee et al., 1977). Nutrient agar or broth do not seem to be as useful because, as claimed by some, they promote the production of capsule, which will mask the fimbriae (de Graaf et al., 1980b; Isaacson, 1980). Aeration stimulates the production of K99 fimbriae (de Graaf et al., 1980b; Isaacson, 1980).

Bacteria possessing K99 fimbriae agglutinate erythrocytes, in particular those of sheep or horses (Morris et al., 1980a, 1982; Orskov et al., 1975). Hemagglutination is not inhibited by mannose (Morris et al., 1980a, 1982). *Escherichia coli* possessing the genes for the production of the K99 fimbrial protein express this substance *in vivo* and will stick to the brush borders of the epithelial cells of the jejunum and ileum of the lamb, calf, and pig (Burrows et al., 1976; Francis, 1983; Isaacson et al., 1978a; Runnels et al., 1980; Deneke et al., 1984).

The degree of hydrophobicity imparted to bacteria expressing K99 fimbriae is similiar to that imparted by the K88 fimbria (Lindahl et al., 1981). It would be expected that bacteria expressing K99 fimbriae would be at the same degree of risk to phagocytosis as those expressing K88 fimbriae, but this has not been determined.

The distribution of K99-positive strains of *E. coli* is such that most come from calves, though some isolates of enterotoxigenic *E. coli* expressing K99 fimbriae have come from pigs that are less than 2 weeks of age (Guinee and Jansen, 1979; Isaacson et al., 1978b; Moon et al., 1976, 1980). There is a positive correlation between the expression of the K99 fimbria and the ability to produce enterotoxin (Guinee and Jansen, 1979; Isaacson et al., 1978b; Moon et al., 1976; Myers and Guinee, 1976).

Antibodies to the antigenic determinants expressed by K99 fimbriae prevent bacteria that express this adhesin from hemagglutinating or sticking to intestinal epithelial cells (Burrows et al., 1976; Isaacson et al., 1978a). Immunization of cows (heifers) or ewes with products containing K99 fimbriae result in the passive transfer of antibodies to this adhesin with protection of the calf or lamb from disease produced by K99-expressing strains of enterotoxigenic *E. coli*. Calves or lambs ingesting colostrum from immunized dams show better weight gains, less depression, and have diarrhea for a shorter period of time than control animals following challenge with K99-possessing enterotoxigenic *E. coli*. Furthermore, death losses among offspring of vaccinates are insignificant when compared to controls (Acres et al., 1979, 1982;

Morris et al., 1980b; Nagy, 1980; Sherman et al., 1983; Sojka et al., 1978). Similiar results are seen with baby pigs nursing sows vaccinated (as gilts) with K99 fimbriae (Morgan et al., 1978). Passive protection is directly correlated with the titer of specific IgG in colostrum (Acres et al., 1979; Morris et al., 1980b). Animals ingesting antibodies to K99 fimbriae possessed fewer bacteria expressing K99 fimbriae (usually in numbers so low as to be undetectable) in their small bowel as compared to those not ingesting specific antibody (Morgan et al., 1978). There is evidence that the capsule may play some role in the pathogenesis of diarrhea induced by enterotoxigenic E. coli (expressing K99 fimbriae). Ewes vaccinated with K99 fimbriae transfer antibodies to this protein, but lambs from vaccinated ewes, when challenged with a mucoid strain (heavily encapsulated) of K99-expressing, enterotoxigenic E. coli, were sicker (Sojka et al., 1978).

4. 987P Fimbriae

Shortly after the adhesins K88 and K99 were described, a strain of E. coli without either adhesin was isolated from the small intestine of a baby pig with diarrhea. This strain, number 987, adhered to the epithelia of the ileum and the jejunum (Nagy et al., 1976; Isaacson et al., 1977). Subsequently, strain 987 was shown to possess a new, undescribed fimbria termed 987P (Nagy et al., 1976, 1977). This fimbria does not hemagglutinate erythrocytes from guinea pigs and only weakly agglutinates chicken erythrocytes, but it forms a pellicle in liquid media, a trait displayed by most, if not all, fimbrianated bacteria (Aning et al., 1983; Isaacson et al., 1977; Nagy et al., 1977).

The 987P fimbria is rod-shaped, 7 nm in diameter, and morphologically similiar to type 1 fimbriae (Isaacson et al., 1977; Isaacson and Richter, 1981). The subunit has a molecular weight of 20,000 (Isaacson and Richter, 1981).

Production of the fimbria in vitro is best demonstrated if the E. coli is cultured in Minca broth with isovitalex, or E broth, though blood-containing agar is satisfactory (Francis et al., 1982).

Bacteria expressing 987P fimbriae are enriched in the small intestine of the baby pig (Nagy et al., 1977). This is due to the production of the fimbria in vivo and subsequent adhesion and growth (Francis, 1983; Isaacson et al., 1978a; Nagy et al., 1976).

Antibodies to 987P fimbriae block adhesion of bacteria expressing this protein to ileal and jejunal epithelial cells (Isaacson et al., 1978a). Baby pigs ingesting colostrum from sows vaccinated as gilts with products containing 987P will have, following challenge, better weight gain, shorter duration of diarrhea, a very low incidence of mortality, and a decrease in the adherence and duration of shedding of the challenge strain (Morgan et al., 1987; Nagy et al., 1978). Baby pigs are not protected following challenge with enterotoxigenic *E. coli* expressing 987P fimbriae if sows are vaccinated with K99 fimbriae (Morgan et al., 1978).

5. F41 Fimbriae

Escherichia coli strain B41, isolated from a calf with diarrhea, possesses K99 fimbriae. If, however, fimbriae are isolated from B41 and subjected to electrophoresis, two different proteins are observed; one anionic, the other cationic. The cationic protein was found to be the K99 fimbria, the anionic protein, at that time, had not been described (Morris et al., 1978, 1980a). The anionic protein was different from the K99 fimbria, being serologically unrelated (Morris et al., 1982). It was shown that this protein was another adhesin, subsequently named F41. In addition, strains expressing F41 are almost totally restricted to the 09 and 0101 serogroups (Morris et al., 1980a).

The F41 fimbria is about 3 nm in diameter and filamentous in morphology (de Graaf and Roordan, 1982; To, 1984). The subunit size is 29,500 MW with an isoelectric point of 4.6, thereby explaining its anionic behavior (de Graaf and Roorda, 1982).

Escherichia coli expresses F41 *in vitro* when grown at 37°C on E or Minca media (de Graaf and Roorda, 1982). The synthesis of F41 is repressed at 18°C and in the presence of alanine (de Graaf and Roorda, 1982).

Strains expressing F41 display hemagglutinating activity with guinea pig and human (type A) erythrocytes and weak activity with equine and ovine cells (de Graaf and Roorda, 1982; Morris et al., 1980a). The hemagglutinating activity is not inhibited with mannose (Morris et al., 1980a).

Enterotoxigenic *E. coli* expressing F41 are isolated most frequently from the small intestine of calves with diarrhea (Morris et al., 1980a, 1983; To, 1984). Most of these strains also express K99 fimbriae, though strains expressing only F41 have been isolated from pigs (Morris et al., 1983). *Escherichia coli* expressing F41 fimbriae adhere to epithelial cells from the jejunum and ileum of the calf and pig (Morris et al., 1982; To, 1984).

6. CFA Fimbriae

Adhesins that mediate adherence of enterotoxigenic *E. coli* to human small intestinal epithelial cells are called "colonization factor antigens" or CFA. CFA/I, the originally discovered adhesin, was demonstrated on enterotoxigenic *E. coli* strain H-10407, which was isolated from the feces of a human affected with a diarrheal disease. There are three serologically distinct varieties of CFA: CFA/I, CFA/II, and CFA/III (Honda *et al.*, 1984).

The adhesin CFA/I, perhaps the most well studied, is a fimbria 7 nm in diameter, composed of subunits originally described to be between 14,000 and 23,800 MW but shown by amino acid sequence analysis to be 15,058 MW (Evans *et al.*, 1979; Klemm, 1979, 1982). There is little homology between the amino acid sequences of type 1, K88, and the CFA fimbriae (Klemm, 1979, 1982). On the other hand, evidence suggests that there may be some relationship between K99 and CFA fimbriae. For example, GM_2-glycoconjugates inhibit hemagglutination mediated by K99 and CFA fimbriae and a monoclonal antibody made against the CFA/I fimbria will react with K99 fimbriae (Worobec *et al.*, 1983; Faris *et al.*, 1980).

The genes encoding CFA fimbriae are carried on conjugal plasmids (Evans *et al.*, 1975; 1977b; McConnell *et al.*, 1981; Smith *et al.*, 1979). These plasmids appear to prefer some bacterial hosts to others, an observation reflected in the limited number of serotypes expressing CFA fimbriae (Evans and Evans, 1978; Orskov and Orskov, 1977). Strains of enterotoxigenic *E. coli* expressing CFA/I fimbriae and ST carry a single plasmid encoding for ST production and for CFA/I expression (Evans *et al.*, 1977a; McConnell *et al.*, 1981).

Expression of CFA fimbriae is temperature dependent, occurring optimally at 37°C, and not at 18°C (Evans *et al.*, 1977b, 1978a). The best medium appears to be one containing casamino acids and yeast extract, called CFA medium (Evans *et al.*, 1977b; Cheney *et al.*, 1983), although some recommend peptone water (Evans *et al.*, 1978a).

The CFA fimbria mediates agglutination of human (type A), bovine, chicken, and guinea pig erythrocytes, whereas CFA/II hemagglutinates bovine but not human (type A) cells (Evans *et al.*, 1979; Evans and Evans, 1978). No hemagglutination has been observed with CFA/III (Honda *et al.*, 1984). When hemagglutination occurs, it is not inhibited by mannose, but by GM_2-glycoconjugates (Faris *et al.*, 1980; Evans and Evans, 1978; Evans *et al.*, 1979).

The relative hydrophobicity imparted to strains expressing CFA fimbriae is the most of all fimbriae studied (Faris *et al.*, 1981; Lindahl *et al.*, 1981). This is due to the high proportion of hydrophobic amino acids present in the protein subunits of this fimbria (Evans *et al.*, 1979; Klemm, 1979, 1982; Honda *et al.*, 1984).

CFA fimbriae mediate adherence to intestinal epithelial cells of the small intestine (Cheney and Boedeker, 1983). Enterotoxigenic *E. coli* without CFA will not cause sickness in humans, but diarrhea will result following ingestion of enterotoxigenic *E. coli* expressing CFA (Evans *et al.,* 1978b). *Escherichia coli* expressing CFA are isolated from intestinal, but not from extraintestinal sources, e.g., urinary tract, cerebral spinal fluid, or blood (Cravioto *et al.,* 1979).

Enterotoxigenic *E. coli* expressing CFA are usually the cause of diarrhea suffered by travelers and newborn infants, though a limited number of common source outbreaks have been reported to be caused by these strains (Evans and Evans, 1978; Evans *et al.,* 1977a, 1978a; Wood *et al.,* 1983; Ryder *et al.,* 1976; Changchawalit *et al.,* 1984; Pickering *et al.,* 1977; Sack *et al.,* 1977; Shore *et al.,* 1974).

7. Miscellaneous Adhesins

Members of the genus *Salmonella,* as well as invasive strains of *E. coli,* seem to have an affinity for certain target cells, i.e., epithelial cells of the lower small bowel and the upper large bowel. It has been difficult, however, to identify special, virulence-determining adhesins on the surface of these microorganisms.

Invasive strains of *E. coli,* isolated most often from tissue of lambs and calves, possess certain qualities that allow survival and multiplication within the circulatory system and tissues of the host. In addition, these strains possess a plasmid, termed vir, encoding for adhesins responsible for adherence to the surface of the intestinal epithelial cells prior to invasion (Lopez–Alvarez and Gyles, 1980; Weinstein and Silverblatt, 1983; Smith, 1962). Since the vir genes are necessary for pathogenicity, it must be assumed that adhesion to the epithelial cell is also necessary.

Members of the genus *Salmonella* have adhesins. There is disagreement in the literature as to whether type 1 fimbriae or another, as yet to be described, mannose-resistant adhesin is responsible for adherence to epithelial cells prior to initiation of disease. Disease is produced subsequent to the secretion of both an enterotoxin-like exotoxin that deregulates cyclic nucleotide synthesis and an exotoxin that interrupts protein synthesis of the target cell (a cytoxin) (Koupal and Deibel, 1975; Koo *et al.,* 1984; Sedlock *et al.,* 1978). In any event, adhesion seems to be an important first step for production of disease by salmonellae (Golderman and Rubinstein, 1982; Jones and Richardson, 1981; Jones *et al.,* 1981; Mintz *et al.,* 1983).

Adherence Factor/Rabbit number 1 (AF/R1) is the name proposed for the fimbria expressed by *E. coli,* notably *E. coli* strain REDEC-1, that attach, destroy, but do not invade, rabbit, small intestinal, epithelial cells (Berendson *et al.,* 1983; Cheney *et al.,* 1983). Strain RE-

DEC-1 is not enterotoxigenic. It is noninvasive, and does not produce a detectable toxin (Cantey and Blake, 1977). Following attachment, patchy in distribution in the ileum and diffuse in the cecum and colon, the epithelial cells of the ileum are destroyed (effaced) (Moon *et al.*, 1983; Takeuchi *et al.*, 1978; Cantey and Blake, 1977).

AF/R1 is a fimbria 5 nm in diameter, 190–820 nm in length, with a subunit size of 19,000 MW (Berendson *et al.*, 1983). This fimbria is responsible for a mannose-inhibitable adherence of *E. coli* strain REDEC-1 to ileal epithelial cells of the rabbit (Berendson *et al.*, 1983; Cheney *et al.*, 1979). Bacterial cells expressing this fimbria adhere best to rabbit epithelial cells and poorly to those of rats, guinea pigs, and humans (Berendson *et al.*, 1983; Cheney *et al.*, 1980). Such strains do not attach to epithelial cells obtained from the small intestine of the pig, but adhere to colonic cells of the pig without producing disease (Moon *et al.*, 1983; Deneke *et al.*, 1984).

The genes responsible for the production of AF/R1 are located on a conjugal plasmid that is 85 MDa in size (Cheney *et al.*, 1983).

AF/R1 fimbriae are expressed best when strain REDEC-1 is grown in penassay broth in 37°C without shaking (Berendson *et al.*, 1983; Cheney *et al.*, 1983). Adherence to epithelial cells is temperature and pH dependent, suggesting an active process (Cheney *et al.*, 1979).

III. The Epithelial Cell Surface

The epithelial cells of the gastrointestinal tract serve at least two functions with respect to the interaction of the host with the microbial world. The most important, from the standpoint of establishing a relationship between the host and the normal flora, is providing receptors for adhesins that might be present on the surface of bacteria destined to be members of the normal flora. The epithelial cell also displays structures that serve as receptors for fimbriae expressed by enteropathogenic strains of bacteria.

The receptors on the surface of epithelial cells for both the adhesins of the nonpathogenic and pathogenic strains of microbes are chemically similiar, i.e., they are composed of carbohydrates that are a part of the glycoproteins in the epithelial cell membrane. However, they are specific for each of the different fimbriae (Isaacson *et al.*, 1978a).

The receptor for type 1 fimriae is a trisaccharide that binds to hydrophobic portions of the fimbriae (Firon *et al.*, 1984). Studies utilizing various carbohydrates as inhibitors of adhesion between bacteria expressing type 1 fimbriae and epithelial cells have shown that Man α(1→3)-Man β(1→4)-Glc-NAc (Man, mannose; Glc-NAc, N-acetylglucosamine) and other mannose-containing, branched oligosaccharides are 20 times more efficient inhibitors of binding than methyl-α-D-mannoside (Firon et al., 1984; Ofek and Beachey, 1978). That the receptor for the common or type 1 fimbria would contain mannose is not unexpected, because of the mannose sensitivity of the hemagglutination reaction observed with this fimbria. It is reassuring, however, that a range of cell types, including epithelial cells lining various mucosal surfaces, possess mannose residues on their surfaces (Podolsky and Weiser, 1973: Sharon and Lis, 1972).

It has been more difficult to ascertain the structure of the receptor for the mannose-resistant group of adhesins. This group, as discussed above, contains fimbriae responsible for adhesion to the surface of target epithelial cells. A variety of carbohydrates and glycoproteins have been found to interfere with the adhesion of bacteria expressing mannose-resistant hemagglutinins to the epithelial cell surface. The most inhibitory substances are glycoproteins composed of N-acetylglucosamine, N-acetylgalactosamine, or β-D-galactosyl-bearing glycoproteins for K88 fimbriae-bearing bacteria, and GM_2-like glycoconjugates for CFA/I and K99 fimbriae-bearing microbes (Anderson et al., 1980; Faris et al., 1980; Gibbons et al., 1975). The sialic acid, N-acetylneuraminic acid, plays an essential role in the adhesion of CFA/I and K99 fimbriae (Faris et al., 1980; Lindahl and Wadstrom, 1984). The receptor for K99 has recently been characterized (Smit et al., 1984).

Receptors on the surface of epithelial cells play just as important a role in the initiation of disease as the adhesin on the surface of the enteropathogen. If an epithelial cell does not express the appropriate receptor, adhesion between the pathogen and target cell is not possible. It has been noted for many years that certain herds of pigs seem to have a lower incidence of diarrheal disease than others, and, in addition, the offspring of certain sires or dams within a herd seem to be more resistant to diarrheal disease than littermates or herdmates (Sweeney, 1968; Wijeratne et al., 1970). These observations led to the discovery that baby pigs that are resistant to diarrheal disease produced by K88-expressing, enterotoxigenic E. coli lacked the receptor on the target epithelial cell for this particular fimbria (Kearns and Gibbons, 1979; Kobata and Ginsberg, 1972; Rutter et al., 1975). This phenomenon was found to be related to the possession of one of two alleles located at a single chromosomal locus; the allele encoding information for the expression of the receptor being dominant, and segregating in simple Mendelian fashion (Sellwood et al., 1975). Since this discovery, five different pig phenotypes have been described, depending upon the specificity for each of the three variants of the K88 fimbria, i.e., K88ab, K88ac, or K88ad (Bijlsma et al., 1982). A simple genetic relationship between host cell receptor and other fimbriae has not been found in swine or any other species of animal.

The presence or absence of an appropriate receptor, or expression of a sufficient number, is important from an epidemiological standpoint. Some receptors are expressed only during the first few days following birth, whereas others are made throughout the life of the animal. The receptors for the K99 fimbria are found on the surface of calf and lamb target epithelial cells in the jejunum and ileum during the first days of life (Runnels et al., 1980). Very few receptors are demonstrable after 2 days. The receptors for K88 fimbriae are found on target epithelial cells in the jejunum and ileum of very young pigs (1 day of age) as well as on epithelial cells from pigs 6 weeks of age. As a result, E. coli expressing K88 fimbriae adhere to the epithelial cells taken from very young pigs (1 day of age) and also to cells taken from older pigs (6 weeks of age) (Runnels et al., 1980).

Expression of the receptors for the K99 fimbriae on epithelial cells of the lamb appears to be influenced by levels of thyroid hormone present at the time of birth (Cabello et al., 1983). Increased thyroid hormone secretion by the lamb prior to birth is postulated to account for lower numbers of receptors as compared to lambs born prematurely. Premature lambs are more susceptible to enterotoxigenic diarrhea; this may be due to the abundance of receptors on target epithelial cells brought about by the lower levels of thyroid hormone (Cabello et al., 1983).

IV. Fimbriae in the Clinical Setting (A Summary Statement)

Newborn animals acquire enterotoxigenic *E. coli* at birth from their environment. Sources include the feces of the dam and/or infected and symptomatic new born animals on the farm.

Enterotoxigenic *E. coli* adhere to the receptors on epithelial cells of the ileum and jejunum by way of fimbriae, and multiply to numbers approaching 10^8 to 10^9 per ml of lumenal contents. Enterotoxin secreted by the adhering bacteria deregulates cyclic nucleotide synthesis, resulting in secretion of fluid and electrolytes. If the animal survives, enterotoxigenic *E. coli* are shed in large numbers into the environment.

Diagnosis is based upon suspicion that the disease is due to enterotoxigenic *E. coli*. Clues include (1) lack of evidence of inflammation or invasion of the intestinal epithelial cells (absence of white blood cells, red blood cells, or cellular debris in the feces), (2) finding an increase in pH of the feces (due to increase secretion of bicarbonate ions), (3) a metabolic acidosis, (4) a hyperkalemia, and (5) an increase in packed cell volume. Fever is not present (Merrit, 1980).

Verification of the clinical impression that enterotoxigenic *E. coli* are the cause of the disease is based upon the demonstration of large numbers of fimbriae-expressing, toxin-secreting *E. coli* in the small intestine (Moon *et al.*, 1976). The most difficult is demonstration of toxin-secreting *E. coli*. The tests for toxin production are difficult, tedious, and expensive to run, requiring special reagents, cell culture, and/or animal inoculation. The least troublesome and least invasive procedure (also the least reliable) is to demonstrate large numbers of fimbriae-expressing *E. coli* in the feces, since most animals with disease produced by enterotoxigenic *E. coli* will excrete large numbers of such organisms (Moon *et al.*, 1968, 1976, 1980; Smith and Halls, 1968). This entails plating the fecal sample onto selective media so that the number of fimbrianated bacteria can be determined. Unfortunately, fimbriae are expressed very poorly on selective media, such as MacConkey agar (Guinee *et al.*, 1976). Therefore, a number of colonies have to be taken from such an agar and subcultured onto media that will promote the expression of the various fimbriae: for K88, E medium; for K99, Minca medium; for 987P, Minca medium; and for F41, E or Minca medium (Francis *et al.*, 1982; Guinee *et al.*, 1977; de Graaf and Roorda, 1982). Slide agglutination tests are performed on colonies by using appropriately specific antisera to determine whether fimbriae-bearing *E. coli* are present. This method is based upon the assumption that a large number of the offending strain will be present in the feces. Finding a few such colonies, or none at all, makes interpretation of the results of this test very difficult. An enzyme-linked immunosorbant assay has been developed to measure the presence of K88 fimbriae-expressing bacteria in the feces (Mills *et al.*, 1983). Such a method eliminates many of the problems inherent in the analysis of feces for fimbrianated bacteria.

The reliability of correctly substantiating the diagnosis of enterotoxigenic diarrhea by examining the feces for fimbriae-expressing *E. coli* is substantially reduced if the herd to which the sick animal belongs is not affected. In such situations, the incidence of fimbriae-expressing, nonenterotoxigenic *E. coli* is higher than is the case if the sick animal comes from a herd in which the disease is endemic (Myers *et al.*, 1984).

A more reliable method to verify the clinical diagnosis of enterotoxigenic *E. coli*-induced diarrhea is to quantitate the number of *E. coli* in the small intestine (Francis, 1983; Lariviere *et al.*, 1975; Isaacson *et al.*, 1978b). Since there should be very few *E. coli* in such sites, especially in the jejunum, the finding of large numbers of such microbes in these locations is highly suggestive that enterotoxigenic *E. coli* are present (Lariviere *et al.*, 1975; Smith and Orcutt, 1925). Samples are plated onto various media choosen to promote the expression of fimbriae, and colonies are picked and tested with appropriate antisera. Examination of stained smears of the contents of the small intestine is another method based upon the multiplication of enterotoxigenic *E. coli* in this location (Lariviere *et al.*, 1975). Though this method lacks specificity, it strengthens the diagnosis.

Using fluorescent labeled antibody techniques is the easiest, and probably the most reliable, of the methods used except for assaying for the toxin (Francis, 1983). In this method, smears of scrapings taken from the small intestine are flooded with antisera that are specific for the various fimbriae. After applying fluorescent labeled secondary antiserum, preparations are examined for fluorescently labeled bacteria adhering to the epithelial cells.

After the diagnosis is substantiated, action should be taken to prevent future occurrence of the disease. These decisions are made with the knowledge that prevention of adherence of enterotoxigenic *E. coli* to target epithelial cells is the ultimate goal. Elimination of enterotoxigenic *E. coli* from a herd is not practical.

The immune system of the newborn animal is neither sufficiently mature nor experienced to produce an active response in time for protection. Protection is acquired passively from the dam by way of immunoglobulins in colostrum and milk. These immunoglobulins must be specific for the antigenic determinants on the surface of the fimbriae. For this reason it is imperative that, prior to parturition, expectant mothers be exposed to organisms that will be in the environment of their newborn offspring (Kohler, 1974; Kohler *et al.*, 1975). This can be achieved by placing the mother-to-be into the environment several weeks prior to parturition. If this is impossible, then active immunization of the dam is necessary. Active immunization entails feeding the dam live strains of the expected pathogen, or vaccination with products that contain either the purified fimbrial protein or killed bacterial suspensions that have fimbriae on their surface. Passive protection can be achieved artificially by orally giving antibody to the appropriate fimbrial protein to the newborn animals (Sherman *et al.*, 1983).

There are a number of novel methods that have been devised or suggested for prevention of enterotoxigenic *E. coli*-induced disease. Bacterial competition is one such method. Orally administered, live, nontoxigenic *E. coli* possessing the genes for K88 fimbriae has been used successfully to exclude enterotoxigenic, *E. coli*-expressing K88 fimbriae from target cells and thereby preventing disease (Davidson and Hirsh, 1975, 1976). Likewise, live *Streptococcus faecium* administered orally has been shown to prevent diarrhea induced by enterotoxigenic *E. coli,* presumably by bacterial competition (Underdahl *et al.,* 1982).

Theoretically, carbohydrates that are structurally similar or identical to the receptor on the target cell could be fed to susceptible animals. The binding of these carbohydrates to the fimbriae would prevent enterotoxigenic *E. coli* from adhering to the target cell. Likewise, chemicals that alter the receptor on the epithelial cell might be useful for preventing attachment (Sugarman *et al.,* 1983).

References

Abraham, S. N., Hasty, D. L., Simpson, A., and Beachey, E. H. (1983). *J. Exp. Med.* **158,** 1114–1128.
Abrams, G. D., and Bishop, J. E. (1966). *J. Bacteriol.* **92,** 1604–1608.
Acres, S. D., Forman, A. J., and Kapitany, R. A. (1982). *Am. J. Vet. Res.* **43,** 569–575.
Acres, S. D., Isaacson, R. E., Babiuk, L. A., and Kapitany, R. A. (1979). *Infect. Immun.* **25,** 121–126.
Adegbola, R. A., and Old, D. C. (1983). *J. Gen. Microbiol.* **129,** 2175–2180.
Anderson, M. J., Whitehead, J. S., and Kim, Y. S. (1980). *Infect. Immun.* **29,** 897–901.
Anderson, T. F. (1949). *Symp. Gen. Microbiol.* **1,** 76–94.
Aning, K. G., Thomlinson, J. R., Wray, C., Sojka, W. J., and Coulter, J. (1983). *Vet. Rec.* **112,** 251.
Arbuckle, J. B. R. (1970). *J. Med. Microbiol.* **3,** 333–340.
Bak, A. L., Christiansen, G., Christiansen, C., and Stenderup, A. (1972). *J. Gen. Microbiol.* **73,** 373–385.
Bar-Shavit, Z., Ofek, I., Goldman, R., Mirelman, D., and Sharon, N. (1977). *Biochem. Biophys. Res. Commun.* **78,** 455–460.
Bar-Shavit, Z., Goldman, R., Ofek, I., Sharon, N., and Mirelman, D. (1980). *Infect. Immun.* **29,** 417–424.
Berendson, R., Cheney, C. P., Schad, P. A., and Boedeker, E. C. (1983). *Gastroenterology* **85,** 837–845.
Bergeim, O. (1940). *J. Infect. Dis.* **66,** 222–234.
Bergeim, O., Hanzen, A. H., Pincussen, L., and Weiss, E. (1941). *J. Infect. Dis.* **69,** 155–166.
Bertschinger, H. U., Moon, H. W., and Whipp, S. C. (1971). *Infect. Immun.* **5,** 595–605.
Bijlsma, I. G. W., De Nijs, A., Van Der Meer, C., and Frik, J. F. (1982). *Infect. Immun.* **37,** 891–894.
Bjorksten, B., and Wadstrom, T. (1982). *Infect. Immun.* **38,** 298–305.
Brinton, C. C. (1959). *Nature (London)* **183,** 782–786.
Brinton, C. C. (1965). *Trans. N.Y. Acad. Sci.* **27,** 1003–1054.

Brinton, C. C., and Baron, L. S. (1960). *Biochim. Biophys. Acta* **42,** 298–311.
Brinton, C. C., Gemski, P., Falkow, S., and Baron, L. S . (1961). *Biochem. Biophys. Res. Commun.* **5,** 293–298.
Brinton, C. C., Gemski, P., and Carnahan, J. (1964). *Proc. Natl. Acad. Sci. U.S.A.* **52,** 776–783.
Burgess, M. N., Bywater, R. J., Cowley, C. M., Mullan, N.A., and Newsome, P. M. (1978). *Infect. Immun.* **21,** 526–531.
Burgess, M. N., Mullan, N. A., and Newsome, P. M. (1980). *Infect. Immun.* **28,** 1038–1040.
Burrows, M. R., Sellwood, R., and Gibbons, R. A. (1976). *J. Gen. Microbiol.* **96,** 269–275.
Cabello, G., Lerieux, D., Girardeau, J. P., and Lefairre, J. (1983). *Res. Vet. Sci.* **35,** 242–244.
Cantey, J. R., and Blake, R. K. (1977). *J. Infect. Dis.* **135,** 454–462.
Carpenter, C. M., and Woods, G. (1924). *Cornell Vet.* **14,** 218–225.
Chan, R., Acres, S. D., and Costerton, J. W. (1982). *Infect. Immun.* **37,** 1170–1180.
Changchawalit, S., Echeverria, P., Taylor, D. N., Leksomboon, U., Tirapat, C., Eampokalap, B., and Rowe, B. (1984). *Infect. Immun.* **45,** 525–527.
Cheney, C. P., and Boedeker, E. C. (1983). *Infect. Immun.* **39,** 1280–1284.
Cheney, C. P., Boedeker, E. C., and Formal, S. B. (1979). *Infect. Immun.* **26,** 736–743.
Cheney, C. P., Schad, P.A., Formal, S. B., and Boedeker, E. C. (1980). *Infect. Immun.* **28,** 1019–1027.
Cheney, C. P., Formal, S. B., Schad, P. A., and Boedeker, E. C. (1983b). *J. Infect. Dis.* **147,** 711–723.
Clements, J. D., Yancey, R. J., and Finkelstein, R. A. (1980). *Infect. Immun.* **29,** 91–97.
Collier, W. A., and De Miranda, J. C. (1955). *Antonie van Leeuwenhoek* **21,** 133–140.
Collier, W. A., and Jacoeb, M. (1955b). *Antonie van Leeuwenhoek* **21,** 113–123.
Collier, W. A., Wong, S. T., and De Miranda, J. C. (1955). *Antonie van Leeuwenhoek* **21,** 124–140.
Constable, F. L. (1956). *J. Pathol. Bacteriol.* **72,** 133–136.
Craven, J. A., Miniats, O. P., and Barnum, D. A. (1971). *Am. J. Vet. Res.* **32,** 1775–1779.
Cravioto, A., Gross, R. J., Scotland, S. M., and Rowe, B. (1979). *FEMS Microbiol. Lett.* **6,** 41–44.
Davidson, J. N., and Hirsh, D. C. (1975). *Infect. Immun.* **12,** 134–136.
Davidson, J. N., and Hirsh, D. C. (1976). *Infect. Immun.* **13,** 1773–1774.
de Graaf, F. K., and Roorda, I. (1982). *Infect. Immun.* **36,** 751–758.
de Graaf, F. K., Klaasen-Boor, P., and Van Hees, J. E. (1980a). *Infect. Immun.* **30,** 125–128.
de Graaf, F. K., Wientjes, F. B., and Klaasen-Boor, P. (1980b). *Infect. Immun.* **27,** 216–221.
de Graaf, F. K., Klemm, P., and Gastra, W. (1981). *Infect. Immun.* **33,** 877–833.
de Graaf, F. K., Krenn, B. E., and Klaasen, P. (1984). *Infect. Immun.* **43,** 508–514.
Deneke, C. F., Mc Gowan, K., Larson, A. D., and Gorbach, S. C. (1984). *Infect. Immun.* **45,** 522–524.
Dixon, J. M. S. (1960). *J. Pathol. Bacteriol.* **79,** 131–140.
Dodd, D. C., and Eisenstein, B. I. (1982). *Infect. Immun.* **38,** 764–773.
Drucker, M. M., Yeivin, R., and Sacks, T. G. (1967). *Isr. J. Med. Sci.* **3,** 445–452.
Duguid, J. P. (1959). *J. Gen. Microbiol.* **21,** 271–286.
Duguid, J. P., and Gillies, R. R. (1957). *J. Pathol. Bacteriol.* **74,** 397–411.
Duguid, J. P., and Gillies, R. R. (1958). *J. Pathol. Bacteriol.* **75,** 519–520.
Duguid, J. P., Smith, I. W., Dempster, G., and Edmunds, P. N. (1955). *J. Pathol. Bacteriol.* **70,** 335–348.

Duguid, J. P., Anderson, E. S., and Campbell, I. (1966). *J. Pathol. Bacteriol.* **92,** 107-138.
Duguid, J. P., Anderson, E. S., Alfredsson, G. A., Barker, R., and Old, D. C. (1975). *J. Med. Microbiol.* **8,** 149-166.
Duguid, J. P., Darekar, M. R., and Wheater, D. W. F. (1976). *J. Med. Microbiol.* **9,** 459-473.
Duguid, J. P., Clegg, S., and Wilson, M. (1979). *J. Med. Microbiol.* **12,** 213-227.
Edebo, L., Hed, J., Kihlstrom, E., Magnusson, K.-E., and Stendahl, O. (1980). *Scand. J. Infect. Dis. Suppl.* **24,** 93-99.
Eshdat, Y., Silverblatt, F. J., and Sharon, N. (1981). *J. Bacteriol.* **148,** 308-314.
Evans, D. G., and Evans, D. (1978). *Infect. Immun.* **21,** 638-647.
Evans, D. G., Silver, R. P., Evans, D. J., Chase, D. G., and Gorbach, S. L. (1975). *Infect. Immun.* **12,** 656-667.
Evans, D. G., Evans, D. J., and Du Pont, H. L. (1977a). *J. Infect. Dis.* **136,** S118-S123.
Evans, D. G., Evans, D. J., and Tjoa, W. (1977b). *Infect. Immun.* **18,** 330-333.
Evans, D. G., Evans, D. J., Tjoa, W. S., and Du Pont, H. L. (1978a). *Infect. Immun.* **19,** 727-736.
Evans, D. G., Satterwhite, T. K., Evans, D. J., and Du Pont, H. L. (1978b). *Infect. Immun.* **19,** 883-888.
Evans, D. G., Evans, D. J., Clegg, S., and Pauley, J. A. (1979). *Infect. Immun.* **25,** 738-748.
Fader, R. C., Arots-Arotins, A. E., and Davis, C. P. (1979). *Infect. Immun.* **25,** 729-737.
Fader, R. C., Duffy, L. K., Davis, C. P., and Kurosky, A. (1982). *J. Biol. Chem.* **257,** 3301-3305.
Faris, A., Lindahl, M., and Wadstrom, T. (1980). *FEMS Microbiol. Lett.* **7,** 265-269.
Faris, A., Wadstrom, T., and Freer, J. H. (1981). *Curr. Microbiol.* **5,** 67-72.
Firon, N., Ofek, I., and Sharon, N. (1984). *Infect. Immun.* **43,** 1088-1090.
Francis, D. H. (1983). *Am. J. Vet. Res.* **44,** 1884-1888.
Francis, D. H., Remmers, G. A., and De Zeeuw, P. S. (1982). *J. Clin. Microbiol.* **15,** 181-183.
Gaastra, W., Klemm, P., Walker, J. M., and de Graaf, F. K. (1979). *FEMS Microbiol. Lett.* **6,** 15-18.
Gibbons, R. A., Jones, G. W., and Sellwood, R. (1975). *J. Gen. Microbiol.* **86,** 228-240.
Gill, D. M., and Richardson, S. H. (1980). *J. Infect. Dis.* **141,** 64-70.
Golderman, L., and Rubinstein, E. (1982). *Isr. J. Med. Sci.* **18,** 1032-1036.
Guinee, P. A. M., and Jansen, W. H. (1979). *Zentralbl. Bakteriol. Parasitenkd. Infektionskr. Hyg. Abt.*1:*Orig. Reihe A* **243,** 245-257.
Guinee, P. A. M., Jansen, W. H., and Agterberg, C. M. (1976). *Infect. Immun.* **13,** 1369-1377.
Guinee, P. A. M., Veldkamp, J., and Jansen, W. H. (1977). *Infect. Immun.* **15,** 676-678.
Guyot, G. (1908). *Zentralbl. Bakteriol. Parasitenkd. Infektjonskr.* **47,** 640-653.
Gyles, C., So, M., and Falkow, S. (1974). *J. Infect. Dis.* **130,** 40-49.
Hentges, D. J. (1969). *J. Bacteriol.* **97,** 513-517.
Hentges, D. J., and Maier, B. R. (1970). *Infect. Immun.* **2,** 364-370.
Hohmann, A., and Wilson, M. R. (1975). *Infect. Immun.* **12,** 866-880.
Holmgren, J. P., Fredman, P., Lindblad, M., Svennerholm, A.-M., and Svennerholm, L. (1982). *Infect. Immun.* **38,** 424-433.
Honda, T., Arita, M., and Miwatani, T. (1984). *Infect. Immun.* **43,** 959-965.
Horwitz, M. A., and Silverstein, S. C. (1980). *J. Clin. Invest.* **65,** 82-94.
Houwink, A. L., and Van Iterson, W. (1950). *Biochim. Biophys. Acta* **5,** 10-44.
Hull, R. A., Gill, R. E., Hsu, P., Minshew, B. H., and Falkow, S. (1981). *Infect. Immun.* **33,** 933-938.

Ikari, N. S., Kenton, D. M., and Young, V. M. (1969). *Proc. Soc. Exp. Biol. Med.* **130,** 1280.
Impey, C. S., Mead, G. C., and George, S. M. (1982). *J. Hyg.* **89,** 479–490.
Isaacson, R. E. (1977). *Infect. Immun.* **15,** 272–279.
Isaacson, R. E. (1980). *Infect. Immun.* **28,** 190–194.
Isaacson, R. E., and Richter, P. (1981). *J. Bacteriol.* **146,** 784–789.
Isaacson, R. E., Nagy, B., and Moon, H. W. (1977). *J. Infect. Dis.* **135,** 531–539.
Isaacson, R. E., Fusco, R. C., Brinton, C. C., and Moon, H. W. (1978a). *Infect. Immun.* **21,** 392–397.
Isaacson, R. E., Moon, H. W., and Schneider, R. A. (1978b). *Am. J. Vet. Res.* **39,** 1750–1755.
Isaacson, R. E., Colmenero, J., and Richter, P. (1981). *FEMS Microbiol. Lett.* **12,** 229–232.
Johns, M., Skehill, A., and Mc Cabe, W. R. (1983). *J. Infect. Dis.* **147,** 57–67.
Jones, G. W., and Richardson, L. A. (1981). *J. Gen. Microbiol.* **127,** 361–370.
Jones, G. W., and Rutter, J. M. (1972). *Infect. Immun.* **6,** 918–927.
Jones, G. W., and Rutter, J. M. (1974). *J. Gen. Microbiol.* **84,** 135–144.
Jones, G. W., Richardson, L. A., and Uhlman, D. (1981). *J. Gen. Microbiol.* **127,** 351–360.
Kauffmann, F. (1943). *Acta Pathol. Microbiol. Scand.* **20,** 21–44.
Kauffmann, F. (1948). *Acta Pathol. Microbiol. Scand.* **25,** 502–506.
Kearns, M. J., and Gibbons, R. A. (1979). *FEMS Microbiol. Lett.* **6,** 165–168.
Kehoe, M., Sellwood, R., Shipley, P., and Dougan, G. (1981). *Nature (London)* **291,** 122–126.
Kehoe, M., Winther, M., Dowd, G., Morrissey, P., and Dougan, G. (1982). *FEMS Microbiol. Lett.* **14,** 129–132.
Kelen, A. E., Campbell, S. G., and Barnum, D. A. (1959). *Can. J. Comp. Med.* **23,** 216–228.
Klemm, P. (1979). *FEBS Lett.* **108,** 107–110.
Klemm, P. (1981). *Eur. J. Biochem.* **117,** 617–627.
Klemm, P. (1982). *Eur. J. Biochem.* **124,** 339–348.
Knutton, S., Williams, P. H., Lloyd, D. R., Candy, D. C. A., and McNeish, A. S. (1983). *Infect. Immun.* **44,** 599–608.
Kobata, A., and Ginsberg, V. A. (1972). *J. Biol. Chem.* **247,** 1525–1529.
Kohler, E. M. (1974). *Am. J. Vet. Res.* **35,** 331–338.
Kohler, E. M., Cross, R. F., and Bohl, E. H. (1975). *Am. J. Vet. Res.* **36,** 757–764.
Konstantinov, G., Karacholeva, M., Eskenazy, M., Ivanova, R., Vassileva, J., Naumova, F., Tekelieva, R., and Strahilov, D. (1982). *Ann. Immunol. (Paris)* **133,** 71–76.
Koo, F. C. W., Peterson, J. W., Houston, C. W., and Molina, N. C. (1984). *Infect. Immun.* **43,** 93–100.
Korhonen, T. K. (1979). *FEMS Microbiol. Lett.* **6,** 421–425.
Korhonen, T. M., Lounatmaa, K., Ranta, H., and Kuusi, N. (1980). *J. Bacteriol.* **144,** 800–805.
Koupal, L. R., and Deibel, R. H. (1975). *Infect. Immun.* **11,** 14–22.
Lariviere, S., Lallier, R., and Morin, M. (1975). *Am. J. Vet. Res.* **40,** 130–134.
Leunk, R. D., and Moon, R. J. (1982). *Infect. Immun.* **36,** 1168–1174.
Levine, M. M., Black, R. E., Brinton, C. C., Clements, M. L., Fusco, P., Hughes, T. P., O'Donnell, S., Robins-Brown, R., Wood, S., and Young, C. R. (1982). *Scand. J. Infect. Dis. Suppl.* **33,** 83–95.
Lindahl, M., and Wadstrom, T. (1984). *Vet. Microbiol.* **9,** 249–257.
Lindahl, M., Faris, A., Wadstrom, T., and Hjerten, S. (1981). *Biochim. Biophys. Acta* **677,** 471–476.

Lopez-Alvarez, J., and Gyles, C. L. (1980). *Am. J. Vet. Res.* **41,** 769–774.
McConnell, M. M., Smith, H. R., Willshaw, G. A., Field, A. M., and Rowe, B. (1981). *Infect. Immun.* **32,** 927–936.
McMichael, J. C., and Ou, J. T. (1979). *J. Bacteriol.* **138,** 976–983.
Magnusson, K.-E., and Stjernstrom, I. (1981). *Immunology* **45,** 239–248.
Magnusson, K.-E, Stendahl, O., Stjernstrom, I., and Edebo, L. (1978). *Acta Pathol. Microbiol. Scand. Sect. B: Microbiol.* **86,** 113–120.
Magnusson, K.-E., Stendahl, O., Stjernstrom, I., and Edebo, L. (1979). *Immunology* **36,** 439–447.
Magnusson, K.-E, Davies, J., Grundstrom, T., Kihlstrom, E., and Normark, S. (1980). *Scand. J. Infect. Dis. Suppl.* **24,** 135–140.
Merrit, A. M. (1980). In "Veterinary Gastroenterology" (N. V. Anderson, ed.), pp. 463–522. Lea & Febiger, Philadelphia.
Meynell, G. G. (1963). *Br. J. Exp. Pathol.* **44,** 209–219.
Middlebrook. J. L., and Dorland, R. B. (1984). *Microbiol. Rev.* **48,** 199–221.
Mills, K. W., Tietze, K. L., and Phillips, R. M. (1983). *Am. J. Vet. Res.* **44,** 2188–2189.
Mintz, C. S., Cliver, D. O., and Deibel, R. H. (1983). *Can. J. Microbiol.* **29,** 1731–1735.
Mooi, F. R., and de Graaf, F. K. (1979). *FEMS Microbiol. Lett.* **5,** 17–20.
Mooi, F. R., Harms, N., Bakker, D., and de Graaf, F. K. (1981). *Infect. Immun.* **32,** 1155–1163.
Mooi, F. R., Wijfjes, A., and de Graaf, F. K. (1983). *J. Bacteriol.* **154,** 41–49.
Moon, H. W., Sorensen, D. K., and Sautter, J. H. (1968). *Can. J. Comp. Med.* **32,** 493–497.
Moon, H. W., Whipp, S. C., and Skartredt, S. M. (1976). *Am. J. Vet. Res.* **37,** 1025–1029.
Moon, H. W., Kohler, E. M., Schneider, R. A., and Whipp, S. C. (1980). *Infect. Immun.* **27,** 222–230.
Moon, H. W., Whipp, S. C., Argenzio, R. A., Levine, M. M., and Giannella, R. A. (1983). *Infect. Immun.* **41,** 1340–1351.
Morgan, R. L., Issacson, R. E., Moon, H. W., Brinton, C. C., and To, C.-C. (1978). *Infect. Immun.* **22,** 771–777.
Morris, J. A., Stevens, A. E., and Sojka, W. J. (1978). *J. Gen. Microbiol.* **107,** 173–175.
Morris, J. A., Thorns, C. J., and Sojka, W. J. (1980a). *J. Gen. Microbiol.* **118,** 107–113.
Morris, J. A., Wray, C., and Sojka, W. J. (1980b). *J. Med. Microbiol.* **13,** 265–271.
Morris, J. A., Thorns, C., Scott, A. C., Sojka, W. J., and Wells, G. A. (1982). *Infect. Immun.* **36,** 1146–1153.
Morris, J. A., Thorns, C. J., Wells, G. A. H., Scott, A. C., and Sojka, W. J. (1983). *J. Gen. Microbiol.* **129,** 2753–2759.
Morrison, D. C. (1983). *Rev. Infect. Dis.* **5,** s733–s747.
Myers, L. L., and Guinee, P. A. M. (1976). *Infect. Immun.* **13,** 1117–1119.
Myers, L. L., Firehammer, B. D., Border, M. M., and Shoop, D. S. (1984). *Am. J. Vet. Res.* **45,** 1544–1548.
Nagy, B. (1980). *Infect. Immun.* **27,** 21–24.
Nagy, B., Moon, H. W., and Isaacson, R. E. (1976). *Infect. Immun.* **13,** 1214–1220.
Nagy, B., Moon, H. W., and Isaacson, R. E. (1977). *Infect. Immun.* **16,** 344–352.
Nagy, B., Moon, H. W., Isaacson, R. E., To., C.-C., and Brinton, C. C. (1978). *Infect. Immun.* **21,** 269–274.
Nomura, M. (1967). *Annu. Rev. Microbiol.* **21,** 257–284.
Ofek, I., and Beachey, E. H. (1978). *Infect. Immun.* **22,** 247–254.
Ofek, I., Mirelman, D., and Sharon, N. (1977). *Nature (London)* **265,** 623–625.
Ohmann, L., Hed, J., and Stendahl, O. (1982). *J. Infect. Dis.* **146,** 751–757.

Orskov, I., and Orskov, F. (1966). *J. Bacteriol.* **91,** 69–75.Orskov, I., and Orskov, F. (1977). *Med. Microbiol. Immunol.* **163,** 99–110.

Orskov, I., and Orskov, F. (1983). *In* "Progress in Allergy" (L. A. Hanson, P. Kallos, and O. Westphal, eds.), pp. 80–105. Kavger, Basel.

Orskov, I., Orskov, F., Sojka, W. J., and Leach, J. M. (1961). *Acta Pathol. Microbiol. Scand. Sect. B:* Microbiol. **53,**404–422.

Orskov, I., Orskov, F., Sojka, W. J., and Witting, W. (1964). *Acta Pathol. Microbiol. Scand.* **62,** 439–447.

Orskov, I., Orskov, F., Smith, H. W., and Sojka, W. J. (1975). *Acta Pathol. Microbiol. Scand. Sect. B: Microbiol.* **83,** 31–36.

Orskov, I., Orskov, F., Jann, B., and Jann, K. (1977). *Bacteriol. Rev.* **41,** 667–710.

Paranchych, W., Frost, L. S., and Carpenter, M. (1978). *J. Bacteriol.* **134,** 1179–1181.

Pearce, W. A., and Buchanan, T. M. (1980). *In* "Bacterial Adherence" (E. H. Beachey, ed.), pp. 289–344. Chapman and Hall, London.

Perers, L., Andaker, L., Edebo, L., Stendahl, O., and Tagesson, C. (1977). *Acta Pathol. Microbiol. Scand. Sect. B: Microbiol.* **85,** 308–316.

Perry, A., and Ofek, I. (1984). *Infect. Immun.* **43,** 257–262.

Perry, A., Ofek, I., and Silverblatt, F. J. (1983). *Infect. Immun.* **39,** 1334–1345.

Pickering, L. K., Du Pont, H. L., Evans, D. G., Evans, D. J., and Olarte, J. (1977). *J. Infect. Dis.* **135,** 1003–1005.

Podolsky, D. K., and Weiser, M. M. (1973). *J. Cell Biol.* **58,** 497–500.

Porter, P., and Linggood, M. A. (1983). *J. Infect.* **6,** 111–121.

Pruzzo, C., Dainelli, B., and Ricchetti, M. (1984). *Infect. Immun.* **43,** 189–194.

Rosenthal, L. (1943). *J. Bacteriol.* **45,** 545–550.

Rottini, G., Cian, F., Soranzo, M. R., Albrigo, R., and Patriarca, P. (1979). *FEBS Lett.* **105,** 307–312.

Runnels, P. L., Moon, H. W., and Schneider, R. A. (1980). *Infect. Immun.* **28,** 298–300.

Rutter, J. M., and Jones, G. W. (1972). *Nature (London)* **242,** 531–532.

Rutter, J. M., Burrows, M. R., Sellwood, R., and Gibbons, R. A. (1975). *Nature (London),* **257,** 135–136.

Rutter, J. M., Jones, G. W., Brown, G. T. H., Burrows, M. R., and Luther, P. D. (1976). *Infect. Immun.* **13,** 667–676.

Ryder, R. W., Wachsmuth, I. K., Buxton, A. E., Evans, D. G., Du Pont, H. L., Mason, E., and Barrett, F. F. (1976). *New Engl. J. Med.* **295,** 849–853.

Sack, R. B., Sack, D. A., Mehlman, I. J., Orskov, F., and Orskov, I. (1977). *J. Infect. Dis.* **135,** 313–317.

Salit, I. E., and Gotschlich, E. C. (1977a). *J. Exp. Med.* **146,** 1182–1194.

Salit, I. E., and Gotschlich, E. C. (1977b). *J. Exp. Med.* **146,** 1169–1181.

Saunders, C. N., Stevens, H. J., Spence, J. B., and Sojka, W. (1963). *Res. Vet. Sci.* **4,** 333–346.

Savage, D. C. (1970). *Am. J. Clin. Nutri.* **23,** 1495–1501.

Savage, D. C. (1972). *In* "Microbial Pathogenicity in Man and Animals" (H. Smith and J. H. Pearce, eds.), pp 25–57. Cambridge University Press, London.

Savage, D. C. (1980). *In* "Bacterial Adherence" (E. H. Beachey, ed.), pp 31–59. Chapman and Hall, London.

Schreil, W., and Schleich, F. (1955). *Z. Hyg.* **141,** 576–584

Sedlock, D. M., Koupal, L. R., and Deibel, R. H. (1978). *Infect. Immun.* **20,** 375–380.

Sellwood, R., Gibbons, R. A., Jones, G. W., and Rutter, J. M. (1975). *J. Med. Microbiol.* **8,** 405–411.

Sharon, N., and Lis, H. (1972). *Science* **177,** 949–959.

Sherman, D. M., Acres, S. D., Sadowski, P. L., Springer, J. A., Bray, B., Raybould, T. J. G., and Muscoplat, C. C. (1983). *Infect. Immun.* **42,** 653–658.
Shipley, P. L., Gyles, C. L., and Falkow, S. (1978). *Infect. Immun.* **20,** 559–566.
Shore, E. G., Dean, A. G., Holik, K. J., and Davis, B. R. (1974). *J. Infect. Dis.* **129,** 577–582.
Silverblatt, F. J., Dreyer, J. S., and Schauer, S. (1979). *Infect. Immun.* **24,** 218–226.
Smit, H., Gaastra, W., Kamerling, J. P., Vliegenthart, J. F. G., and de Graaf, F. K. (1984). *Infect. Immun.* **46,** 578–584.
Smith, H. R., Cravioto, A., Willshaw, G. A., Mc Connell, M. M., Scotland, S. M., Gross, R. J., and Rove, B. (1979). *FEMS Microbiol. Lett.* **6,** 255–260.
Smith, H. W. (1962). *J. Pathol. Bacteriol.* **84,** 147–168.
Smith, H. W. (1972). *J. Med. Microbiol.* **5,** 345–352.
Smith, H. W. (1974). *J. Gen. Microbiol.* **83,** 95–111.
Smith, H. W., and Gyles, C. L. (1970). *J. Med. Microbiol.* **3,** 387–401.
Smith, H. W., and Halls, S. (1967). *J. Pathol. Bacteriol.* **93,** 499–529.
Smith, H. W., and Halls, S. (1968). *J. Med. Microbiol.* **1,** 45–59.
Smith, H. W., and Jones, J. E. T. (1963). *J. Pathol. Bacteriol.* **86,** 387–412.
Smith, H. W., and Linggood, M. A. (1971). *J. Med. Microbiol.* **4,** 467–484.
Smith, H. W., and Linggood, M. A. (1972). *J. Med. Microbiol.* **5,** 243–250.
Smith, T., and Orcutt, M. L. (1925). *J. Exp. Med.* **41,** 89–106.
Smyth, C. J., Jonsson, P., Olsson, E., Soderlind, O., Rosengren, J., Hjerten, S., and Wadstrom, T. (1978). *Infect. Immun.* **22,** 462–472.
Sojka, W. J., Wray, C., and Morris, J. A. (1978). *J. Med. Microbiol.* **11,** 493–499.
Stendahl, O., Tagesson, C., and Edebo, L. (1973). *Infect. Immun.* **8,** 36–41.
Stendahl, O., Tagesson, C., and Edebo, L. (1974). *Infect. Immun.* **10,** 316–319.
Stenhadl, O., Normann, B., and Edebo, L. (1979). *Acta Pathol. Microbiol. Scand. Sect B: Microbiol* **87,** 85–91.
Stirm, S., Orskov, F., Orskov, I., and Birch-Andersen, A. (1967a). *J. Bacteriol.* **93,** 740–748.
Stirm, S., Orskov, F., Orskov, I., and Mansa, B. (1967b). *J. Bacteriol.* **93,** 731–739.
Stjernstrom, I., Magnusson, K.-E., Stendahl, O., and Tagesson, C. (1977). *Infect. Immun.* **18,** 261–265.
Sugarman, B., Epps, L. R., and Stenback, W. A. (1983). *Proc. Soc. Exp. Biol. Med.* **173,** 588–597.
Svendsen, J., and Wilson, M. R. (1971). *Am. J. Vet. Res.* **32,** 899–904.
Sweeney, E. J. (1968). *Ir. Vet. J.* **22,** 42–46.
Takeuchi, A., Inman, L. R., O'Hanley, P. D., Cantey, J. R., and Lushbaugh, W. B. (1978). *Infect. Immun.* **19,** 686–694.
Tavendale, A., Jardine, C. K. H., Old, D. C., and Duguid, J. P. (1983). *Med. Microbiol.* **16,** 371–380.
Thornley, M. J., and Horne, R. W. (1962). *J. Gen. Microbiol.* **28,** 51–56.
To, S. C.-M., Moon, H. W., and Runnels, P. L. (1984). *Infect. Immun.* **43,** 1–5.
Underdahl, N. R., Torres-Medina, A., and Doster, A. R. (1982). *Am. J. Vet. Res.* **43,** 2227–2232.
Van Embden, J. D. A., de Graaf, F. K., Schouls, L. M., and Teppema, J. S. (1980). *Infect. Immun.* **29,** 1125–1133.
Van Oss, C. J., and Gillman, C. F. (1972). *J. Reticuloendothel. Soc.* **12,** 283–292.
Watts, T. H., Sastry, P. A., Hodges, R. S., and Paranchych, W. (1983). *Infect. Immun.* **42,** 113–121.
Weinstein, R., and Silverblatt, F. J. (1983). *J. Infect. Dis.* **147,** 882–889.

Weir, D. M., and Ogmundsdottir, H. M. (1977). *Clin. Exp. Immunol.* **30,** 323–329.
Wijeratne, W. V. S., Crossman, P. J., and Gould, C. M. (1970). *Br. Vet. J.* **126,** 94–99.
Williams, D. J., and Becker, E. L. (1984). *J. Leukocyte Biol.* **35,** 71–90.
Wilson, M. R., and Hohmann, A. W. (1974). *Infect. Immun.* **10,** 776–782.
Wittig, W. (1965). *Zentralbl. Bakteriol. Parasiterkd. Infektionskr. Hyg.* **197,** 487–499.
Wood, L. V., Wolfe, W. H., Ruiz-Palacios, G., Foshee, W. S., Corman, L. I., McCleskey, F., Wright, J. A., and Du Pont, H. L. (1983). *Infect. Immun.* **41,** 931–934.
Worobec, E. A., Shastry, P., Smart, W., Bradley, R., Singh, B., and Paranchych, W. (1983). *Infect. Immun.* **41,** 1296–1301.

Atrophic Rhinitis in Swine

J. M. RUTTER

*Agricultural and Food Research Council
Institute for Research on Animal Diseases
Compton, Newbury, Berkshire, England*

I.	Introduction	240
II.	Occurrence and Importance	242
	Economic Significance	243
III.	Clinical and Pathological Features	244
	A. Clinical Signs	244
	B. Pathological Changes	245
IV.	Etiology	246
	A. Heredity	246
	B. Nutrition	247
	C. Infection	247
	D. Environment and Management	248
V.	Pathogenesis	249
	A. *B. bronchiseptica*	249
	B. *P. multocida*	254
VI.	Epidemiology	259
VII.	Diagnosis	262
	A. Clinical	262
	B. Pathological	262
	C. Cultural	263
	D. Value of Cultural and Serological Tests	265
VIII.	Control	266
	A. Eradication	266
	B. Monitoring	267
	C. Environment and Management	267
	D. Medication	267
IX.	Immunity and Vaccination	268
	A. *B. bronchiseptica*	269
	B. *P. multocida*	271
X.	Conclusions	274
	References	275

I. Introduction

The first description of atrophic rhinitis in pigs (synonyms: infectious atrophic rhinitis, chronic atrophic rhinitis) was published in Germany (Franque, 1830). Since then there have been numerous papers from all parts of the world on the etiology, pathogenesis, and control of the disease, yet these topics are still the subject of debate and controversy. Part of the problem is the wide range of clinical signs attributed to this complex disease. These include partial or complete atrophy of one or both of the turbinate bones (nasal conchae), shortening or twisting of the snout, sneezing, nasal discharges and epistaxis, pneumonia, and reduced growth rates. In severe outbreaks all the above signs are present, whereas in some herds a relatively mild degree of turbinate damage may be the only manifestation of disease. This variation in the severity of clinical signs raises the question, when does turbinate atrophy become atrophic rhinitis?

The etiology of the changes outlined above has been attributed to a number of infectious, genetic, metabolic, and nutritional factors; this has contributed to a divergence of views on the cause and nature of the disease. In 1958, Gwatkin referred to the severe clinical signs and concluded that "It is difficult to accept the idea that many different types of organisms can reproduce such a consistent set of signs and pathological findings." Subsequently, Switzer and Farrington (1975) stated that *Bordetella bronchiseptica* is the principal cause of atrophic rhinitis. Others have argued that such a complex disease cannot be an "all or none" condition (Goodwin, 1980) and that "a search for *the* cause of atrophic rhinitis is a hopeless quest based on unsound logic" (Done, 1981). The latter view considers that atrophic rhinitis is a multifactorial disease and suggests that turbinate atrophy is "the product of a severe persistent inflammatory reaction in the nose of the young very rapidly growing pig which is etiologically non-specific" (Done, 1983a). This difference of opinion is more than just a semantic argument. There are important practical implications, such as whether a herd with mild turbinate atrophy is likely to become severely affected, or whether "severe disease" can be transmitted by purchasing pigs from unaffected herds that provide a missing infectious component in a complex link.

Recent research findings help to elucidate these vexed questions. It is generally agreed that the most important signs of atrophic rhinitis are severe and persistent turbinate atrophy, snout deformation, and reduced growth rate. There is now good evidence that two bacteria, *B.*

bronchiseptica and *Pasteurella multocida,* are each capable of causing turbinate atrophy in pigs but the severity and persistence of the changes they produce are different. In the case of *P. multocida,* the changes can be produced in germ-free pigs by the parenteral injection of toxin, indicating that severe, persistent, inflammatory changes in the nasal mucosa are not an essential prerequisite for the lesion (Rutter and Mackenzie, 1984). Research in Europe has also led, for the first time, to the consistent reproduction of the progressive changes associated with atrophic rhinitis in specific pathogen-free (SPF) (Pedersen and Barfod, 1981, 1982) and gnotobiotic pigs (Rutter and Rojas, 1982; Rutter, 1983). The above results have led to an explanation for the wide variation in severity of clinical signs of the disease (Pedersen and Barfod, 1982; Rutter and Rojas, 1982; Schöss, 1982; Rutter, 1983). This proposes that infections with *B. bronchiseptica* and perhaps nontoxigenic strains of *P. multocida* cause "atrophic rhinitis" in herds where clinical signs are limited to moderately severe nonprogressive turbinate damage, whereas infection with toxigenic *P. multocida* causes severe turbinate atrophy and snout changes (which accounts for outbreaks of progressive disease). Although this important distinction may help to resolve some of the previous anomalies, the picture is complicated by the observation that, in germ-free pigs, infection with *B. bronchiseptica* assists colonization by toxigenic *P. multocida* and leads to more severe lesions, as compared to infection with either organism alone (Rutter and Rojas, 1982; Rutter, 1983). Furthermore, Pedersen and Barfod (1982) considered that other predisposing factors may be important in assisting toxigenic *P. multocida,* because *B. bronchiseptica* could not be found in all herds with atrophic rhinitis. Thus, it is probably useful to continue to regard atrophic rhinitis as a single disease complex, even though the latest edition of "Diseases of Swine" has separate chapters on Bordetellosis (Switzer, 1981) and Pasteurellosis (Farrington, 1981).

An early assessment of the role of *P. multocida* in atrophic rhinitis was published in this series (Gwatkin, 1958) and, since then, there have been a number of reviews of atrophic rhinitis (Switzer and Farrington, 1975; Schuller, 1980; Goodwin, 1980; Pedersen and Nielsen, 1983), Bordetellosis (Goodnow, 1980; Switzer, 1981), vaccination against atrophic rhinitis (Giles and Smith, 1983), and Pasteurellosis (Farrington, 1981). This article will not retrace the same ground. Instead, aspects of work up to August, 1984 will be interpreted in the light of the new proposals for the etiology of atrophic rhinitis.

II. Occurrence and Importance

Atrophic rhinitis occurs throughout the world in areas with an intensive swine-rearing industry (Switzer, 1981). Infection of pig herds with *B. bronchiseptica* appears to be virtually universal and, because this organism causes turbinate atrophy, it is not surprising that "atrophic rhinitis" has been reported from most countries. However, if progressive disease is caused by toxigenic *P. multocida*, then its distribution might be more limited and this could explain some previous findings. For example, a rhinitic condition of pigs had been recognized in the United Kingdom since the 1850s (Done *et al.*, 1964), but the apparent introduction of classical atrophic rhinitis in 1954 was associated with the importation of Swedish Landrace stock (Anon, 1954) and might have been attributable to the introduction of toxigenic *P. multocida*. Similarly, Hodges (1981) reported that a mild form of atrophic rhinitis might be more common in New Zealand than was generally realized; this might mean that *B. bronchiseptica*, but not toxigenic *P. multocida*, was present in that country. Surveys carried out in various countries indicate that up to 30% of pigs can be affected with progressive disease (Table I). Toxigenic *P. multocida* has been demonstrated in most of these countries, but it is not possible to conclude that this organism is invariably associated with severe disease until its distribution has been more clearly established.

Atrophic rhinitis became more prevalent and more serious during the 1960s and 1970s (Penny and Mullen, 1975; de Jong, 1983a). This may be attributable to factors such as increased herd size, changes in housing conditions, and more pig movements. Surprisingly, however, results from Denmark indicate that the incidence of severely affected pigs showed little change between 1916 and 1983 (Nielsen, 1983).

TABLE I

PREVALENCE OF ATROPHIC RHINITIS IN DIFFERENT COUNTRIES

Country	Percentage of pigs with severe turbinate atrophy/ clinical disease	Reference
United Kingdom	17.5	Penny and Mullen (1975)
United States	14.4	Switzer (1981)
Denmark	6–8	Nielsen (1983)
France	6.5–12	Kobisch and Madec (1983)
Netherlands	3–4	de Jong (1983a)
Germany	10–30	Schöss (1983)

Economic Significance

Franque (1830) stated that pigs with atrophic rhinitis did not fatten and this has been confirmed in a number of subsequent reports. For example, the depression in growth rate associated with severe turbinate atrophy has been estimated to be in the range of 5–25% (Schuman and Earl, 1956; Hasebe, 1971; Muirhead, 1979). King (1981) stated that atrophic rhinitis accounted for approximately 12% of the total losses due to pig diseases in the United States, while Muirhead (1979) estimated that the total cost of a severe outbreak in a 100-sow herd in the United Kingdom in 1976 was £5000. Furthermore, Goodnow et al, (1979) claimed that pigs vaccinated with a *B. bronchiseptica* bacterin in a herd with mild and in another with severe atrophic rhinitis reached 100 kg in a significantly faster time than controls.

The direct and indirect costs of disease are now a crucial factor in pig rearing and contrary reports that atrophic rhinitis has little effect on growth rates and production costs have significant implications for the economic importance of this disease. Thus, Young et al. (1959) and Pearce and Roe (1967) reported that atrophic rhinitis had no effect on mean daily gains, while Bendixen (1971) and Straw et al. (1983) noted that in trials with pigs reared from 20 to 25 kg until slaughter, the degree of turbinate atrophy at slaughter was not associated with reduced weight gains. On the other hand, in experimental infections, Nielsen et al. (1976) reported that infection with *B. bronchiseptica* had no effect on growth rates, whereas *P. multocida* produced "growth retarding atrophic rhinitis." Pedersen and Barfod (1981) demonstrated a 5% reduction in growth rates of pigs that were infected with toxigenic *P. multocida* and had developed severe turbinate atrophy.

In view of the accepted economic importance of atrophic rhinitis, these conflicting results with regard to reductions in productivity need further investigation. The mechanisms involved and the relationship between severity of disease and profitability are inadequately understood, but new knowledge of the etiological agents may help in the design of future studies. In particular, efforts should be made to identify the relative contributions made by individual pathogens, or combinations, to turbinate atrophy and pneumonia, together with the effects of these clinical signs on growth rates.

In addition to reduced growth rates, there may be other significant costs associated with clinical disease, e.g., costs of medication, penalties at slaughter, or inability of breeding or multiplying herds to sell stock (Nielsen, 1983).

III. Clinical and Pathological Features

A. CLINICAL SIGNS

The clinical signs of atrophic rhinitis include sneezing, nasal discharge and epistaxis, shortening or twisting of the snout, dark crescent-shaped stains below the medial canthus of the eye, pneumonia, and reduced growth rates. Atrophy of the turbinate bones will be apparent in live animals by endoscopy or X-radiography and in snout sections at slaughter. In severe outbreaks of disease, all of the changes described above will be seen in some pigs and some of the changes will be apparent in others. However, all the changes may be attributable to more than one causal factor and could occur independently.

Sneezing is a good example of this complex relationship. The original name for atrophic rhinitis was "Schnuffelkrankheit" or sniffing disease (Franque, 1830) because sneezing and sniffling were the first signs noticed in affected piglets (Switzer and Farrington, 1975). A harsh inspiration of air occurs in severely affected pigs suggesting that the nasal cavity is blocked, but when cut in cross section the turbinate bones are invariably absent. Schöss (1983) stated that violent sneezing was frequently present in pigs with severe atrophic rhinitis, while Kobisch (1983) noted that sneezing and coughing were most noticeable 5–30 days after intranasal infection with *B. bronchiseptica*. On the other hand, Switzer and Farrington (1975) observed that acute sneezing in piglets may subside in a few weeks with no turbinate atrophy developing. In the author's laboratory, experimental infection of gnotobiotic pigs with *B. bronchiseptica* and *P. multocida,* in which all developed severe turbinate atrophy and some showed snout deformation, has not been associated with persistent sneezing. Thus, the development of these lesions is not associated *a priori* with sneezing, which can also occur as a result of infection with other agents, or from dust in the environment.

Similarly, snout deformation is not pathognomic of atrophic rhinitis. Brachygnathia superior can now be produced by infection with, or injection of, the toxin of *P. multocida,* but it is also a breed-associated characteristic which occurs in herds without the disease (Duthie, 1947; Done, 1983a; Schöss, 1983). Dark tear staining below the medial canthus of the eye is frequently observed in pigs with atrophic rhinitis, but also occurs in herds without the disease. Pneumonia can be caused by *Mycoplasma hyopneumoniae, B. bronchiseptica, P. multocida,* or *Haemophilus* spp. in herds without atrophic rhinitis, and turbinate atrophy can be produced independently by *B. bronchiseptica* and *P. multocida.*

The complexity of these relationships raises the question, what is atrophic rhinitis? At a recent symposium it was generally agreed that the three most important signs of atrophic rhinitis as a herd problem are progressive turbinate atrophy, snout deformation, and poor growth rates (Pedersen and Nielsen, 1983). Once snout deformation and turbinate damage have occurred, they do not regress; thus, the disease is chronic but does not cause significant mortality.

B. Pathological Changes

The gross pathological and histopathological changes of atrophic rhinitis (Schofield and Jones, 1950; Björklund, 1958; Pearce and Roe, 1966; Switzer and Farrington, 1975), as well as those seen with the electron microscope (Fetter and Capen, 1971; Fetter et al., 1975), have been well documented. Atrophy of the turbinate bones can vary from slight atrophy of the inferior scroll of one of the ventral turbinates to complete bilateral atrophy of the dorsal and ventral turbinates. This gradation of changes raises the question of whether they are (1) progressive manifestations of the same cause, (2) attributable to different causes, or (3) a combination of the two. In some, but not all animals, with severe turbinate atrophy the snout is distorted, the lower mandible protrudes, and the skin covering the snout becomes heavily wrinkled. The snout is shortened and turned upward or to one side. Snout changes have been observed in piglets aged 3 weeks (Braend and Flatla, 1954), but usually appear between 6 and 12 weeks. The nasal septum may show lateral deviation, but other bony structures in the nasal cavity generally remain intact. In severe cases, extension of lesions to the sinus walls has been described (Duthie, 1947).

Histopathological changes include hyperplasia and metaplasia of the nasal epithelium with the development of a stratified cuboidal type, and marked thickening of the arterial walls in the lamina propria, with a dense infiltration of the submucosa with neutrophils, lymphocytes, and fibrous tissue. There is also resorption of the osseous trabeculae of the turbinate bones, with replacement by a shrunken mass of fibrous tissue. In an electron microscopic study, Fetter and Capen (1971) noted severe degenerative changes of osteoblasts and osteocytes and suggested that the lesion was caused by reduced formation of organic matrix.

Comparatively little attention has been paid to changes in other tissues due to atrophic rhinitis. Björklund (1958) concluded that the changes he observed in the facial bones were comparable with those that gave rise to severe atrophy of the conchae. He also noted that sections from the shaft of the radius showed disturbance in bone formation, indicating that the lesions may not be localized to the facial bones. In addition, he reported dilated excretory ducts, fibrosis in the lacrimal glands, and less conspicuous changes in the salivary glands which he likened to mucoviscidosis in children.

More recently, Yoshikawa and Hanada (1981) reported chondrolytic and necrotizing changes in the matrix of epiphyseal cartilage at various sites in pigs with atrophic rhinitis and retarded growth. There is little evidence of significant hematological or plasma changes in outbreaks of atrophic rhinitis (MacNabb, 1948a), or in growing pigs infected with *B. bronchiseptica* (Baetz et al., 1974). As might be predicted, a significant leukocytosis developed in gnotobiotic pigs that were given *B. bronchiseptica* (Rutter et al., 1982) or injected with *P. multocida* toxin (J. M. Rutter and A. Mackenzie, unpublished).

IV. Etiology

Numerous etiological agents and factors have been associated with atrophic rhinitis. They can be broadly classified into hereditary, nutritional, and infectious, and the evidence for their roles has frequently been contradictory.

A. HEREDITY

An hereditary influence on atrophic rhinitis was first suggested by Franque (1830) and estimates of the heritability of the disease have ranged from 0.06 to 0.61 (reviewed by Smith, 1983). It has also been reported that the offspring of affected parents became more seriously affected than those of nonaffected parents within the same herd (Bugnowski, 1973), and that atrophic rhinitis could be eradicated by culling affected dams (Elias and Hamori, 1975). Some authors noted that short-nosed pigs had a more serious disease (Franque, 1830; Radtke, 1938), while others found no relationship between facial conformity and the severity of atrophic rhinitis (Gendrau, 1948; Gilman, 1949; MacNabb, 1948b; Flatla and Braend, 1953). Lundeheim (1979) and Done (1962) suggested that Landrace pigs were more commonly and more severely affected; Smith (1983) observed that outbreaks were more severe in herds using Large White boars, and Björklund (1958) reported that Landrace and Large White pigs were equally susceptible to atrophic rhinitis.

One interpretation of these conflicting findings is that heredity plays no role in the etiology of atrophic rhinitis. However, different authors may have been referring to various syndromes and, now that the infectious nature of atrophic rhinitis has been clarified, it should be possible to investigate hereditary influences in a more systematic way. Infection experiments in gnotobiotic piglets, for example, suggest little variation in their susceptibility to *B. bronchiseptica,* but some variation in colonization by toxigenic *P. multocida* has been noted in older pigs (J. M. Rutter, unpublished); whether this is attributable to age or to a genetic influence has not been investigated.

B. Nutrition

The role of nutrition in the etiology of atrophic rhinitis has been the subject of much debate. Hering (1842 cited by Switzer, 1955) suggested that facial deformity resulted from rickets and that it could be cured in its early stage by feeding bone salts and cod liver oil. Bendixen (1957) discussed vitamin A and D deficiencies as predisposing factors in atrophic rhinitis, as well as faulty calcium/phosphorus ratios in the feed. The latter view was expanded by Brown *et al.* (1966), who proposed that an imbalance of calcium and phosphorus in the diet induced hyperparathyroidism, of which turbinate hypoplasia was one manifestation. However, numerous reports, e.g., Peo *et al.* (1967), Baustad *et al.* (1967), Kemeny *et al.* (1970), concluded that calcium deficiency, or an imbalance of calcium and phosphorus, was not the cause of atrophic rhinitis. One reason for suggestions that atrophic rhinitis was caused by nutritional imbalances was the presence of more generalized changes in other bones and tissues (Björklund, 1958; Brown *et al.,* 1966). The demonstration that the toxin of *P. multocida* produces changes in tissues other than the turbinate bones (Rutter and Mackenzie, 1984) may help to explain some of these anomalies.

C. Infection

Most authors have stated that atrophic rhinitis behaves like a contagious disease, and the early work was summarized by Switzer (1955). These studies implicated bacteria (*Pseudomonas, Actinomyces, Sphaerophorus, Corynebacterium,* or *Mycoplasmas*), viruses (cytomegalovirus), and trichomonads as etiological agents. One of the main problems, however, has been to reproduce the disease with pure cultures of these microorganisms. Successful results were reported with crude suspensions from the nasal cavity of affected pigs (Radtke, 1938; Phillips *et al.,* 1948), but these were frequently not repeated in experiments with filtrates or pure cultures (Jones, 1947; MacNabb,

1948a; Phillips et al., 1948). Current evidence indicates that only two bacteria, *B. bronchiseptica* and *P. multocida,* consistently produce a significant degree of turbinate atrophy in pigs. The effect of *B. bronchiseptica* was first demonstrated (as *Alcaligenes* spp.) by Switzer (1956) and by Cross and Claflin (1962), and that of *P. multocida* by Gwatkin et al. (1953) and Braend and Flatla (1954). Much work was done in the United States during the 1960s on the role of *B. bronchiseptica* in atrophic rhinitis, and this organism was said to be the principal cause of the disease (Switzer and Farrington, 1975). However, the results of Braend and Flatla (1954), together with the significance of the observation that experimental infection with *B. bronchiseptica* did not cause severe progressive lesions (Duncan et al., 1966), may not have been adequately appreciated.

Meanwhile in Germany, Schöss (1971) found *P. multocida* was frequently present in affected herds and reproduced the progressive disease with these strains (Dirks et al., 1973). In the United Kingdom, infection with *B. bronchiseptica* was widespread, but the prevalence of progressive disease was more restricted (Giles et al., 1980).

One explanation for discrepant results in different countries could be variations in virulence of the organisms concerned. This has been reported for isolates of *B. bronchiseptica* in the United States (Ross et al., 1967; Skelly et al., 1980), Canada (Miniats and Johnson, 1980), and the United Kingdom (Collings, 1983). However, even the most virulent of 10 United Kingdom isolates did not cause progressive turbinate atrophy or significant snout deformation in experimental infections (Rutter et al., 1982). More importantly, strains isolated in the United Kingdom from herds with or without progressive disease all caused nonprogressive lesions of similar severity (Rutter et al., 1982; Smith, cited by Giles and Smith, 1983). Thus, there is strong evidence that, although there are differences in the virulence of isolates of *B. bronchiseptica,* the severe lesions of atrophic rhinitis cannot be attributed to this organism.

In contrast, a major difference associated with toxin production has been identified in the virulence of porcine isolates of *P. multocida* (Ilina and Zasukhin, 1975; de Jong et al., 1980; Pedersen and Barfod, 1981; Rutter and Rojas, 1982; Rutter, 1983). This has led to the view that toxigenic strains of *P. multocida* are the key microorganisms in progressive atrophic rhinitis.

D. Environment and Management

Several reports state that atrophic rhinitis is more severe under conditions of bad ventilation and poor management. In particular, high stocking densities and continuous throughput in farrowing houses and weaner accommodation have been identified as important factors (de Jong, 1983a; Smith, 1983). Presumably, increased stocking rates facilitate the spread of infection within large groups of pigs, while continuous throughput increases the weight of infection in the environment. Increased prevalence of atrophic rhinitis in litters born during late winter and spring (see Smith, 1983) might be attributable to reduced ventilation rates during these periods, when heat is being conserved. Furthermore, the presence of noxious gases, e.g., ammonia in the environment, can exacerbate the severity of turbinate atrophy produced by *B. bronchiseptica* (Drummond *et al.*, 1981).

V. Pathogenesis

There are three important stages in the pathogenesis of most infectious diseases: (1) evasion of the nonspecific and specific defense mechanisms of the host by the pathogen; (2) establishment and multiplication of the pathogen; (3) production of toxic factors which are responsible, directly or indirectly, for the clinical signs of disease. A defect at any of these three stages can result in a strain being rendered avirulent or poorly virulent. There is now good evidence that variations in colonization and toxicity are the most important determinants of virulence for *B. bronchiseptica* and *P. multocida*.

A. *B. bronchiseptica*

The biology of *B. bronchiseptica* has been reviewed by Goodnow (1980). This organism is related to *Bordetella pertussis,* the cause of whooping cough in children, and is a common cause of respiratory disease in pigs, dogs, cats, and laboratory animals. *B. bronchiseptica* has been associated with disease in man (Ghosh and Tranter, 1979; Byrd *et al.*, 1981), but it is not a frequent isolate from ruminants.

1. *Attachment and Colonization*

There is evidence that *B. bronchiseptica* becomes closely associated with the ciliated epithelium of the respiratory tract of the pig (Yokomizo and Shimizu, 1979), dog (Bemis *et al.*, 1977b), and rabbit (Matsuyama and Takino, 1980). However, the properties of this organism are influenced by phase variation (Leslie and Gardner, 1931) and antigenic modulation (Lacey, 1960), which are fascinating features of the genus *Bordetella. B. bronchiseptica,* when cultured on Bordet Gengou medium, exhibits several distinct colonial morphologies, each characteristically associated with the presence or absence of a number of bacterial products. These morphological differences are not apparent on blood agar or media without blood. Four distinct phases (I, II, III, and IV) have been recognized (Nakase, 1957a), phase I being virulent for mice (Nakase, 1957b) and phases I and II for guinea pigs (Nakagawa et al., 1971).

The role of phase variation in the etiology and pathogenesis of disease has been studied mainly with nonporcine isolates and laboratory animal or canine models of *B. bronchiseptica* infection (Nakase, 1957b; Thompson et al., 1976; Bemis et al., 1977a). However, Yokomizo and Shimizu (1979) demonstrated that phase I organisms of porcine strains of *B. bronchiseptica* adhered *in vitro* to nasal epithelial cells from pigs, whereas phase III variants exhibited feeble adherence; similar results were obtained *in vivo* in piglets killed 4 days after infection with these organisms.

The potential significance of differences in the virulence of *B. bronchiseptica* in the pathogenesis of atrophic rhinitis has been mentioned earlier, and particular attention has been paid to phase variation in the author's laboratory (Rutter et al., 1982; Collings, 1983; Collings and Rutter, 1985) in order to determine whether phase I variants are associated with progressive disease, and phase III or IV variants with less severe lesions. This research has shown that phase variation occurs in porcine strains of *B. bronchiseptica in vivo* as well as *in vitro*. Strains dissociated *in vitro* from phase I to III or IV, a change which was accelerated by culture in broth medium or retarded by growth on Bordet Gengou medium. Reversion to phase I was not observed. Intranasal infection of gnotobiotic pigs with phase I organisms gradually produced phase III isolates, particularly in the pharynx and feces and less frequently in the nasal cavity, trachea, and lungs. An unexpected result was that infection of pigs with phase III variants resulted in the appearance of phase I organisms in the nasal cavity after a few days.

There were numerous differences between organisms in phase I and III. Those in phase I produced fimbriae, capsules, hemagglutinin, hemolysin, heat-labile toxin, and adenylate cyclase, whereas those in phase III did not, apart from capsule production by one phase III variant. Phase I organisms colonized the nasal cavity of pigs better than those in phase III and, when reversion to phase I occurred *in vivo*, it was accompanied by enhanced colonization by the phase I variant. Phase IV cultures colonized poorly and failed to revert *in vivo*.

The attachment of porcine isolates of *B. bronchiseptica* to the respiratory mucosa (Yokomizo and Shimizu, 1979) may be caused by fimbriae of variable length and 3–4 nm in diameter (Blom et al., 1983;

Collings, 1983) and which are hemagglutinins. However, additional factors, e.g., capsules and the specificity of fimbriae, may also be involved in colonization of the porcine nasal cavity. Evidence for this is that a capsulate, nonfimbriate phase III variant colonized better than noncapsulate, nonfimbriate variants, and porcine phase I isolates persisted in larger numbers in the nasal cavity than phase I isolates from other species (Collings, 1983; Collings and Rutter, 1985).

Although the above observations raise interesting questions about the control of bacterial phase variation *in vitro* and *in vivo,* this phenomenon appears to be unimportant in relation to progressive atrophic rhinitis. Virtually all strains isolated in the author's laboratory from commercial pig herds with or without a history of progressive disease have been in phase I, and attempts to recover phase III organisms from the pharynx of slaughtered pigs in a herd with endemic infection were unsuccessful (Collings, 1983). Perhaps phase III organisms compete poorly with the commensal flora, and their ready detection in the infection experiments described above was attributable to the use of gnotobiotic animals. Nevertheless, reversible phase variation could be an effective mechanism for bacterial conservation and survival *in vivo* and might influence the epidemiology of *B. bronchiseptica* infection.

2. Production of Toxins

All members of the genus *Bordetella* produce substances with various biological activities (Munoz, 1971; Morse, 1976). In *B. bronchiseptica,* an intracellular heat-labile toxin, inactivated at 56°C for 30 min, and released by alternate freezing and thawing or by ultrasonic disruption of phase I cells, has been extensively studied. Crude toxin prepared from guinea pig (Nakase, 1957b) or porcine strains (Rutter *et al.,* 1982) is lethal for mice and causes a skin lesion in guinea pigs. Duncan *et al.* (1966) and Fetter *et al.* (1975) suggested that an endotoxin-like substance had a direct effect on bone cells in the turbinates, while Hanada *et al.* (1979) showed that repeated instillation on cotton wool swabs or by spray instillation of cell-free sonicated extracts from phase I strains caused turbinate damage in pigs. On the other hand, Ilina and Zasukhin (1975) reported that repeated instillation of a culture filtrate of *B. bronchiseptica* in the nasal cavity of pigs had no effect on the turbinates, although the growth of the piglets was retarded. Intraperitoneal injection of freeze-dried toxin prepared from sonicated phase I cells of *B. bronchiseptica* was acutely toxic in gnotobiotic piglets (J. M. Rutter and A. Mackenzie, unpublished). A suspension containing 250 μg of toxin killed piglets within 18 hr, with signs of acute toxemia and circulatory collapse, whereas an equivalent amount of *P. multocida* toxin prepared in the same way was not lethal, but caused persistent turbinate atrophy and snout deformation (Rutter and Mackenzie, 1984). When the dose of *B. bronchiseptica* toxin was reduced piglets survived, but no turbinate atrophy was produced with toxin given by this route.

Collings (1983) demonstrated variations in the toxicity of different strains and variants of *B. bronchiseptica* in assays of lethality in mice and in a cell culture test. Preparations from phase I isolates from pigs were significantly more toxic than similar material from phase I organisms isolated from other species, while material from phase III organisms was poorly toxic or nontoxic (Collings and Rutter, 1985). Preliminary results (Collings, 1983) demonstrated no detectable neutralizing activity for the cytotoxin in hyperimmune rabbit serum prepared against whole cells of phases I or III, nor in sera from piglets infected with *B. bronchiseptica* for 30 days, although these sera had high levels of agglutinating activity. Neutralizing activity was first detected in sera from pigs infected for 35 days and the levels increased up to 11 weeks.

These results suggested that the toxin was being produced *in vivo*, although the neutralizing response was slow to develop, possibly because the antigen is an internal product of the bacterial cell. The variations in toxicity demonstrated in different phase I isolates, together with the variations in colonization, explained the differences in severity of turbinate atrophy produced by infection of gnotobiotic piglets (Collings, 1983; Collings and Rutter, 1985). Strains which produced less severe lesions were less toxic and did not colonize the porcine nasal cavity as well as those which produced severe lesions. However, Rutter *et al.* (1982) found that toxin prepared from phase I strains of *B. bronchiseptica* from herds with progressive atrophic rhinitis, or from herds with no history of progressive disease caused similar mean LD_{50} in mice. These results indicated that the production of severe lesions was not attributable to phase I strains with a greater toxicity.

The regulatory enzyme, adenylate cyclase, is produced by phase I but not by phase III cultures of porcine isolates of *B. bronchiseptica* (A. J. Lax and J. M. Rutter, unpublished); however, its relationship to the heat-labile toxin and its effect on turbinate development have not been determined.

The presence of plasmids in *B. bronchiseptica* has also been reported, and the possibility that these are associated with toxins or virulence factors has been investigated. Recent results have indicated that not all phase I strains with comparable virulence in gnotobiotic piglets

(Rutter *et al.*, 1982) have plasmids (A. J. Lax and C. Walker, personal communication), suggesting that determinants of the major biological activities are controlled by chromosomal genes.

3. Lesions

The lesions produced in the nasal cavity of pigs following infection with *B. bronchiseptica* have been well documented (Duncan *et al.*, 1966; Shimizu *et al.*, 1971). In SPF or gnotobiotic pigs a nonprogressive, moderately severe turbinate atrophy is apparent 2–4 weeks after infection, followed frequently by regeneration of the turbinate bones (Duncan *et al.*, 1966; Nielsen *et al.*, 1976; Rutter *et al.*, 1982). The significance of the nonprogressive nature of this lesion has frequently been overlooked.

Histopathological changes include hyperplasia and metaplasia of the nasal epithelium, fibrosis in the lamina propria, and resorption and replacement fibrosis of the osseous core. With the electron microscope, progressive degenerative changes were seen in the osteoblasts and osteocytes of infected pigs (Fetter *et al.*, 1975) and bacteria, believed to be *B. bronchiseptica*, were seen in the cytoplasm of osteoblasts in close proximity to the bone surfaces. Changes observed by scanning electron microscopy included loss and shortening of cilia on the respiratory mucosa, attachment of numerous bacteria to the shortened cilia, and the presence of extruded and shrunken epithelial cells (Yokomizo and Shimizu, 1979).

Infection experiments with *B. bronchiseptica* alone have not resulted in severe persistent turbinate atrophy or significant twisting or shortening of the snout; attempts have been made to enhance the pathogenicity of this organism by mixed infections, e.g., with porcine cytomegalovirus (PCMV) or mycoplasmas. Infection with PCMV was first described by Done (1955) as "inclusion body rhinitis," which caused destruction of acini in the mucous glands of the nasal mucosa and metaplasia of the respiratory epithelium (Plowright, 1979). Although PCMV prejudices the integrity of the mucosa and immunosuppression has been observed following cytomegalovirus infection in mice (Osborn *et al.*, 1968), combined infections of PCMV and *B. bronchiseptica* in pigs did not increase the severity of turbinate atrophy as compared to *B. bronchiseptica* alone (Edington *et al.*, 1976). Further experiments in gnotobiotic pigs indicated that the lesions in combined infections were less severe than with *B. bronchiseptica* alone (J. M. Rutter, W. Plowright, and M. Bew, unpublished). Gois *et al.* (1977) reported "grossly perceptible" turbinate atrophy in gnotobiotic pigs after combined infection with *B. bronchiseptica* and *Mycoplasma hyorhinis;* however, these piglets were killed 32 days after infection and the persistence of lesions was not investigated.

A model for turbinate atrophy in mice was reported by Sawata and Kume (1982). Intranasal instillation of a phase I porcine isolate of *B. bronchiseptica* in mice aged 5 days caused turbinate atrophy in 80% of the mice by 3 weeks of age. If a phase III variant or older mice were used, no lesions were produced.

B. *P. multocida*

P. multocida is an important bacterial pathogen in most animal species and its role in pigs was reviewed by Farrington (1981). Its association with atrophic rhinitis was demonstrated by Gwatkin *et al.* (1953), Flatla and Braend (1953), and Braend and Flatla (1954) but only recently has its role been elucidated. Four types of *P. multocida* (A, B, D, and E) are recognized on the basis of capsular antigens demonstrable by indirect hemagglutination tests (Carter, 1965), while typing systems for the somatic antigens are based on acid agglutination (Namioka, 1978), or gel precipitin tests (Heddleston *et al.*, 1972). Porcine isolates belong mainly to capsular types A and D (Carter, 1967), although type-B isolates have also been reported (Meyeringh *et al.*, 1977).

1. *Attachment and Colonization*

Harris and Switzer (1968) showed that a type-D isolate of *P. multocida* failed to colonize the nasal cavity of pigs, but established and persisted if the animals had been previously infected with *B. bronchiseptica*. Combined infection did not increase the macroscopic severity of turbinate atrophy, but caused an increase in the microscopic severity of the lesions. In a series of experiments with gnotobiotic pigs quantitative results were obtained for colonization by types A and D of *P. multocida* (Rutter and Rojas, 1982; Rutter, 1983). It was found that a nontoxigenic type-A strain of *P. multocida* colonized the nasal cavity poorly during the 11 weeks after infection (mean count $10^{1.5}$ colony-forming units). Colonization by a toxigenic type-D strain was 10–100 times better than the type-A strain, but was 10,000 times better in pigs infected 5 days previously with *B. bronchiseptica;* these higher numbers persisted throughout the period of observation. Some enhancement of growth of the type-A strain occurred as a result of previous infection with *B. bronchiseptica,* but did not persist after 4 weeks. Enhanced colonization by nontoxigenic type-D strains also occurred in combined infections with *B. bronchiseptica* but did not persist beyond 35 days, while colonization by a nonporcine, toxigenic type-D isolate was poor. These results demonstrated quantitatively that *B. bronchiseptica* enhanced colonization by *P. multocida,* particularly colonization by toxigenic type-D strains isolated from pigs.

Recent experiments in SPF pigs (Elling and Pedersen, 1983; Pedersen and Elling, 1984) have shown that two instillations of 0.5 ml of a 1% solution of acetic acid in one side of the nose, followed 3 days later by infection with a toxigenic type-A or type-D strain of *P. multocida,* resulted in colonization of the treated, but generally not the untreated, side of the nasal cavity. Treatment with acetic acid did not produce ultrastructural changes in the epithelium of the turbinates, the lamina propria, or the osseous core, yet clearly assisted colonization by *P. multocida.*

Little research has been done on the mechanisms of enhanced colonization, or on attachment of *P. multocida* to the respiratory epithelium. The organism is nonmotile, but the presence of fimbriae has been reported in a type-A strain isolated from a rabbit and these were thought to assist attachment to respiratory epithelial cells *in vitro* (Glorioso *et al.*, 1982). Since the organism grows relatively poorly on nutrient agar medium, but growth is luxuriant with the addition of blood, it may be significant that infection with *B. bronchiseptica* damages the epithelial tissues (Duncan *et al.*, 1966); this may allow leakage of blood, or other growth-promoting factors for *P. multocida,* across the mucosa. Although enhancement of colonization by *P. multocida* has been produced *in vivo* by *B. bronchiseptica* and by acetic acid, it was not observed in gnotobiotic pigs accidentally contaminated with *Staphylococcus* spp. (Rutter and Rojas, 1982). This suggests that the effect is more than a nonspecific reaction.

2. Production of Toxins

Smith (1957, cited by Carter, 1967) first reported that a heat-labile toxin was produced by some strains of *P. multocida* and was lethal for mice, but the significance of toxin production by porcine strains of *P. multocida* in relation to atrophic rhinitis was first recognized by Ilina and Zasukhin (1975). Filtrates of 30-day-old cultures were lethal for mice and produced turbinate atrophy in piglets after repeated instillation in the nasal cavity. The toxin also produces a dark hemorrhagic zone, called a dermonecrotic reaction, in the skin of guinea pigs after intradermal injection (de Jong *et al.*, 1980); a cytopathic effect in cultures of embryo bovine lung cells (Rutter and Luther, 1984); and persistent turbinate atrophy and snout shortening in germ-free pigs after a single parenteral injection (Rutter and Mackenzie, 1984). The biological activities of *P. multocida* toxin are destroyed at 56°C for 30 min. In a series of experiments, rapid loss of lethal activity occurred between 54 and 56°C (J. M. Rutter, unpublished) but occasionally, a repeated period of heating may be necessary to completely destroy the toxicity. The cytotoxin appears to be produced inside the bacterial cell; it can be detected in the filtrates of sonicated cells after 12–16 hr incubation, but does not appear in the culture supernatants until 20–24 hr (Rutter and Luther, 1984). The latter observation is presumably attributable to the release of toxin from lysing cells, with the result that the lethal and dermonecrotic toxin is demonstrated more reliably in culture supernatants after 48 rather than 24 hr.

Toxin production by porcine isolates of *P. multocida* was first reported in type-D strains and both toxigenic and nontoxigenic isolates of type D are common (de Jong *et al.*, 1980; Rutter and Luther, 1984; Sawata *et al.*, 1984). All type-A strains in these reports were nontoxigenic; however, toxigenic type-A strains have been isolated from herds with atrophic rhinitis in Denmark (Elling and Pedersen, 1983). Preliminary results indicate that, although these strains may be less toxic than type-D strains, some are particularly virulent for gnotobiotic pigs, causing death and turbinate atrophy within 14 days (J. M. Rutter and A. Mackenzie, unpublished). This may be due to production of the hyaluronic acid capsule by type-A strains, in addition to the toxin which may enable them to penetrate host defense mechanisms more effectively and produce toxin in various organs.

Whether the lethal, dermonecrotic, cytotoxic, and osteolytic activities of *P. multocida* are attributable to the same or to different toxins is currently being investigated. All the activities were present in toxigenic and absent in nontoxigenic strains (Rutter and Luther, 1984). Van der Heidjen *et al.* (1983) stated that the dermonecrotic toxin was a protein of at least three components with molecular weights between 80,000 and 110,000 and an isoelectric point at about pH 5. Fractionation of crude toxin by preparative polyacrylamide gel electrophoresis and DEAE Sephadex A50 chromatography has shown that the lethal, cytotoxic, and osteolytic activities in a type-D strain are associated with a polypeptide of a molecular weight of approximately 155,000 (N. Chanter and J. M. Rutter, unpublished data). The biological activities in partially purified fractions seem to be less stable than in crude material.

The crude toxin can be neutralized in pig antisera in the four assays (Rutter and Luther, 1984; Rutter *et al.*, 1984a); however, tests with different sera have indicated that neutralization of the cytotoxic activity can occur with serum that does not neutralize the lethal, dermonecrotic, and osteolytic activities (Rutter et al., 1984a). These results may imply that there is a single toxin, which acts in a different way in different assays. Purification of the toxic substances and analysis by monoclonal antibodies should help to resolve such questions, although the production of monoclonal antibodies is complicated by the extreme toxicity of these preparations for mice.

3. Lesions

Successful production of the progressive lesions of atrophic rhinitis following experimental infection with *P. multocida* was reported by Gwatkin *et al.* (1953), Braend and Flatla (1954), Dirks *et al.* (1973), and Nielsen *et al.* (1976). Others were unable to repeat these findings (Harris and Switzer, 1968; Smith *et al.*, 1973; Nakagawa *et al.*, 1974; and Miniats and Johnson, 1980), but this discrepancy may now be explained by the observation that, in SPF (de Jong *et al.*, 1980; Pedersen and Barfod, 1981) or gnotobiotic (Rutter and Rojas, 1982; Rutter, 1983) pigs, only toxigenic strains of *P. multocida* produce progressive lesions affecting the turbinate bones and snout. There is now field evidence to support this view. Recent results in four commercial herds have indicated that comparatively low numbers of nontoxigenic type-A, nontoxigenic type-D, and toxigenic type-D isolates persisted for at least 16 weeks in the nasal cavity, and that severe turbinate atrophy and brachygnathia superior were associated with the presence of toxigenic type-D strains (Rutter *et al.*, 1984b).

Direct evidence for the effects of *Pasteurella* toxin in pigs is provided by the results of Ilina and Zasukhin (1975), who gave repeated intranasal instillations, and those of Rutter and Mackenzie (1984), who gave a single parenteral injection of toxin to germ-free piglets aged 3 weeks. The latter procedure caused severe turbinate atrophy in all, and snout shortening in a proportion of cases, which persisted for 20 weeks. Histopathologically, the lesions were extensive and could be divided into 5 main categories: degenerative, hyperplastic, obstructive, reactive, and osteolytic. Changes in the ventral turbinates consisted of epithelial hyperplasia, atrophy of mucous glands, osteolysis, and proliferation of mesenchymal cells, which later provided a cellular core that completely replaced bone trabeculae and osteogenic and osteoclastic tissue. Increased osteoclast activity was apparent within the first few days, but histopathological changes comparable with this single injection model were not observed in other osseous tissues, e.g., tail vertebrae, the costochondral junction, and long bones. These changes in the turbinate bones are similar to those described following infection with *B. bronchiseptica* (Duncan et al., 1966), or toxigenic type-A (Elling and Pedersen, 1983) or type-D (Pedersen and Elling, 1984) strains of *P. multocida,* suggesting either that the tissues can only respond in a limited way, or that the toxins produce their effects by similar mechanisms. However, an important difference should be emphasized: turbinate regeneration occurs more readily following infection with *B. bronchiseptica* than after infection with *P. multocida.*

In addition to the lesions produced in the nasal cavity, degenerative hyperplastic and obstructive changes occurred in the liver and urinary tract of germ-free piglets that had been given *P. multocida* toxin (Rutter and Mackenzie, 1984). Larger doses of toxin caused edema of the eyelids, severe jaundice, and death, while smaller doses caused necrosis of liver cells, accumulation of bile pigments, extramedullary hematopoiesis, and hyperplasia of hepatocytes. In the kidneys, hydronephrosis and degeneration of the renal tubules were associated with pronounced hyperplasia of the transitional epithelium of the ureters and bladder.

These observations with the toxin model raise the question of whether comparable changes occur in field outbreaks of the disease. Similar effects can be produced by the injection of toxin in conventional pigs (A. Mackenzie and J. M. Rutter, unpublished), while some germ-free pigs that had been given larger doses of toxin became anorexic and their growth rate decreased. Whether the latter observation could explain growth retardation in field outbreaks remains to be determined. Most descriptions of the pathology of atrophic rhinitis have been confined to changes in the turbinates and facial bones, but it is of interest that Volkova (1975) referred to "dystrophic changes" in the livers of 98/150 and kidneys of 31/150 Large White pigs in which atrophic rhinitis had been diagnosed. Clearly, it would be useful to carry out more extensive histopathological examinations on animals affected with progressive disease.

The toxin model provides a powerful tool for investigating the pathogenesis of the lesions and also for studying the regulatory mechanisms of the cells and tissues affected. Whether all of the changes described in different tissues are attributable to the same toxin is an interesting question. Pig sera appeared to neutralize all of the effects in gnotobiotic pigs (Rutter et al., 1984a), but tests with toxin purified from crude preparations should elucidate this point.

Infection with *P. multocida* or *B. bronchiseptica* causes bronchopneumonia in pigs and the lesions are characteristic for each organism (see Switzer, 1981; Farrington, 1981). However, recent results suggest that severe turbinate atrophy is not invariably associated with severe pneumonia (Straw et al., 1983; Rutter et al., 1984b). Furthermore, bronchopneumonia was rarely observed in experimental infections with toxigenic type-D strains of P. multocida in gnotobiotic piglets (Rutter, 1983), while most isolates from lungs of four commercial herds were nontoxigenic strains of type A (Rutter et al., 1984b). Thus, the role of toxin-producing strains in pneumonia, and the relationship of pneumonia with severe turbinate atrophy are not supported by current evidence.

In summary, toxigenic strains of P. multocida are, at present, the only microorganisms shown to be capable of reproducing the clinical signs of progressive atrophic rhinitis. Whether B. bronchiseptica infection is the main predisposing factor in herd outbreaks remains to be determined. Pedersen and Barfod (1982) considered that other factors were significant because B. bronchiseptica could not be found in all herds with atrophic rhinitis.

VI. Epidemiology

Ways in which a disease is introduced and spreads within a population depends on numerous factors including the nature of the etiological agent, the host, and the structure of the population. In intensive pig rearing, many animals are in close contact and there is often widespread movement of breeding and replacement stock between herds. The main risks of introducing infection are associated with purchased pigs and disease may then spread rapidly within a seronegative herd. Early reports clearly recognized that atrophic rhinitis was introduced by carrier pigs. The disease appeared in many Norwegian herds that had imported pigs, several of which eventually developed severe clinical signs. This led Braend and Flatla (1954) to conclude that "atrophic rhinitis was practically unknown in Norway prior to the last war, after which it has been rather common, most certainly because of importation of pigs from Sweden where the disease is common." It was, therefore, assumed that a new infectious organism had been imported. Similarly, the introduction of atrophic rhinitis into the United Kingdom was attributed to the importation of Swedish stock (Anon, 1954). There are at least two possible explanations for these observations; either that B. bronchiseptica was introduced in infected animals and exacerbated existing infections with toxigenic P. multocida or, more likely, that toxigenic P. multocida was introduced in the imported stock.

B. bronchiseptica colonizes the ciliated mucosa of the porcine respiratory tract very effectively; it is frequently isolated from the tonsils and large numbers (10^6/g) have been found in the intestinal contents of infected gnotobiotic pigs (J. M. Rutter, unpublished). Thus, direct contact, droplet infection, and perhaps ingestion of fecal material are likely to be the main routes of transmission. The cycle of infection appears to be maintained by a small proportion of breeding females. Litters within the farrowing house become infected at an early age, but in the United Kingdom, the major spread seems to occur, after weaning at 3 weeks of age, in large groups on flat decks, when 70–80% of a group can become infected. Infection persists for several months with a gradual reduction in the intensity and rate of infection. The age at which animals first become infected with *B. bronchiseptica* has an important effect on the development of lesions. The most severe lesions occur in nonimmune animals infected during the first week of life (Duncan *et al.*, 1966). Animals infected at 4 weeks show less severe lesions, while those infected at 10 weeks show virtually no lesions (M. F. de Jong, personal communication).

The amount and type of immunity also influence the epidemiology of *Bordetella* infection. The presence of passive antibody in the sera of piglets born to naturally infected dams appeared to provide protection against the development of turbinate lesions (Rutter, 1981), but not against infection. However, vaccination of sows appeared to delay infection in their piglets until 12–16 weeks as compared to nonvaccinated herds in which litters became infected by 2 weeks of age (Rutter *et al.*, 1984b). Heavy and widespread infection occurred in pigs after 12–16 weeks in the vaccinated herds.

B. bronchiseptica has been isolated from most domestic and wild animal species (Goodnow, 1980) and, because it is a ubiquitous pathogen, there is always the risk that infection could be introduced by nonporcine vectors. Most isolates from other species appear to be poorly virulent in pigs, but it is possible that rodents might become infected with pig strains and transmit them. In the United Kingdom virtually every pig herd is infected with *B. bronchiseptica,* and variable amounts of moderately severe turbinate atrophy might be expected in all herds. For this to occur, pigs from nonimmune dams must become infected within the first 4 weeks of life and develop lesions which persist to slaughter. In the field, however, the picture is likely to be more complicated, e.g., there are reports that *Haemophilus parasuis* in combined infections with type-A strains of *P. multocida* can produce mild turbinate lesions (Gois *et al.*, 1983).

The epidemiology of *P. multocida* infection in pigs is less well understood. The organism colonizes the tonsils, but some factor(s), the mechanism of which is not understood, is needed to assist colonization of the nasal mucosa. Nontoxigenic type-A strains can be isolated from the lungs of pigs with pneumonia, but *P. multocida* is much less effective than *B. bronchiseptica* in colonizing the trachea.

P. multocida has also been isolated from most animal species and is well recognized as an important pathogen in cattle, poultry, and turkeys (Carter, 1967). In some studies its distribution in pig herds was limited, e.g., only 9% were infected in one report (Harris *et al.*, 1969), but such results may be attributable to the presence of the commensal flora in the nasal cavity. In most laboratories, selective media and the technique of mouse passage are now used for isolation of the organism. Material from 30 of 30 herds examined in this way in the author's laboratory has yielded nontoxigenic isolates of types A or D and mixed infections with these two types in the same pig often occurred.

In contrast, the distribution of toxigenic isolates of *P. multocida* in the United Kingdom appears to be limited to those herds with progressive atrophic rhinitis, or a history of the disease (J. M. Rutter and R. J. Taylor, unpublished). In Denmark (Pedersen, 1983) and Germany (P. Schöss, personal communication) the picture is similar, suggesting that the majority of herds infected with toxigenic *P. multocida* exhibit clinical signs of progressive disease. In the Netherlands, however, toxigenic *P. multocida* has been isolated from 15% of those herds with no history or clinical signs of progressive disease (M. F. de Jong, personal communication). Only 5% of pigs in these herds were infected, but this is an important observation that needs confirmation in other countries, because it indicates that toxigenic strains may be present in some unaffected herds, and these could transmit progressive disease if infected stock were purchased from them.

The main source of *P. multocida* infection for young pigs appears to be pharyngeal carriage of the organism among breeding stock. Ten to fifteen percent of sows in farrowing houses were infected with toxigenic isolates (M. F. de Jong, personal communication) and piglets became infected with these strains within a week of birth. The age at which piglets first become infected with *P. multocida* affects the severity of the lesions produced but, unlike *B. bronchiseptica* infection, older pigs may still develop lesions. Significant turbinate atrophy occurred in pigs infected with toxigenic *P. multocida* up to 12 weeks of age (M. F. de Jong, personal communication), while Rutter *et al.* (1984b) found that pigs which became naturally infected between 12 and 16 weeks of age had mild turbinate lesions. Injection of *P. multocida* toxin (125 µg/kg) produced significant atrophy in conventional pigs aged 10 weeks (A. Mackenzie and J. M. Rutter, unpublished).

The prevalence of toxigenic *P. multocida* may be related to the extent of clinical disease. The organism was isolated from 50 to 60% of young pigs sampled in a herd in which almost 30% of fattening pigs had twisted snouts. In less severely affected herds, larger numbers of young pigs had to be sampled before toxigenic strains were isolated (J. M. Rutter and R. J. Taylor, unpublished).

The distribution of toxigenic *P. multocida* in other species has still to be determined; Pedersen (1983) reported that dermonecrotic strains occurred in cattle, rabbits, dogs, and cats, while, in the author's laboratory, a toxigenic type-D strain has been identified from a severe outbreak of pasteurellosis in turkeys. The latter strain produced severe turbinate atrophy in gnotobiotic pigs (J. M. Rutter and R. J. Taylor, unpublished data) but a toxigenic strain thought to have been isolated from ovine pneumonia colonized the nasal cavity of pigs poorly, and did not produce significant lesions in combined infection with *B. bronchiseptica* (Rutter, 1983).

VII. Diagnosis

A. Clinical

The clinical signs associated with atrophic rhinitis are not pathognomic. While there may be no difficulty in making a clinical diagnosis when a substantial proportion of fattening pigs are affected with progressive disease, diagnosis is difficult when the signs are sporadic or mild. If the disease occurs as a herd problem, pigs with twisted snouts invariably have severe turbinate atrophy associated with infection by toxigenic *P. multocida*. On the other hand, sporadic cases of snout abnormality do not mean that the pigs have severe turbinate damage or are infected with toxigenic *P. multocida*. The etiology of these changes may be associated with congenital abnormalities or breed characters (Done, 1983a). In an attempt to improve differential diagnosis, X-radiography and endoscopy have been used to examine the condition of the turbinate bones in the living animal. Such procedures are relatively expensive, difficult to perform, and difficult to interpret; they are not now thought to be particularly helpful (Schuller, 1980; Switzer, 1981; Schöss, 1983).

B. Pathological

The main diagnostic criterion for atrophic rhinitis has been the visual examination of snout sections from slaughtered pigs for the presence and severity of turbinate atrophy (Done *et al.*, 1964). The site at which the snout is sectioned (second premolar tooth) is crucial because the size of the turbinate bone reduces anteriorly and may give a false, positive result if the section is taken too far forward. The original method of grading was based on a simple 0–5 system, but, more recently, morphometric and other techniques have been devised to quantify the extent of turbinate atrophy more accurately (Dunn, 1974; Schwartz and Williams, 1975; Done et al., 1982; Rutter et al., 1982; Straw et al., 1983). Such methods are helpful if precise differences in turbinate atrophy are to be compared, but for diagnostic purposes they are laborious and provide little extra information as compared to subjective scoring systems (Done, 1983a).

One problem associated with these methods is that turbinate damage occurs as a continuous spectrum, and it is difficult to judge whether a pig with a grade 3 lesion represents the more severe manifestation of *B. bronchiseptica* infection, which is unlikely to progress further, or an early manifestation of infection with toxigenic *P. multocida*, which could develop into a severe herd problem. Regular monitoring of successive samples of slaughtered pigs provides a "rolling mean value" for turbinate atrophy and it has been suggested that a progressive increase in this figure may provide an early indication of a herd problem (Done, 1983b).

C. Cultural

1. *B. bronchiseptica*

The isolation and culture of *B. bronchiseptica* from nasal swabs, tracheal swabs (which frequently yield a pure culture of the organism from infected animals), and lung material are not difficult. It is not a fastidious organims, but requires 48 hr for colonies to attain a diameter of 1–2 mm on Bordet Gengou agar, a medium on which the typical morphology and phase variation of *B. bronchiseptica* can be seen. The incorporation of selective agents reduces growth of the nasal commensal flora and various selective media have been described (see Goodnow, 1980). In the author's laboratory, a selective Bordet Gengou medium containing penicillin, streptomycin, furaltadone, spectinomycin, and fungizone (Rutter, 1981) has proved satisfactory for routine use. The identity of isolates can be confirmed by their characteristic biochemical reactions and by slide agglutination tests with specific antisera (Pedersen, 1975; Rutter, 1981).

2. *P. multocida*

P. multocida grows readily after 18 hr on blood agar medium, but its isolation from nasal swabs is difficult because it is frequently overgrown by the commensal flora. Although selective media for *P. multocida* have been reported (Smith and Baskerville, 1983; Knight et al., 1983), a selective medium which is satisfactory for one herd may be ineffective for another where the antibiotic resistance of the commensal flora is quite different. A selective medium containing neomycin, bacitracin, and cefsulodin has recently been developed (Rutter et al., 1984b) and has proved better than nonselective media in the author's laboratory and in Denmark (K. B. Pedersen, personal communication).

The most sensitive method for recovering *P. multocida* is by passage of material through mice (Pedersen, 1983; Rutter, et al., 1984b). In the author's laboratory, nasal swabs prepared from calcium alginate are used and placed in charcoal transport medium for several hours, during which the swabs dissolve. The transport medium is then suspended in 7 ml phosphate-buffered saline and 0.2–0.5 ml volumes are injected by the intraperitoneal route into mice. The mice die, or are killed after 24 and 48 hr, and cultures are made from the liver on selective or nonselective blood agar medium. Other organisms from the nasal swab are often recovered from the livers of mice using this method, including *B. bronchiseptica,* but relatively pure cultures of *P. multocida* are frequently obtained from swabs which give an overgrowth of contaminant organisms on primary culture. Pedersen (1983) reported recovery of *P. multocida* from 7.3% of 602 nasal swabs by direct culture, as compared to 33.7% by mouse inoculation. With the technique described above, *P. multocida* was isolated from 13.8% of 283 nasal swabs by direct culture on selective medium, as compared to 46.3% by mouse passage (R. J. Taylor and J. M. Rutter, unpublished). The numbers of *P. multocida* in the original material cannot be counted if the mouse inoculation technique is used, because it is an enrichment method.

Tests for confirmation of the identity of *P. multocida* include failure to grow on MacConkey agar, indirect fluorescent antibody staining, and identification of capsular and somatic antigens by serology. Acriflavine and hyaluronidase tests are useful for rapid identification of types A and D (Carter and Subronto, 1973; Carter and Rundell, 1975). Differentiation of toxigenic from nontoxigenic strains involves assays of lethality in mice, skin tests in guinea pigs, or cytopathic activity in cell cultures. Thus, the isolation and characterization of strains of *P. multocida* can be a lengthy procedure.

3. Serological

Serological diagnosis of *B. bronchiseptica* infection generally involves agglutination tests (Harris and Switzer, 1969; Jenkins, 1978; Farrington and Switzer, 1979; Shashidar et al., 1983). *B. bronchisep-*

tica is a good antigen and agglutinating antibodies can be detected in serum within 10 days of infection in conventional (Kemeny, 1973) and gnotobiotic pigs (Collings, 1983). The majority of animals in herds with endemic infection have detectable antibodies, although it appears that some breeding stocks have not been exposed to infection and do not transmit passive antibody to their litters (Rutter, 1981).

There are few reports of serological tests for *P. multocida* in pigs. Early attempts were unsuccessful (Gwatkin, 1958), while in experimentally infected gnotobiotic piglets (Rutter, 1983), somatic but not capsular antibodies were detected. Although it was possible to differentiate gnotobiotic pigs infected with types A and D of *P. multocida*, there were extensive cross-reactions when the same test was used with sera from conventional pigs. These results are not surprising because commercial pigs may become infected with strains of both types. Furthermore, close antigenic similarity was found between some toxigenic and nontoxigenic strains with the Heddleston gel precipitin test (J. M. Rutter and P. Curtis, unpublished), suggesting that these tests are unlikely to differentiate pigs infected with toxigenic *P. multocida*. Although antitoxin was detected in sera from a proportion of experimentally infected pigs (Rutter, 1983), sera from severely affected pigs in field outbreaks of the disease did not contain significant amounts of antitoxin. Thus, the development of sensitive ELISA, or radioimmunoassays, to detect toxin or antitoxin in sera appears to be the next logical step for the identification of animals infected with toxigenic *P. multocida*.

D. Value of Cultural and Serological Tests

All the above tests are labor intensive and their value in the diagnosis of atrophic rhinitis needs to be critically assessed. Isolations of *B. bronchiseptica* and *P. multocida* are currently being used as herd tests to determine whether those infected with toxigenic *P. multocida* develop more serious signs of disease. However, the predictive value of these results in individual pigs needs careful interpretation. Isolation of *B. bronchiseptica* from a young pig does not imply that it will develop turbinate lesions, since it can be protected by passive antibody (Rutter, 1981), whereas pigs infected with toxigenic *P. multocida* appear likely to develop turbinate lesions of varying severity, depending on the age at which they become infected. Thus, screening of pigs for toxigenic *P. multocida* may have predictive value, while screening of breeding stock by taking nasal or pharyngeal swabs may identify carriers of *B. bronchiseptica* and toxigenic *P. multocida*. If a sensitive serological test were developed for toxigenic *P. multocida,* then purchased stock might also be screened more reliably for evidence of infection.

On the basis of present knowledge, identification of *B. bronchiseptica* or nontoxigenic *P. multocida* has no particular significance for the diagnosis of progressive disease, whereas isolation of toxigenic *P. multocida* gives an indication of the potential severity of disease that might develop.

VIII. Control

The principal methods of controlling atrophic rhinitis are by local eradication schemes, i.e., by deriving SPF herds, or by mitigating the effects of disease by medication, vaccination, or improvements in environment and management.

A. Eradication

Early attempts to control atrophic rhinitis were based on the eradication of *B. bronchiseptica,* but many herds became reinfected (Switzer and Farrington, 1975). However, if the criterion of success is the absence of progressive disease, then eradication schemes have been effective. In Denmark, atrophic rhinitis appears to have been largely controlled by an SPF scheme, while in the United Kingdom, the Pig Health Control Association runs a pilot scheme with designated herds free of atrophic rhinitis. This scheme is based on regular examinations of the snouts of a proportion of slaughtered pigs and only those herds with a mean snout score below a predefined low, but arbitrary, limit are eligible for the pilot list (Goodwin and Whittlestone, 1983).

All SPF schemes depend on close monitoring for the appearance of disease, particularly in herds selling breeding or replacement stock. Breakdowns can occur (see Pedersen, 1983), and at present it is not always clear how toxigenic *P. multocida* has been introduced. Furthermore, infection in herds that exhibit no signs of disease would represent a potential threat because little is known of the factors and conditions that precipitate a severe outbreak of disease. Important questions that need answers include how many animals need to be sampled to guarantee that a herd is free of toxigenic *P. multocida,* what action should be taken if a breeding herd becomes infected with toxigenic *P. multocida,* and, if depopulation and repopulation with clean stock is undertaken, can reinfection be prevented.

In view of the central role now being proposed for toxigenic *P.*

multocida in atrophic rhinitis, the development of specific and sensitive tests for the detection of infected animals would be helpful. The prevalence of such animals in some herds may be limited and their removal might be sufficient to break the cycle of infection.

B. Monitoring

Attention is now being directed to monitoring systems that could act as "early warning" systems for atrophic rhinitis, because the disease can have severe consequences for the profitability of pig production. The selection of the parameters to be measured and ways of handling the information have been discussed by Done (1983b).

C. Environment and Management

There is general agreement that atrophic rhinitis is associated with increased herd size, poor hygiene, and poor management. Improvements generally involve several changes, e.g., better ventilation, smaller group sizes, and perhaps medication, but it is not clear which specific factors or combinations are important in breaking the cycle. Nevertheless, it has been claimed that attention to environment, management, and hygiene can reduce the prevalence of clinical disease in some, but not all, herds (Muirhead, cited by Smith, 1983). There is little evidence regarding the relative importance of contact infection or airborne spread in the transmission of *B. bronchiseptica* and *P. multocida* infections, so control measures in this area are essentially empirical. Furthermore, improvements in hygiene and management may be difficult to sustain in large herds over long periods and, in these herds, the main emphasis for control of atrophic rhinitis has been medication and vaccination.

D. Medication

B. bronchiseptica and *P. multocida* are sensitive to a number of antimicrobial agents *in vitro* and drugs are commonly used to treat atrophic rhinitis. The antibiotic sensitivity patterns of isolates depends on numerous factors including the method of testing, the amount of antibiotic in the test, and the use of antibiotics in the herd from which the strain was isolated. Thus, it is advisable to check the antibiogram of isolates before devising selective media or recommending feed medication.

Switzer (1963) reported that *B. bronchiseptica* was sensitive to sulfonamides and showed that incorporation of these antibiotics in the feed was effective in controlling infection in the nasal cavity of pigs; subsequently, 85% of isolates of *B. bronchiseptica* were reported to have developed resistance to sulfonamides (Switzer, 1981). Similar results were obtained in the United Kingdom (Smith *et al.*, 1980; Rutter, 1981). In the latter study, isolates from herds with progressive disease in which sulfonamide medication was used without beneficial effect were resistant, whereas isolates from unmedicated, unaffected herds were sensitive. Plasmids coding for transmissible antibiotic resistance occur in *B. bronchiseptica* (Terakado *et al.*, 1973; Hedges *et al.*, 1974) and, in one study, 86% of strains carried R factors capable of transfer by conjugation (Terakado *et al.*, 1974).

Isolates of *P. multocida* are sensitive to many antibiotics *in vitro* and this causes problems when attempting to devise selective media. Most strains are sensitive to penicillin, tetracyclines, and chloramphenicol, but show some resistance to streptomycin and sulfamethoxydin (Chang and Carter, 1976; Sisak *et al.*, 1978). In disk diffusion tests, most pig isolates from the United Kingdom are resistant to lincomycin (2 μg) and some show resistance to streptomycin (10 μg), tylosin (25 μg) and sulfadimidine (100 μg) (J. M. Rutter, unpublished).

Egoshin *et al.* (1965) and de Jong and Oosterwoud (1977) recommended treatment of atrophic rhinitis with tetracyclines. In the author's experience, feed medication containing oxy- or chlortetracycline alone, or in combination with penicillin and sulfonamides, has generally given a beneficial effect in reducing the clinical signs of progressive disease (Rutter, 1981). This treatment did not reduce the prevalence or intensity of *B. bronchiseptica* infection even though clinical signs of the disease disappeared. Furthermore, resistance to tetracyclines in *B. bronchiseptica* and *P. multocida* does not seem to have become a problem in medicated herds.

The reasons for the success of tetracycline medication have not been elucidated. It is possible that high levels of the antibiotic find their way into nasal secretions and reduce the numbers of toxigenic *P. multocida* on the nasal mucosa. On the other hand, tetracyclines can be retained at sites of new bone formation (Wade, 1977), and there may be subtle effects associated with bone metabolism which contribute to the control of clinical signs of atrophic rhinitis by these antibiotics.

IX. Immunity and Vaccination

In one of the first attempts to vaccinate against atrophic rhinitis, Eber and Meyn (1934, cited by Switzer, 1955) reported favorable results with a bacterin prepared from *Bordetella pyocyaneus*. Daugherty (1941, cited by Giles and Smith, 1983) used a killed *B. bronchiseptica* vaccine in pigs and Gwatkin (1958) reported that *P. multocida* vaccines were ineffective. However, during the late 1970s a commercial vaccine consisting of inactivated *B. bronchiseptica* became available (Switzer, 1981). This type of vaccine has been used throughout the world and, although it has been reported to reduce the prevalence of clinical atrophic rhinitis in herds where the disease is endemic, the extent of the improvements has varied considerably (Giles and Smith, 1983). In the light of current knowledge, it might be expected that an effective vaccine against *B. bronchiseptica* would (1) reduce the severity of turbinate atrophy caused by this organism; (2) reduce the severity of clinical disease in herds where *B. bronchiseptica* was playing an important initiating role for toxigenic *P. multocida;* and (3) have no effect in herds where other factors were responsible for enhancing toxigenic *P. multocida*. Thus, variable results could be explained on this basis.

As in most diseases of intensive livestock production, it is necessary to protect the unweaned as well as the weaned animal, and this involves vaccinating the dam to provide passive protection for the piglets and then stimulating active immunity in the young animal. Some of the problems associated with these needs will now be considered in more detail.

A. *B. bronchiseptica*

The extensive literature on vaccination and immunity against *B. bronchiseptica* infection has been reviewed (Goodnow, 1980; Giles and Smith, 1983). Taking account of the mechanisms of pathogenicity of *B. bronchiseptica* (Section V,A), prevention of colonization of the nasal mucosa might be achieved by the use of killed or live avirulent *Bordetella* vaccines, while turbinate atrophy might be prevented by toxoid vaccines. Different classes of antibody might be needed for these two approaches. Local IgA production might be necessary to control colonization of the mucosal surface, while systemic IgG might be needed for neutralization of the toxic products.

Resistance to reinfection by *B. bronchiseptica* of the nasal cavity of pigs was first demonstrated by Harris and Switzer (1969), who later showed that accelerated clearance of a virulent porcine strain was induced by subcutaneous vaccination with a sonicated strain of *B. bronchiseptica* or a *Bordetella pertussis* vaccine (Harris and Switzer, 1972). Koshimizu *et al.* (1973) reported that vaccination of pregnant sows resulted in colostral transfer of antibodies to newborn pigs which enabled them to resist establishment of *B. bronchiseptica* in the nasal cavity. Pedersen (1975) showed close antigenic relationships existed between *B. bronchiseptica* isolates from pigs, and these results suggested there should be good protection from vaccines containing appropriate antigens. Various commercial *B. bronchiseptica* vaccines have been used during the last 10 years in the field, but the results have been rather variable. Some reports stated that vaccination of sows and/or piglets was successful or moderately successful in reducing turbinate atrophy (Nakase et al., 1976; Pedersen and Barfod, 1977; Keller and Loretz, 1980; Giles, 1981), or improving weight gains (Goodnow, 1977; Goodnow et al., 1978). Others reported disappointing results (Bercovich and Oosterwoud, 1977; de Jong and Rondhuis, 1982). However, it is now apparent that discrepant results could probably be attributed to the relative importance of *B. bronchiseptica* in different herds, either as the cause of turbinate atrophy, or as the predisposing factor for infection with toxigenic *P. multocida*.

Vaccination of young pigs has been reported to reduce colonization of the nasal mucosa and turbinate atrophy (reviewed by Giles and Smith, 1983), but there are some reports that vaccination produced no differences in (1) the prevalence or intensity of *B. bronchiseptica* infection, or (2) the severity of clinical disease and turbinate atrophy in natural outbreaks (Giles, 1981) or in experimental infections (Smith et al., 1982).

Until recently, little attention had been directed to the effects of passive colostral antibodies on active vaccination of piglets, even though the procedure has been recommended (Nakase et al., 1976; Goodnow, 1977). As might be expected, the active immune response is reduced in piglets that have received passive antibodies in colostrum from vaccinated sows, and Giles (1981) concluded that vaccination of sows and piglets had no advantage as compared to vaccination of the sow alone.

Similarly, little attention has been paid to the mechanisms and isotype(s) involved in protection. IgG and IgA are present in nasal and tracheal secretions of piglets aged 1 week (Morgan and Bourne, 1981) and IgG, IgM, and IgA can be flushed from the nasal cavity within 4 hr of birth (Smith, cited by Giles and Smith, 1983). Parenteral vaccination of sows to provide passive transfer of colostral antibodies, or active vaccination of piglets is most likely to stimulate IgG, and the success of these procedures in reducing colonization at the nasal mucosa may be due to leakage of this immunoglobulin across the mucosa. Attempts to stimulate local immunity with live avirulent *B. bronchiseptica* resulted in a reduction in the numbers of *B. bronchiseptica* at subsequent challenge, but gave disappointing protection against turbinate atrophy (Wisecarver and Goodnow, 1980).

Clearly, there are conflicting views about the efficacy of *B. bronchiseptica* vaccines in the field and little information is available on their mode of action. Present evidence suggests that, even if complete immunological control of *B. bronchiseptica* were to be achieved, it would be unlikely to prevent the progressive lesions of atrophic rhinitis, and an effective combined *Bordetella/Pasteurella* vaccine would seem essential.

B. *P. multocida*

In contrast to the extensive literature on vaccination with *B. bronchiseptica* there is comparatively little published information on vaccination of pigs with *P. multocida*. This organism causes serious disease in many animal species (Carter, 1967), but effective vaccines are still being sought (Collins, 1977). Combined vaccines of *Bordetella* and *Pasteurella* have been used in attempts to control atrophic rhinitis, but their efficacy appears to be limited. For example, Schöss (1980), Schuller et al., (1980), Wittowski et al. (1980), and Baars et al. (1982) reported that combined vaccines reduced the prevalence of atrophic rhinitis but failed to eliminate the condition. More recently, Pedersen and Barfod (1982) showed that vaccination of pregnant sows with *P. multocida* toxin reduced snout distortion in piglets experimentally infected with *B. bronchiseptica* and toxigenic *P. multocida* from 47 to 18%; reduced severe turbinate lesions from 43 to 4%; reduced colonization by toxigenic *P. multocida* in the offspring of vaccinated sows at weaning; and improved growth rates as compared to nonvaccinated controls.

Consideration of the mechanisms of pathogenicity of *P. multocida* suggests three possible methods of raising immunity: (1) parenteral vaccination with killed vaccines that stimulate antibacterial antibodies to prevent colonization of the nasal mucosa; (2) live attenuated vaccines, perhaps nontoxigenic strains, to prevent colonization; and (3) toxin or toxoid vaccines to prevent the harmful effects of toxin. Most attention is now being paid to the third method. In developing vaccine regimes it should be remembered that *P. multocida* can produce lesions in older pigs; thus, the importance of providing passive antibodies from the dam, together with active production of immunity by the piglet, is probably greater than for *B. bronchiseptica*.

Although Pedersen and Barfod (1982) reported beneficial results in piglets following dam vaccination with toxin, their findings did not include the measurement of antitoxin. Toxin vaccines are unlikely to be acceptable commercially and results in the author's laboratory suggest that there may be problems in developing toxoid vaccines. The toxin itself appears to be a poor antigen in natural infections. Only 7 of 14 gnotobiotic pigs infected with toxigenic *P. multocida* alone, or with *B. bronchiseptica,* produced antitoxin (Rutter, 1983), even though high titers of antibodies to the somatic antigen of *P. multocida* were detected by acid agglutination tests with sera from all of these animals. Furthermore, significant amounts of antitoxin were not detected in sera from severely affected pigs in the field. Antitoxin can be raised by vaccination with a formalinized bacterin or with toxoid, but this can cause toxicity problems. Injection of the toxin (de Jong, 1983b; Rutter and Mackenzie, 1983), or toxoid, or formalinized bacterin produced significant turbinate atrophy in young pigs (J. M. Rutter, unpublished). The results of the latter experiments are summarized in Table II. Germ-free piglets aged 1 week were vaccinated intramuscularly with formalinized bacterin or toxoid combined with Freund's Incomplete Adjuvant; the *Pasteurella* toxoid was no longer lethal when injected into mice. The piglets were boosted with bacterin or toxoid alone 4 weeks later, then all groups were challenged intranasally 2 weeks later with the vaccine strain of *B. bronchiseptica,* followed by the toxigenic strain of *P. multocida.* Five piglets in the four groups vaccinated with the *Pasteurella* toxoid or bacterin that died following vaccination (Table II) showed characteristic signs of *Pasteurella* toxicity, including moderately severe turbinate atrophy graded 2–3. Vaccination with the single or combined *Bordetella* bacterin produced high levels of antibodies and significantly reduced colonization of the nasal cavity by *B. bronchiseptica,* as compared to unvaccinated groups in both experiments. There was a significant reduction in turbinate atrophy in the groups vaccinated with the *Bordetella* bacterin alone, even though small numbers of the toxigenic strain of *P. multocida* established for 28 days in the nasal cavity of the vaccinated group in Experiment 1 (Table II). Vaccination with *P. multocida* toxoid or bacterin produced good titers of antibodies that were detectable in the acid agglutination test, but demonstrated low levels of antitoxin in the cytotoxin test and no neutralizing activity in the mouse lethal test. Vaccination did not reduce colonization of the nasal cavity by *P. multocida* (colonization was enhanced in three of the four groups given *P. multocida* vaccines as compared to the control animals), and severe turbinate atrophy was present 56 days after infection in all the pigs vaccinated with *P. multocida.*

The piglets in these experiments were aged 7 weeks when chal-

TABLE II

VACCINATION AGAINST TOXIGENIC *P. multocida*[a]

| Experiment number | Group | Number of pigs | Preinfection titers | | | Mean bacterial counts in nasal swabs (log$_{10}$ CFU/g) | | | | Mean grade of turbinate atrophy |
| | | | Bb[b,c] | Pm[b,d] | Pm antitoxin[e] | Bb | | Pm | | |
						1–28[f]	29–56	1–28[f]	29–56	
1	Control	3	<10	<10	<10	6.9	6.0	1.6	0	1.7
	Bb bacterin	3	10,240	<10	<10	4.3	4.6	3.3	0	0.3
	Pm toxoid	3(2)[g]	<10	10,240	40	7.8	5.8	6.6	2.8	5.0
	Bb bacterin + Pm toxoid	3(1)[g]	10,240	10,240	20	4.6	4.4	0.9	0	5.0
2	Control	3	<10	<10	<10	5.9	3.1	1.8	0	0.7
	Bb bacterin	3	10,240	<10	<10	3.8	4.6	0	0	0.0
	Pm bacterin	2(1)[g]	<10	2,560	10	5.2	7.1	3.4	0	4.0
	Bb bacterin + Pm bacterin	3(2)[g]	10,240	400	<10	4.2	4.4	3.5	0	4.0

[a]J. M. Rutter (unpublished data).
[b]Bb, *B. bronchiseptica*; Pm, *P. multocida*.
[c]Agglutination test.
[d]Acid agglutination test.
[e]Cytotoxin neutralization test.
[f]Days after infection.
[g]Number of surviving piglets at challenge.

lenged. This did not affect colonization by *B. bronchiseptica,* but presumably accounted for the mild lesions produced by *Bordetella* infection in the control group. In contrast, colonization by *P. multocida* in all except the group vaccinated with *P. multocida* toxoid alone was poor, particularly in the control groups. It was not clear whether the latter effect was related to the age of the pigs or to genetic differences.

Different results might be obtained in conventional pigs, but on the basis of these results it would seem that more research is needed to develop *P. multocida* toxoid vaccines of sufficient antigenicity and without toxic side effects. Whether such vaccines would completely control the clinical signs of progressive atrophic rhinitis, and whether they would cross-protect against toxin from type-A strains or toxin from nonporcine isolates remains to be determined.

Little attention has been paid to the presence or effect of antibacterial antibodies to prevent establishment of *P. multocida* in the nasal cavity. The organism persists in the nasal cavity and throat of infected pigs (Pedersen and Barfod, 1982; Rutter, 1983), suggesting that immunity may not be readily achieved. Furthermore, nontoxigenic strains of type D are present in most herds with progressive disease, suggesting that there is little or no cross-protection against toxigenic strains. Because of the difficulties outlined above, the efficacy of *P. multocida* vaccines must be critically evaluated both in experimental and field studies. If a vaccine can be shown to be effective in one of the experimental challenge models then it should be effective against that organism in the field.

X. Conclusions

Atrophic rhinitis is a complex disease. *B. bronchiseptica* or *P. multocida* alone can reproduce turbinate atrophy in experimental infections, but suggestions that *B. bronchiseptica* is the cause of progressive disease have been shown to be inadequate. Current evidence indicates that toxigenic strains of *P. multocida* are responsible for severe turbinate atrophy, snout deformation, and probably for reduced growth rates, which are the main lesions associated with progressive disease. The wide variation in severity of clinical signs in field outbreaks could be explained by separate or combined infections with *B. bronchiseptica,* or by toxigenic or nontoxigenic strains of *P. multocida,* together with variations in immunity and age at infection. Various factors, including other microorganisms, may cause rhinitis as opposed to atrophic rhinitis. This may contribute to mild turbinate lesions, or assist toxigenic *P. multocida* to colonize the nasal cavity and produce severe lesions. Genetics, environment, management, and hygiene may all contribute to the severity of the lesions.

Control of atrophic rhinitis can be achieved by SPF schemes, but breakdowns occur. Complete control has not yet been achieved by immunization. Future research should have as its main objectives: (1) confirmation of the key role proposed for toxigenic *P. multocida;* (2) identification of factors that lead to growth retardation in affected animals; (3) characterization of *P. multocida* toxin and the development of sensitive tests to detect infected animals; and (4) development and evaluation of effective combined vaccines for atrophic rhinitis.

REFERENCES

Anon. (1954). *Vet. Rec.* **66**, 337–338.
Baars, J. C., Jong, M. F. de., Storm, P. K., Willems, H., and Pennings, A. (1982). *Proc. Congr. Int. Pig. Vet. Soc. 7th, Mexico City,* p. 121.
Baetz, A. L., Kemeny, L. J., and Graham, C. K. (1974). *Am. J. Vet. Res.* **35**, 451–453.
Baustad, B., Teige, J., Jr., and Tollersrud, S. (1967). *Acta Vet. Scand.* **8**, 369–389.
Bemis, D. A., Greisen, H. A., and Appel, M. J. G. (1977a). *J. Clin. Microbiol.* **5**, 471–480.
Bemis, D. A., Greisen, H. A., and Appel, M. J. G. (1977b). *J. Infect. Dis.* **135**, 753–762.
Bendixen, H. C. (1957). *Dtsch. Tieraerztl. Wochenschr.* **64**, 330–333.
Bendixen, H. C. (1971). *Nord. Veterinaermed.* **23**, (Suppl. I), 171.
Bercovich, Z., and Oosterwoud, R. A. (1977). *Tijdschr. Diergeneeskd.* **102**, 485–494.
Björklund, N. E. (1958). "Atrophic Rhinitis of Pigs: A Morphologic Study Including Some Aetiological Aspects," p. 100. State Veterinary Medical Institute, Stockholm.
Blom, J., Hansen, G. A., and Poulsen, F. M. (1983). *Infect. Immun.* **42**, 308–317.
Braend, M., and Flatla, J. L. (1954). *Nord. Veterinaermed.* **6**, 81–122.
Brown, W. R., Krook, L., and Pond, W. G. (1966). *Cornell Vet.* **56** (Suppl. 1), 1–107.
Bugnowski, H. (1973). *Monatsh. Veterinaermed.* **28**, 17–24.
Byrd, L. H., Anama, L., Gutkin, M., and Chmel, H. (1981). *J. Clin. Microbiol.* **14**, 232–233.
Carter, G. R. (1965). *Vet. Rec.* **75**, 1264.
Carter, G. R. (1967). *Adv. Vet. Sci. Comp. Med.* **11**, 321–379.
Carter, G. R., and Rundell, S. W. (1975). *Vet. Rec.* **96**, 343.
Carter, G. R., and Subronto, P. (1973). *Am. J. Vet. Res.* **34**, 293–294.
Chang, W. H., and Carter, G. R. (1976). *J. Am. Vet. Med. Assoc.* **169**, 710–712.
Collings, L. A. (1983). Ph.D. thesis, University of Reading, England.
Collings, L. A., and Rutter, J. M. (1985). *J. Med. Microbiol.* **19**, 247–255.
Collins, F. M. (1977). *Cornell Vet.* **67**, 103–138.
Cross, R. F., and Claflin, R. M. (1962). *J. Am. Vet. Med. Assoc.* **141**, 1467–1468.
de Jong, M. F. (1983a). *In* "Atrophic Rhinitis in Pigs" (K. B. Pedersen and N. C. Nielsen, eds.), pp. 52–60. Commission of the European Communities, Luxembourg.
de Jong, M. F. (1983b). *In* "Atrophic Rhinitis in Pigs" (K. B. Pedersen and N. C. Nielsen, eds.), pp. 136–146. Commission of the European Communities, Luxembourg.
de Jong, M. F., and Oosterwoud, R. A. (1977). *Tijdschr. Diergeneeskd.* **102**, 266–273.
de Jong, M. F., and Rondhuis, P. R. (1982). *Proc. Congr. Int. Pig Vet. Soc. 7th Mexico City,* p. 118.

de Jong, M. F., Oei, H. L., and Testenburg, G. J. (1980). *Proc. Congr. Int. Pig Vet. Soc. 6th Copenhagen*, p. 211.
Dirks, C., Schöss, P., and Schimmelpfennig, H. (1973). *Dtsch. Tieraerztl. Wochenschr.* **80**, 342–345.
Done, J. T. (1955). *Vet. Rec.* **67**, 525–527.
Done, J. T. (1962). *N. Z. Vet. J.* **10**, 71–78.
Done, J. T. (1981). *Vet. Rec.* **109**, 23.
Done, J. T. (1983a). *In* "Atrophic Rhinitis in Pigs" (K. B. Pedersen and N. C. Nielsen, eds.), pp. 3–12. Commission of the European Communities, Luxembourg.
Done, J. T. (1983b). *In* "Atrophic Rhinitis in Pigs" (K. B. Pedersen and N. C. Nielsen, eds.), pp. 193–199. Commission of the European Communities, Luxembourg.
Done, J. T., Richardson, M., and Hebert, C. N. (1964). *In* "Animal Disease Surveys," No. 3, pp. 29–48. HMSO, London.
Done, J. T., Upcott, D. H., and Lund, L. J. (1982). *Proc. Congr. Int. Pig Vet. Soc. 7th Mexico City*, p. 111.
Drummond, J. G., Curtis, S. G., Meyer, R. C., Simon, J., and Norton, H. W. (1981). *Am. J. Vet. Res.* **42**, 963–968.
Duncan, J. R., Ross, R. F., Switzer, W. P., and Ramsey, F. K. (1966). *Am. J. Vet. Res.* **27**, 457–466.
Dunn, J. W. (1974). Ph.D. thesis, University of Nebraska.
Duthie, R. C. (1947). *Can. J. Comp. Med.* **11**, 250–259.
Edington, N., Smith, I. M., Plowright, W., and Watt, R. G. (1976). *Vet. Rec.* **98**, 42–45.
Egoshin, I. S., Shergin, Yu.K., and Vidomskii, E. V. (1965). *Veterinariya (Moscow)* **42**, No. 10, pp. 36–38.
Elias, B., and Hamori, D. (1975). *Magy. Allatorv. Lapja* **30**, 535–539.
Elling, F., and Pedersen, K. B. (1983). *In* "Atrophic Rhinitis in Pigs" (K. B. Pedersen and N. C. Nielsen, eds.), pp. 123–135. Commission of the European Communities, Luxembourg.
Farrington, D. O. (1981). *In* "Diseases of Swine" (A. D. Leman, R. D. Glock, W. L. Mengeling, R. H. C. Penny, E. Scholl, and B. Straw, eds.), 5th ed., pp. 378–385. Iowa State Univ. Press, Ames.
Farrington, D. O., and Switzer, W. P. (1979). *Am. J. Vet. Res.* **40**, 1347–1351.
Fetter, A. W., and Capen, C. C. (1971). *Lab. Invest.* **24**, 392–403.
Fetter, A. W., Switzer, W. P., and Capen, C. C. (1975). *Am. J. Vet. Res.* **36**, 15–22.
Flatla, J. L., and Braend, M. (1953). *Proc. Int. Vet. Congr. XVth* (Part 1), p. 180.
Franque, L. W. (1830). *Dtsch. Z. Tierheilkd.* **1**, 75–77.
Gendreau, L. A. (1948). *Can. J. Comp. Med.* **12**, 291–294.
Ghosh, H. K., and Tranter, J. (1979). *J. Clin. Pathol.* **32**, 546–548.
Giles, C. J. (1981). Ph.D. thesis, University of London, England.
Giles, C. J., and Smith, I. M. (1983). *Vet. Bull. (London)* **53**, 327–338.
Giles, C. J., Smith, I. M., Baskerville, A. J., and Brothwell, E. (1980). *Vet. Rec.* **106**, 25–28.
Gilman, J. W. P. (1949). *Can. J. Comp. Med.* **13**, 266–274.
Glorioso, J. C., Jones, G. W., Rush, H. G., Pentler, L. J., Darif, C. A., and Coward, J. E. (1982). *Infect. Immun.* **35**, 1103–1109.
Gois, M., Kuksa, F., and Siśak, F. (1977). *Zentralbl. Veterinaermed. Reihe B* **24**, 89–96.
Gois, M., Barnes, H. J., and Ross, R. F. (1983). *Am. J. Vet. Res.* **44**, 372–378.
Goodnow, R. A. (1977). *Vet. Med. Small Anim. Clin.* **72**, 1210–1212.
Goodnow, R. A. (1980). *Microbiol. Rev.* **44**, 722–738.
Goodnow, R. A., Lehr, C. D., and McLennan, J. (1978). *Vet. Med. Small Anim. Clin.* **73**, 1187–1188.

Goodnow, R. A., Shade, F. J., and Switzer, W. P. (1979). *Am. J. Vet. Res.* **40,** 58–60.
Goodwin, R. F. W. (1980). *In Pract.* **2,** 5–11.
Goodwin, R. F. W., and Whittlestone, P. (1983). *Vet. Rec.* **113,** 411–412.
Gwatkin, R. (1958). *Adv. Vet. Sci. Comp. Med.* **4,** 211–234.
Gwatkin, R., Dzenis, L., and Byrne, J. L. (1953). *Can. J. Comp. Med.* **17,** 215–217.
Hanada, M., Shimoda, K., Tomita, S., Nakase, Y., and Nishiyama, Y. (1979). *Jpn. J. Vet. Sci.* **41,** 1–8.
Harris, D. L., and Switzer, W. P. (1968). *Am. J. Vet. Res.* **29,** 777–785.
Harris, D. L., and Switzer, W. P. (1969). *Am. J. Vet. Res.* **30,** 1161–1166.
Harris, D. L., and Switzer, W. P. (1972). *Am. J. Vet. Res.* **33,** 1975–1984.
Harris, D. L., Ross, R. F., and Switzer, W. P. (1969). *Am. J. Vet. Res.* **30,** 1621–1624.
Hasebe, H. (1971). *Bull. Nippon Vet. Zootech. Coll.* **19,** 92–102.
Heddleston, K. L., Gallagher, J. E., and Rebers, P. A. (1972). *Avian Dis.* **16,** 925–936.
Hedges, R. W., Jacob, A. E., and Smith, J. T. (1974). *J. Gen. Microbiol.* **84,** 199–204.
Hodges, R. T. (1981). *N. Z. Vet. J.* **29,** 142–143.
Ilina, Z. M., and Zasukhin, M. I. (1975). *Sb. Nauchn. Rab. Sib. Nauchn. Issled. Vet. Inst. Omsk* **25,** 76–86.
Jenkins, E. M. (1978). *Can. J. Comp. Med.* **42,** 286–292.
Jones, T. L. (1947). *Agric. Inst. Rev.* **2,** 274–279.
Keller, H., and Loretz, H. (1980). *Schweiz. Arch. Tierheilkd.* **122,** 541–551.
Kemeny, L. J. (1973). *Cornell Vet.* **63,** 130–137.
Kemeny, L. J., Littledike, E. T., and Cheville, N. F. (1970). *Cornell Vet.* **60,** 502–517.
King, B. (1981). *Am. J. Vet. Res.* **42,** 1093–1108.
Knight, D. P., Paine, J. E., and Speller, D. C. E. (1983). *J. Clin. Pathol.* **36,** 591–594.
Kobisch, M. (1983). *In* "Atrophic Rhinitis in Pigs" (K. B. Pedersen and N. C. Nielsen, eds.), pp. 177–192. Commission of the European Communities, Luxembourg.
Kobisch, M. and Madec, F. (1983). *In* "Atrophic Rhinitis in Pigs" (K. B. Pedersen and N. C. Nielsen, eds.), pp. 43–45. Commission of the European Communities, Luxembourg.
Koshimizu, K., Kodama, Y., Ogata, M., Kino, T., Sanbyakuda, S., and Mimura, M. (1973). *Jpn. J. Vet. Sci.* **35,** 411–418.
Lacey, B. W. (1960). *J. Hyg.* **58,** 57–93.
Leslie, P. H. and Gardner, A. D. (1931). *J. Hyg.* **31,** 423–434.
Lundeheim, N. (1979). *Acta Agric. Scand.* **29,** 209–215.
MacNabb, A. L. (1948a). *Rep. Ont. Vet. Coll.* , 12–13.
MacNabb, A. L. (1948b). *Rep. Ont. Vet. Coll.* 64–66.
Matsuyama, T., and Takino, T. (1980). *J. Med. Microbiol.* **13,** 159–161.
Meyeringh, H., Dirks, C., Schöss, P., and Schimmelpfennig, H. (1977). *Dtsch. Tieraerztl. Wochenschr.* **84,** 266–268.
Miniats, O. P., and Johnson, J. A. (1980). *Can. J. Comp. Med.* **44,** 358–365.
Morgan, K. L., and Bourne, F. J. (1981). *Res. Vet. Sci.* **31,** 40–42.
Morse, S. I. (1976). *Adv. Appl. Microbiol.* **20,** 9–26.
Muirhead, M. R. (1979). *Br. Vet. J.* **135,** 497–508.
Munoz, J. (1971). *In* "Microbial Toxins" (S. Kadis, T. C. Montie, and S. A. Aje, eds.), Vol. 2A, pp. 271–300. Academic Press, New York.
Nakagawa, M., Muto, T., Yoda, H., Nakano, T., and Imaizumi, K. (1971). *Jpn. J. Vet. Sci.* **33,** 53–60.
Nakagawa, M., Shimizu, T., and Motoi, Y. (1974). *Natl. Inst. Anim. Health Q.* **14,** 61–71.
Nakase, Y. (1957a). *Kitasato Arch. Exp. Med.* **30,** 73–78.
Nakase, Y. (1957b). *Kitasato Arch. Exp. Med.* **30,** 79–84.
Nakase, Y., Kimura, M., and Shimoda, K. (1976). *Proc. Congr. Int. Pig Vet. Soc. 4th, Ames,* p. 8.

Namioka, S. (1978). *In* "Methods in Microbiology" (T. Bergan and J. R. Norris, eds.), Vol. 10, pp. 271–292. Academic Press, London.
Nielsen, N. C. (1983). *In* "Atrophic Rhinitis in Pigs" (K. B. Pedersen and N. C. Nielsen, eds.), pp. 35–42. Commission of the European Communities, Luxembourg.
Nielsen, N. C., Riising, H. J., and Bille, N. (1976). *Proc. Congr. Int. Pig Vet. Soc. 4th, Ames,* p. 1.
Osborn, J. E., Blazkovec, A. A., and Walker, D. L. (1968). *J. Immunol.* **100,** 835–844.
Pearce, H. G., and Roe, C. K. (1966). *Can. Vet. J.* **7,** 243–251.
Pearce, H. G., and Roe, C. K. (1967). *Can. Vet. J.* **8,** 186–188.
Pedersen, K. B. (1975). *Acta Pathol. Microbiol. Scand. Sect. B* **83,** 590–594.
Pedersen, K. B. (1983). *In* "Atrophic Rhinitis in Pigs" (K. B. Pedersen and N. C. Nielsen, eds.), pp. 22–31. Commission of the European Communities, Luxembourg.
Pedersen, K. B., and Barfod, K. (1977). *Nord. Veterinaermed.* **29,** 369–375.
Pedersen, K. B., and Barfod, K. (1981). *Nord. Veterinaermed.* **33,** 513–522.
Pedersen, K. B., and Barfod, K. (1982). *Nord. Veterinaermed.* **34,** 293–302.
Pedersen, K. B., and Elling, F. (1984). *J. Comp. Pathol.* **94,** 203–214.
Pedersen, K. B., and Nielsen, N. C. (eds.) (1983). "Atrophic Rhinitis in Pigs," p. 201. Commission of the European Communities, Luxembourg.
Penny, R. H. C., and Mullen, P. A. (1975). *Vet. Rec.* **96,** 518–521.
Peo, E. R., Jr., Andrews, R. P., Libal, G. W., Dunn, J. W., and Vipperman, P. E., Jr. (1967). *J. Anim. Sci.* **26,** 910.
Phillips, C. E., Longfield, H. F., and Miltimore, J. E. (1948). *Can. J. Comp. Med.* **12,** 268–273.
Plowright, W. (1979). *Proc. Munich Symp. Microbiol. 4th,* pp. 163–171.
Radtke, G. (1938). *Arch. Wiss. Prakt. Tierheilkd.* **72,** 371–423.
Ross, R. F., Switzer, W. P., and Duncan, J. R. (1967). *Can. J. Comp. Med.* **31,** 53–57.
Rutter, J. M. (1981). *Vet. Rec.* **108,** 451–454.
Rutter, J. M. (1983). *Res. Vet. Sci.* **34,** 287–295.
Rutter, J. M., and Luther, P. D. (1984). *Vet. Rec.* **114,** 393–396.
Rutter, J. M., and Mackenzie, A. (1983). *In* "Atrophic Rhinitis in Pigs" (K. B. Pedersen and N. C. Nielsen, eds.), p. 147. Commission of the European Communities, Luxembourg.
Rutter, J. M., and Mackenzie, A. (1984). *Vet. Rec.* **114,** 89–90.
Rutter, J. M., and Rojas, X. (1982). *Vet. Rec.* **110,** 531–535.
Rutter, J. M., Francis, L. M. A., and Sansom, B. F. (1982). *J. Med. Microbiol.* **15,** 105–116.
Rutter, J. M., Mackenzie, A., and Rolley, N. (1984a). *Proc. Congr. Int. Pig Vet. Soc. 8th, Ghent,* p. 156.
Rutter, J. M., Taylor, R. J., Crighton, W. G., Robertson, I. B., and Benson, A. J. (1984b). *Vet. Rec.* **115,** 615–619.
Sawata, A., and Kume, K. (1982). *Am. J. Vet. Res.* **43,** 1845–1847.
Sawata, A., Nakai, T., Tuji, M., and Kume, K. (1984). *Jpn. J. Vet. Sci.* **46,** 141–148.
Schofield, F. W., and Jones, T. L. (1950). *J. Am. Vet. Med. Assoc.* **116,** 120–123.
Schöss, P. (1971). *Dtsch. Tieraerztl. Wochenschr.* **78,** 371–374.
Schöss, P. (1980). *Proc. Congr. Int. Pig Vet. Soc. 6th, Copenhagen,* p. 204.
Schöss, P. (1982). *Dtsch. Tieraerztl. Wochenschr.* **89,** 176–181.
Schöss, P. (1983). *In* "Atrophic Rhinitis in Pigs" (K. B. Pedersen and N. C. Nielsen, eds.), pp. 13–21. Commission of the European Communities, Luxembourg.
Schuller, W. (1980). *Pig News Inf.* **1,** 77–80.
Schuller, W., Trubrich, H., Kosztolich, O., Flatscher, J., and Jahn, J. (1980). *Zentralbl. Veterinaermed. Reihe B* **27,** 125–130.

Schwartz, W. L., and Williams, J. D. (1975). *Vet. Med. Small Anim. Clin.* **70,** 1213–1216.
Shashidar, B. Y., Underdahl, N. R., and Socha, T. E. (1983). *Am. J. Vet. Res.* **44,** 1123–1125.
Shimizu, T., Nakagawa, M., Shibata, S., and Suzuki, K. (1971). *Cornell Vet.* **61,** 696–705.
Shuman, R. D., and Earl, F. L. (1956). *J. Am. Vet. Med. Assoc.* **129,** 220–224.
Siśak, F., Gois, M., and Kuksa, F. (1978). *Vet. Med. (Prague)* **23,** 531–540.
Skelly, B. J., Pruss, M., Pellegrino, R., Andersen, D., and Abruzzo, G. (1980). *Proc. Congr. Int. Pig Vet. Soc. 6th, Copenhagen,* p. 210.
Smith, W. J. (1983). *In* "Atrophic Rhinitis in Pigs" (K. B. Pedersen and N. C. Nielsen, eds.), pp. 151–162. Commission of the European Communities, Luxembourg.
Smith, I. M., and Baskerville, A. J. (1983). *Br. Vet. J.* **139,** 476–486.
Smith, I. M., Hodges, R. T., Betts, A. O., and Hayward, A. H. S. (1973). *J. Comp. Pathol.* **83,** 307–321.
Smith, I. M., Oliphant, J., Baskerville, A. J., and Giles, C. J. (1980). *Vet. Rec.* **106,** 462–463.
Smith, I. M., Giles, C. J., and Baskerville, A. J. (1982). *Vet. Rec.* **110,** 488–494.
Straw, B. E., Bürgi, J., Hilley, H. D., and Leman, A. D. (1983). *J. Am. Vet. Med. Assoc.* **182,** 607–611.
Switzer, W. P. (1955). *J. Am. Vet. Med. Assoc.* **127,** 340–348.
Switzer, W. P. (1956). *Am. J. Vet. Res.* **17,** 478–484.
Switzer, W. P. (1963). *Vet. Med. Small Anim. Clin.* **58,** 571–575.
Switzer, W. P. (1981). *In* "Diseases of Swine" (A. D. Leman, R. D. Glock, W. L. Mengeling, R. H. C. Penny, E. Scholl, and B. Straw, eds.), 5th ed., pp. 497–507. Iowa State Univ. Press. Ames.
Switzer, W. P., and Farrington, D. O. (1975). *In* "Diseases of Swine" (H. W. Dunne and A. D. Leman, eds.), 4th ed., pp. 687–711. Iowa State Univ. Press, Ames.
Terakado, N., Azechi, H., Ninomiya, T., and Shimizu, T. (1973). *Antimicrob. Agents. Chemother.* **3,** 555–558.
Terakado, N., Azechi, H., Nonomiya, T., Fukuyasu, T., and Shimizu, T. (1974). *Jpn. J. Microbiol.* **18,** 45–48.
Thompson, H., McCandlish, I. A. P., and Wright, N. G. (1976). Res. Vet. Sci. **20,** 16–23.
Van der Heijden, P. J., Van Es, C. D. M., Kamp, E. M., and Pals-van Dam, J. W. (1983). *In* "Atrophic Rhinitis in Pigs" (K. B. Pedersen and N. C. Nielsen, eds.), pp. 114–120. Commission of the European Communities, Luxembourg.
Volkova, A. M. (1975). *Sb. Nauchn. Tr. Mosk. Vet. Akad.* **79,** 124–130.
Wade, A. (ed.) (1977). "Martindale. The Extra Pharmacopoeia," 27th ed., p. 1189. Pharmaceutical Press, London.
Wisecarver, J. L., and Goodnow, R. A. (1980). *Proc. Congr. Int. Pig Vet. Soc. 6th, Copenhagen,* p. 205.
Wittowski, G., Horner, M., and Tenhumberg, H. (1980). *Berl. Muench. Tieraerztl. Wochenschr.* **93,** 214–218.
Yokomizo, Y., and Shimizu, T. (1979). *Res. Vet. Sci.* **27,** 15–21.
Yoshikawa, T., and Hanada, T. (1981). *Jpn. J. Vet. Sci.* **43,** 221–231.
Young, G. A., Caldwell, J. D., and Underdahl, N. R. (1959). *J. Am. Vet. Med. Assoc.* **134,** 231–233.

Selected Animal Herpesviruses: New Concepts and Technologies

ROBERT A. CRANDELL

*Texas Veterinary Medical Diagnostic Laboratory
College Station, Texas*

I.	Introduction	281
II.	Equine Rhinopneumonitis	283
	A. Introduction and History	283
	B. Clinical Signs	284
	C. Epizootiologic Features	286
	D. Diagnosis	293
	E. Prevention and Control	294
III.	Pseudorabies (Aujeszky's Disease, Mad Itch)	295
	A. Introduction and History	295
	B. Clinical Signs	296
	C. Epizootiologic Features	300
	D. Diagnosis	314
	E. Prevention and Control	316
	F. Vaccines	318
	References	319

I. Introduction

The herpesvirus family, Herpesviridae (Roizman *et al.*, 1981), includes many viruses of economical importance. I have selected two common herpesvirus diseases, pseudorabies and equine rhinopneumonitis, to review. The discussions to follow are primarily concerned with the application of newer concepts and technologies as they may relate to the epizootiology, diagnosis, prevention, and control of these viral diseases. These viruses are distributed worldwide and do

TABLE I

Provisional Designation and Classification of Selected Viruses of Mammals Belonging to the Family Herpesviridae[a]

Provisional designation	Common name	Subfamily
Alcelaphine herpesvirus 1	Malignant catarrhal fever virus of wildebeest	Gammaherpesvirinae (?)
Alcelaphine herpesvirus 2	Hartebeest herpesvirus	Gammaherpesvirinae (?)
Bovine herpesvirus 1	Infectious bovine rhinotracheitis/infectious pustular vulvovaginitis	Alphaherpesvirinae
Bovine herpesvirus 2	Bovine mammilitis virus, Allerton virus, pseudo-lumpy skin disease virus	Alphaherpesvirinae
Bovine herpesvirus 3	Bovine "orphan" herpesvirus	Alphaherpesvirinae
Canid herpesvirus 1	Dog herpesvirus	Alphaherpesvirinae
Caprine herpesvirus 1	Sheep herpesvirus	
Caprine herpesvirus 2	Domestic goat herpesvirus	Alphaherpesvirinae
Equid herpesvirus 1	Equine rhinopneumonitis virus, equine abortion virus	Alphaherpesvirinae
Equid herpesvirus 2	Slow-growing "cytomegalovirus"-like virus	Betaherpesvirinae (?)
Equid herpesvirus 3	Coital-exanthema virus	Alphaherpesvirinae
Felid herpesvirus 1	Cat herpesvirus, infectious rhinotracheitis virus	Alphaherpesvirinae
Felid herpesvirus 2	Cat cytomegalovirus	Betaherpesvirinae (?)
Suid herpesvirus 1	Pseudorabies virus, Aujeszky's disease	Alphaherpesvirinae
Suid herpesvirus 2	Inclusion body rhinitis, pig cytomegalovirus	Betaherpesvirinae

[a]From Roizman et al. (1981). *Intervirology* **16**, 201–217.

not recognize geographic boundaries. Selected viruses of mammals belonging to the herpesvirus family are listed in Table I.

Pseudorabies (PRV) infections continue to be a worldwide problem for the swine industry. Some concepts to control PRV such as vaccination, eradication, and "live with it" are controversial and have caused much dialogue in the United States since 1975. Deliberations on vaccination have continued, despite the fact that extensive vaccination programs in Europe did not stop the spread of the PRV virus. On the other hand, vaccination against bovine rhinotracheitis and equine rhinopneumonitis has been practiced for decades in the United States.

Equine rhinopneumonitis was chosen because it continues to be a major virus disease of horses. Infections with this herpes virus received worldwide attention during the spring of 1983 when a severe outbreak occurred in the famed Lippizaner horses in the Piber stud farm in Austria (Anon., 1983). Following central nervous system involvement mares aborted and died.

During the past decade, molecular biologists have made significant advances in techniques for cleavaging DNA and cloning fragments of herpesvirus DNA, opening avenues for studying the organization and function of viral DNA. With the introduction of the enzymatic method using restriction endonucleases for DNA analysis of herpes simplex virus (Hayward et al., 1975), a new and exciting era in the molecular study of the herpesviruses began. The technique is useful for the application of molecular "epidemiology" to herpesvirus infections (Buchman et al., 1978; Buchman et al., 1980). One strain of virus can be unambiguously distinguished from another; therefore, the method is useful in determining the source of virus in disease outbreaks. The analysis of viral DNA is applied to epidemiological investigations of pseudorabies outbreaks, studying latency, comparing subtype 1 and subtype 2 isolates of equine herpesvirus 1, and vaccine development. These studies are discussed later in the respective virus section.

II. Equine Rhinopneumonitis

A. Introduction and History

Equine rhinopneumonitis is a virus disease of horses manifested by either a respiratory infection, abortion, or neonatal deaths and neurological disorders. The diseases described in the 1930s and 1940s as equine influenza and equine abortion virus are now known to be viral rhinopneumonitis of horses and are caused by the same virus. Equid herpesvirus 1 has been proposed as the name of the virus (Roizman et al., 1981).

Dimock and Edwards (1932) were the first to describe abortion in mares caused by the virus now known as equine herpesvirus 1 (EHV 1). They observed outbreaks of abortions in mares without clinical evidence of illness on breeding farms in Kentucky. Although the condition was first believed to be noninfectious, Dimock and Edwards (1933) later demonstrated that the abortions were caused by a filterable agent. They experimentally induced abortion in mares by intravenous inoculation and the feeding of filtered material from aborted fetuses.

In 1939, Army veterinarians at the U.S. Army Remount Depot, Front Royal, Virginia, encountered the respiratory form of the disease in horses and mules. Although the etiologic agent was shown to be a filterable virus (Jones and Maurer, 1943; Jones et al., 1948), its relationship to the equine abortion virus of Dimock and Edwards (1933) was not recognized. Because of the influenza-like syndrome in the horses, the disease was called equine influenza.

In 1941, equine viral abortion was reported as a naturally occurring disease of horses in Hungary and Austria. European investigators observed a febrile respiratory illness in mares inoculated with suspensions of infected fetal tissue, and demonstrated immunity against the so-called influenza agent in horses previously inoculated with the equine abortion virus. It was then proposed that the equine influenza virus and equine abortion virus were the same agent, and that abortion in mares was a clinical manifestation of the influenza virus. Doll and Kintner (1954) compared the abortion virus, the Army 183 influenza strain (Jones et al., 1948), and the Grayson I virus (Doll and Wallace, 1954) serologically and found them to be identical viruses. The knowledge of viral abortions and diseases of the equine respiratory tract was further elucidated when Doll et al. (1957) isolated the equine arteritis virus. Although both viruses were serologically distinct and produced different clinical signs and lesions in horses, they both caused abortions in pregnant mares. The name equine rhinopneumonitis virus was then proposed to include the equine abortion virus and influenza virus strain 183. Equine herpesvirus is used throughout this section to designate these viruses.

Abortions had been associated with a neurological syndrome (Dimock et al., 1947) and, in 1966, EHV 1 was isolated from the brain and spinal cord of a stallion with paralysis in the lumbar region (Saxegaard, 1966). During the 1970s a number of outbreaks of equine paresis due to EHV 1 were described from different countries (Jackson and Kendrick, 1971; Little, 1974; Dinter and Klingeborn, 1976; Crowhurst et al., 1981). The disease also occurred in vaccinated animals (Liu and Castleman, 1977; Thomson et al., 1979), possibly as a result of vaccination with one particular vaccine, which was subsequently withdrawn from the market (Eugster and Jones, 1977).

B. Clinical Signs

Like the other viruses of this group, the clinical character of the natural respiratory illness of rhinopneumonitis is more severe than that of the experimentally induced infection. The natural disease of the respiratory tract is characterized by fever, anorexia, cough, rhinitis, and in the young horse there is frequently pulmonary involvement. The incubation period varies from 2 to 10 days. The temperature is between 38.8 and 41.1°C and, in uncomplicated cases, persists for 1 to 7 days. In some cases the fever is diphasic.

A catarrhal rhinitis is evident and in some cases becomes mucopurulent. There may be edema and swelling of the mandibular lymph nodes, and occasionally the tendon sheaths and joint capsules exhibit a transient swelling.

A transient leukopenia is a hematologic feature of this disease (Doll and Bryans, 1962a; Purdy et al., 1978; Bumgardner et al., 1982). In general, a leukopenia develops within several days after infection and may persist up to 8 days. Later, in severe cases, an abrupt increase in the polymorphonuclear cells may occur during the secondary temperature rise and the total white blood cell count may exceed 30,000 cm, with over 90% of the cells being neutrophiles. The neutrophile count drops rapidly during convalescence. During convalescence, a moderate lymphocytosis or monocytosis may occur (Maurer and Jones, 1943). In uncomplicated cases, recovery is complete within 1 to 2 weeks.

Complications, which sometimes occur, are the result of secondary bacterial infections. A mucopurulent rhinitis with coughing may persist for 1 to 2 months. The most common complication is suppuration of the submaxillary and parapharyngeal lymph nodes. Pneumonia is a frequent and serious complication where large numbers of horses are assembled.

Although there are no signs of impending abortion, mares may abort 1 to 4 months following respiratory infection with the virus (Doll and Bryans, 1962a). Abortions may occur after the fifth month of pregnancy, however, the majority occur from the eighth month to term. Mares go into labor and expel the fetus, as in normal parturition. Abortion occurs shortly after the death of the fetus. Infected foals that are born alive usually die within 36 hr following parturition. The fetal membranes are usually discharged with the fetus or shortly afterward. The genital tract returns to normal, as following a normal parturition. After abortion, mares will breed during the same season and foal normally.

Abortions are usually uncomplicated, but occasionally a paralytic syndrome develops in pregnant mares. A similar condition also occurs in geldings, stallions, and mares following respiratory infections; it is characterized by ataxia which may progress to paralysis, recumbency, and death. Mildly affected animals recover.

C. Epizootiologic Features

1. *Virus Strain Differences*

a. *Biologic.* In addition to EHV 1, there are two other equine herpesviruses; equine herpesvirus 2 (EHV 2), a slow-growing virus, and equine herpesvirus 3 (EHV 3), the cause of equine coital exanthema. EHV 2 was first isolated in England from the nose of a horse with catarrh and coughing (Plummer and Waterson, 1963). EHV 2 has since been shown to persist in a high percentage of horses without causing clinical illness. EHV 3, first isolated by Petzoldt (1967), is venereally transmitted but is not abortigenic. These two viruses and their diseases have been reviewed (Bagust, 1971; Studdert, 1974).

The three equine herpesviruses have been shown to be antigenically distinct (Petzold, 1970; Plummer *et al.*, 1969, 1973; Studdert, 1974), although they share some common antigens (Gutekunst *et al.*, 1978a). Allen *et al.* (1977) reported very little genetic homology between the EHV 1 and EHV 3 viruses.

Although all EHV 1 viruses are believed to belong to one serotype, a number of attempts have been made to demonstrate strain differences. Earlier approaches were directed toward comparing fetal (F) and respiratory (R) isolates with regard to their serological and biological characteristics.

Various studies using rabbit EHV 1 immune serum have demonstrated antigenic differences between the fetal and respiratory isolates by using cross-neutralization tests and by employing the plaque reduction test (Burrows and Goodridge, 1973; Borgen and Ludwig, 1974; Horner, 1981; Turtinen *et al.*, 1981). These studies included virus strains from a wide geographic area, and, in general, clearly separated the fetal and respiratory isolates into two groups. The F isolates are considered as belonging to subgroup 1 and the R isolates belong to subgroup 2. Some antigenic variations exist between viruses within each group, but larger differences were observed between the two groups.

Turtinen *et al.* (1981) compared 2 recent respiratory isolates with the Army 183 and the Kentucky A hamster-adapted (Ky A-ha) strains. The Army 183 strain originally isolated from the respiratory tract had undergone 28 colt, 7 fetal, and 3 cell culture passages. The Ky A-ha strain was a fetal strain which had been passed 400 times in hamsters. Each of the respiratory isolates had been passed 3 times in cell culture. In cross-neutralization tests, the Army 183 antiserum neutralized the 2 respiratory isolates less than the corresponding homologous serum. Likewise, the 2 respiratory sera neutralized the Army 183 virus less than the 2 respiratory isolates. The Ky A-ha strain reacted similarly to the Army 183 strain. In this study, the respiratory isolate (Army 183), which had been serially passed in colts and fetuses, reacted antigenically like the fetal isolate (Ky A-ha). Similar serological results had been observed with the enzyme-linked immunosorbent assay. Earlier, Mayr *et al.* (1965) reported Army 183 virus to be more antigenically related to the Polish fetal isolate RAC, than to Kentucky D (KyD); therefore Army 183 and RAC were classified as subtype 2.

Various strains have been examined for their ability to produce plaques (Borgen, 1972; Borgen and Ludwig, 1974; Studdert and Blackney, 1979) and to replicate in different host cell cultures (Burrows and Goodridge, 1973; Burrows and Goodridge, 1975; Studdert and Blackney, 1979). Although there is a tendency for the F isolates to fall into one group and the R isolates into another, according to their plaquing characteristics, it is not an unequivocal separation. The F strains generally possess a broader host cell range than the R strains and have a greater affinity for cell cultures of bovine origin (Burrows and Goodridge, 1973; Studdert and Blackney, 1979). Fetal strains grew faster and to a higher concentration in organ cultures of foal trachea than did the R strains (Burrows and Goodridge, 1975).

The pathogenicity of F strains and those viruses causing paresis in horses (subtype 1) was compared to that of the R strains (Patel and Edington, 1983). The R strains did not kill 2-day-old mice, nor was virus recovered from mouse tissue following intracerebral inoculation. All subtype 1 strains were pathogenic and could be divided into two subgroups based on their pathogenicity for mice. Mouse inoculation did not distinguish between known paresis and fetal strains.

There is confusion in the literature with regard to the classification of some virus isolates into subtypes. Unfortunately, some cross-neutralization tests have been performed on EHV 1 isolates without using homologous and heterologous antigens and antisera and some data have been misquoted. In the future EHV 1 isolates will be subtyped by their DNA restriction endonuclease patterns, rather than by the source of isolation and differing biological properties.

b. DNA Analysis. The structure and replication of EHV 1 have been thoroughly reviewed (O'Callaghan *et al.*, 1978). The molecular structure of the genome of EHV 1 was recently determined by restriction endonuclease mapping (Henry *et al.*, 1981). The herpesvirus genome is a 92-MDa, linear, double-stranded, DNA molecule consisting of a 71.6-MDa L (long) region and of a 20.4-MDa S (short) region bracketed by inverted repeat sequences. The genome can exist in two molecular arrangements, due to the ability of the S region to invert relative to the fixed L region.

Studies of the nucleotide sequences of the DNAs from fetal and respiratory virus isolates support suggestions, based on biological and serological activity, that strain differences exist. Comparisons of the restriction enzyme digests of various EHV 1 DNAs revealed differences between the two subtypes (Sabine et al., 1981; Studdert et al., 1981; Turtinen et al., 1981; Studdert, 1983; Allen et al., 1983). These investigators showed that the patterns of the respiratory isolates are similar to each other, but are entirely different from those of the fetal isolates. Minor differences exist between viruses belonging to the 2 subtypes. Allen et al. (1983) reported that a greater genetic heterogeneity exists among subtype 2 strains than with subtype 1 isolates. Because of these demonstrated differences in the DNA restriction endonuclease patterns of fetal and respiratory viruses, it was proposed to consider the two EHV 1 as two distinct infectious agents and designate them as equine herpesviruses 1 and 4 (Studdert et al., 1981). An isolate from EHV 1-related neurological disease was indistinguishable from the fetal isolate (Studdert, 1983).

The application of restriction endonuclease analysis provides a valuable and exciting tool for epizootiologic studies of EHV 1 infections in horses. However, the usefulness of fingerprinting EHV 1 DNA for tracing virus spread may be limited because of the lack of sufficient genetic heterogeneity within the virus population of EHV 1 (Allen et al., 1983). Further studies, with additional enzymes, on isolates from other geographic areas may reveal greater genetic diversity in the equine herpesvirus population. The use of the technique for collectiong surveillance information concerning the emergence of genetic and antigenic variants among the EHV 1 viruses would be useful for the development of new vaccines. Allen et al. (1983) proposed the use of fingerprinting as a means of identifying herpesviruses from the upper respiratory tract of horses. They have demonstrated that the two subtypes of EHV 1 and EHV 2 can be identified and differentiated from each other with a single-restriction enzyme. This would overcome some of the difficulties now encountered with the current diagnostic procedures.

Of interest is the demonstration by Studdert (1983) that viruses from Australian epizootics of abortions and perinatal mortality were caused by fetal strains, whereas sporadic abortions may be caused by the respiratory strains. In Britain there has been a substantial increase in the percentage of subtype 1 strains isolated from the respiratory tract of horses since 1979 (Mumford and Bates, 1984). Sixty percent of the upper respiratory disease outbreaks studied have yielded subtype 1 virus strains. Recent data obtained by analysis of viral genomes with restriction endonucleases of EHV 1 suggest that subtype 2 strains are more frequently the cause of overt respiratory tract infections in horses in the United States (Allen *et al.*, 1983).

The Army 183 virus originally isolated from the respiratory tract of horses at a remount station has been fingerprinted as a fetal strain (Turtinen *et al.*, 1981; Studdert, 1983). Although there is a question concerning the actual identity of the virus Studdert (1983) studied, the Army 183 strain used by Turtinen *et al.* (1981) had undergone considerable laboratory manipulations during its 40 years of existence. Since its source was a remount station, which consisted of a population of barren mares and geldings, it seems unlikely that the original Army 183 is of fetal origin. However, during its 28 consecutive passages in young colts, and 7 equine fetal passages (Turtinen *et al.*, 1981), it is possible that contamination with another strain or mutation had occurred. Although the restriction enzyme cleavage patterns of some herpesviruses appear to be stable (Buchman *et al.*, 1979; Thiry *et al.*, 1983), the DNA fingerprints of EHV 1 were altered during passage in rabbit kidney cells (Allen *et al.*, 1983).

It is the opinion of this author that additional studies on the genetic analysis of the subtypes and pathogenesis of abortions are necessary before the abortion and respiratory strains of EHV 1 are considered as separate etiologic agents. Herpesvirus 1, subtype 1, and subtype 2 should satisfy the need for distinction for the present time. In addition, since both EHV 1 subtypes are capable of causing both upper respiratory disease and abortions in horses, the continued use of "respiratory" and "fetal" to describe isolates serves no useful purpose.

2. Host Range

Equine viral rhinopneumonitis is a naturally occurring disease of the Equidae.

EHV 1 has been isolated from tissues of aborted Hereford fetuses on at least two occasions (Crandell *et al.*, 1976a; Smith, 1977). Although the virus has been recovered from bovine species, attempts to infect calves with the virus have been unsuccessful (Jones *et al.*, 1948; Crandell *et al.*, 1979). Bovine isolate 1247 (Crandell *et al.*, 1976a) inoculated either intravenously or subcutaneously into 2.5-year-old cows, which were 5.5 to 7 months pregnant, did not cause an illness or induce abortion (R. A. Crandall, M. R. Mansfield, R. E. Mock, and G. T. Woods, 1979, unpublished data). It is interesting that attempts to experimentally infect cattle failed, even though cell cultures of bovine origin are highly sensitive to the fetal strains.

The Syrian hamster has been the most useful of experimental animal hosts for studying EHV 1. It was first adapted to suckling hamsters by Doll et al. (1953) and propagated on the chorioallantoic membrane of 9- to 11-day-old chicken embryos by Doll and Wallace (1954). The virus has been serially propagated in 12-day-old embryonated eggs inoculated via the yolk and amniotic sacs, and nuclear inclusions were demonstrated in the liver parenchymal cells of some embryos (Randall, 1955). Adaptation of the virus to infant mice (1 to 3 days old) was accomplished by alternating passages from hamsters to mice (Kaschula et al., 1957). The virus has also been adapted to guinea pigs. A local erythema was observed on the skin of rabbits inoculated intradermally (Plummer and Waterson, 1963).

The virus propagates with cytopathic effect in primary cultures and in cell lines originating from a variety of animal species (Bagust, 1971).

3. Pathogenesis

Although the pathogenesis of rhinopneumonitis infections of the respiratory tract of horses appears to be established, the mechanism by which the virus infects the fetuses of immune mares is unknown. The respiratory mucosa is the primary site of infection. Following an initial multiplication in the upper respiratory tract, the virus gains entrance into the capillaries and lymphatics with the development of a viremia and systemic infection. In pregnant mares, infection of the fetus occurs after the virus enters the uterine mucosa and the allantochorion becomes infected (Doll and Bryans, 1962a).

Experimental transmission occurs by contact, intranasal, oral, intratracheal, conjunctival, vaginal, or parenteral routes of inoculation. The experimentally induced infections are similar, both clinically and pathologically, to the natural disease; however, they are less severe and resemble uncomplicated natural cases.

Viremia has been shown to be a feature of EHV 1 infections (Jones et al., 1948; Bryans, 1969). Virus was recovered intermittently from the buffy coat of mares for as long as 20 days after subcutaneous inoculation (Bryans, 1969). T lymphocytes, B lymphocytes, monocytes, and plasma from pony foals were shown to contain virus after experimental infection (Scott et al., 1983). The T lymphocytes were the predominant cell type to harbor the virus. EHV persisted in the mononuclear cells for a period of 14 days and in the nasal secretions for 20 days after infection. EHV 1 was not demonstrated by plaque assay from disrupted leukocytes but was detected in mononuclear cells and subpopulations by the infective center assay developed by Dutta and Myrup (1983). This finding suggests that EHV 1 resides in infected mononuclear cells as a nonproductive or latent form. Purdy et al. (1978) regularly demonstrated attenuated EHV 1 in peripheral leukocytes up to 14 days after vaccination.

Abortions were first experimentally induced in mares by Dimock and Edwards (1933) using intravenous and subcutaneous injections and the feeding of stomach and thoracic fluid, liver, spleen, and membrane scrapings from aborted fetuses. Mares in their seventh and eighth months of gestation aborted between 27 and 32 days following exposure.

Doll and Bryans (1962a) determined the incubation periods for abortions occurring between the seventh and tenth months of gestation. They used different routes of inoculation with suspensions of lung or liver tissue of aborted fetuses (native virus) and hamster-adapted virus. Abortions occurred 3 to 9 days after intrauterine or interfetal inoculation. Incubation periods for abortion in mares receiving native virus intravenously ranged from 14 to 76 days, with a median of 22 days; whereas mares who were receiving hamster-adapted viruses intranasally aborted between 48 and 115 days.

Gleeson and Coggins (1980) reviewed 11 reports concerning transmission studies in pregnant mares and found the number of days to abortion after inoculation varied from 15 to 90. In their study, a pony mare aborted 6 days and a horse mare 36 days after virus challenge. In a study of 80 naturally occurring epizootics, 95.8% of the abortions were observed within 90 days of the first abortion (Doll and Bryans, 1963). These authors suggested that young horses were the principal source of virus infection in mares. The interesting question is, what was the source of infection for those young horses? Was it recrudescent virus from the mares and other older horses on the premises?

Several hypotheses have been advanced for the pathogenesis of EHV 1 abortion in mares. The two most widely accepted are that reinfection of mares occurs, and, alternatively, it has been suggested that carriers and latent infections occur. In support of the first, mares with circulating antibodies have become reinfected, resulting in infections of the fetus, as well as abortion (Doll, 1961), paralysis (Jackson and Kendrick, 1971; Jackson et al., 1977), and viremia (Bryans, 1969; Gleeson and Coggins, 1980).

Studies by Gleeson and Coggins (1980) and Scott et al. (1983) support the suggestion by Bryans and Prickett (1970) that the virus may reach the fetus via virus-infected leukocytes. Additional studies are needed to further delineate the mechanism involved with this method of virus transport across the placenta. There is evidence to indicate that this infection of the leukocytes represents a nonproductive or latent state.

Another aspect of the pathogenesis of EHV 1 is its oncogenic potential. Whenever a virus is capable of producing latency in a host, the question of oncogenicity arises. Although there is no evidence to suggest that EHV 1 induces tumors in horses, oncogenic transformation of permissive hamster embryo cells *in vitro* by UV-irradiated EHV 1 has been demonstrated (Robinson et al., 1980). EHV 1 DNA sequences were identified in transformed EHV 1 and tumor cell genomes utilizing cloned EHV 1 viral DNA fragments (Robinson et al., 1981).

4. Latent and Persistent Infection

There is a paucity in the literature concerning attempts to demonstrate latency in the equine. The persistence of EHV 1 in horses on breeding farms has long been recognized as a problem for the effective control of abortions. Latent infections or the virus-carrier state have been demonstrated in pigs (Mock et al., 1981), cattle (Sheffy and Rodman, 1973), and cats (Orr et al., 1978).

Turner et al. (1970) attempted to reactivate EHV in horses by the administration of adrenalin and cortisone, with inconclusive results. Burrows and Goodridge (1984) were also unsuccessful in demonstrating recrudescence of EHV 1 after corticosteroid treatment and latent virus in trigeminal ganglia. Ardans (1982) cited Bryans, who successfully demonstrated the presence of EHV 1 in the trigeminal ganglion of a horse which had died of a ruptured uterus following an abortion. The fetus was infected with EHV 1 which differed genetically from the virus recovered from the mare.

To speculate on the role that lymphocytes play in an EHV 1 infection of the fetus, an assumption of the life span of the leukocyte populations and subpopulations is necessary, since those data are not available for the horse. However, based on the information for man, the B lymphocytes may be viable for 5 to 10 weeks, whereas T lymphocytes may survive as long as 10 years, but, to be conservative, it will be considered that their life span is 5 to 10 weeks, similar to that of the B lymphocytes. The monocytes are generally replaced every 100 days, or at the rate of 1% per day. Therefore if these cellular components harbor the virus as a noninfective or subviral form, as shown by Scott et al. (1983), something must trigger their reactivation, which is then followed by replication. An insult, such as altered hormone levels or stress, may set the reactivation replication mechanism in motion and release free infective virions into the blood stream. Accepting this as a possibility, the delay of 90 days from the onset of the initial viremia to abortion observed in experimental and in natural infections can be explained.

Although there is not a severe reaction in the uterus and placenta, some lesions are evident. The most consistent lesion of the uterus is described as an intense perivascular infiltration of lymphocytes and plasma cells associated with the vessels located beneath the glandular layer of the endometrium. Lesions of the allantochorion consist of an intravillar necrosis, which is characterized by nuclear debris, and a low-grade infiltration of fetal inflammatory cells (Prickett, 1970). A generalized infection occurs in the fetus with characteristic lesions. This differs markedly in the pregnant hamster where abortion through placental infection occurs without fetal infection (Burek et al., 1975). However, cells in the placenta contain infectious EHV 1. Perhaps with a mild degree of placentitis certain physiological changes occur, allowing the virus from the mare's blood to pass through the placental barrier and gain entrance into the fetal circulation. Recrudescence of latent virus in the trigeminals may also provide a source of virus for infecting the leukocytes.

D. Diagnosis

The clinical and pathological features of EHV 1 infections are helpful in obtaining a presumptive diagnosis. EHV 1 should be considered in any sudden outbreak of an upper respiratory disease and in abortions occurring during the late stages of pregnancy.

A definitive diagnosis can be obtained by laboratory procedures. The virus is easily isolated from nasal secretions of horses and tissue suspensions from aborted fetuses by cell culture techniques.

The fluorescent antibody (FA) technique (Smith et al., 1972) is used to detect viral antigens in tissues of aborted fetuses and neonates. The liver, lung, and thymus are the tissues of choice and are also used for virus isolation. The FA technique is also used to identify viral isolates.

Central nervous system infections must be differentiated from rabies, equine encephalitides, toxicosis, and toxoplasmosis. EHV 1 has been isolated from brain and cord tissue from affected horses, but it is not recovered consistently.

The serum neutralization and complement fixation tests are used to measure the specific EHV 1 antibody in the serum of horses with respiratory infections (Doll and Bryans, 1962b; Thomson et al., 1976). Since a rise in antibody titer is evidence of a recent infection, it is necessary to test paired serum samples. Titers on single serum specimens are not of diagnostic significance, nor is serological testing of mares a reliable method for determining the cause of EHV 1-induced abortions. For abortions, the serum neutralization (SN) titers are generally high, particularly in vaccinated mares; however, some mares will abort with a low serum antibody titer. Similar serological observations have been made on mares which foal normally. Serum antibody titers will increase in some mares after abortion, whereas in others they may decrease or remain unchanged.

EHV 1 antibodies are also detected by indirect immunofluorescence (Thomson et al., 1976), hemagglutination inhibition (Yurov and Sologub, 1978), and by the enzyme-linked immunosorbent assay (Dutta et al., 1983).

Serological testing of fetal and neonatal serum is helpful in diagnosing in utero infections of the fetus (Crandell and Angulo, 1984). Blood should be collected from newborn weak foals before they receive colostrum. Some aborted fetuses and stillbirths, in which virus and characteristic lesions could not be demonstrated, possessed significant EHV 1 antibody titers.

Diagnosis may be made from lesions in the aborted fetus in the majority of cases. The most consistent and characteristic gross lesions are excessive fluid in the pleural cavity, pulmonary edema, and hepatic necrosis. Although intranuclear inclusion bodies have been demonstrated in the liver, lung, spleen, thymus, lymph node, and Peyer's patch (Westerfield and Dimock, 1946), they are most frequently found in the hepatic cells near necrotic foci, and in the epithelial cells of the bronchioli and alveoli. The lungs may be severely edematous, with necrosis of the bronchiolar and alveolar epithelium.

E. Prevention and Control

Since the virus is endemic in the horse population, exposure to EHV 1 is almost a certainty before a horse reaches breeding age. Most horses have serological evidence of exposure to the virus after 1 year of age.

There are two types of commercial vaccines (modified-live and inactivated) available to immunize horses against EHV 1. Both types of vaccines are used to control the respiratory form of the disease in young horses (Liu, 1983). Multiple vaccinations with the inactivated product at 5, 7, and 9 months of gestation are recommended for pregnant mares, although some mares will abort in spite of vaccination (Ardans, 1982; Mitchell, 1980). Mares usually abort only once. However, the available evidence clearly indicates that some mares with high levels of antibody will abort EHV 1-infected fetuses. It is further recognized that abortions following an infection with EHV 1 are unpredictable, regardless of class or titer of antibody (Doll and Bryans, 1962b; Lindemann et al., 1967; Bryans and Prickett, 1970).

The cellular and humoral immunity of the resistance of EHV 1 infection is not fully understood (Bumgardner et al., 1982). The cell-mediated immune response of mares is suppressed in the latter stages of gestation with exposure to virulent EHV 1 (Gerber et al., 1977).

Good management practices are recommended to reduce the risk of EHV 1 abortions (Mitchell, 1980). Pregnant mares should not have contact with outside horses, especially during the late stages of gestation. Mares in late pregnancy should be protected from unnecessary stresses. In the event of an EHV 1 abortion, the affected mare should be isolated from other horses and disinfection and strict sanitation practices should be enforced.

III. Pseudorabies (Aujeszky's Disease, Mad Itch)

A. Introduction and History

Pseudorabies (Aujeszky's Disease) is an acute, contagious disease affecting many animal species. Since its recognition as a disease entity by Aujeszky (1902), the disease has become of economic importance worldwide. Aujeszky first described the condition as a naturally occurring, fatal illness in cattle, cats, and dogs in Hungary. The etiologic agent, now known to be a herpesvirus, was experimentally transmitted to rabbits, and the virus was differentiated from rabies by its behavior in that host. The name pseudorabies (PR) was given to the disease because of its similarity to bovine clinical rabies.

There is evidence that the term "mad itch" was used to describe the disease in cattle in America over a century ago. In a historical review of pseudorabies in the United States by Hanson (1954), there are accounts cited from farm journals of "mad itch" occurring in cattle in the early 1800s. Shope (1931) reported that the cause of "mad itch" in cattle in the United States was a virus identical to Aujeszky's pseudorabies virus (PRV). It was later established that PR was highly prevalent as an unrecognized infection in swine in the midwestern region of the United States.

While PRV was becoming entrenched in eastern and central Europe, the disease was being diagnosed in widely scattered areas of the world such as Brazil, Africa, and Denmark. By the early 1940s, PR had become recognized as an economically important disease in Hungary and Russia. The disease soon became a serious problem in other eastern and central European countries. PR also existed in western Europe and, with the increase in the number of swine, the frequency of the disease increased, particularly in Denmark,Holland, Belgium, France, and the Federal Republic of Germany.

PR emerged during the 1960s as a serious disease of swine in the state of Indiana. A decade later, PRV was widespread throughout the swine-raising areas of the midwestern United States. In association with this sudden occurrence of clinical PR in swine was a change in the disease pattern. Prior to this time PRV occurred sporadically, causing CNS signs and deaths in baby pigs and occasional deaths in cattle. The disease is now manifested by abortions, illness, and deaths in sows and feeder pigs. There was also a marked increase in the infection of domestic ruminants, dogs, cats, and wildlife.

During the early to mid 1970s the disease became of economic and scientific interest in most countries of Europe and Mexico, particularly in the areas of dense swine raising. Outbreaks of PR were reported for the first time in countries as distant as New Zealand (Burgess et al., 1976). It is interesting that the results of serological surveys in Canada (Dulac and Binns, 1979), and serological testing and virus isolation attempts in Finland (Veijalainen et al., 1982), were negative for the presence of PRV.

A number of reasons were proposed to explain the sudden appearance of epidemics of an old disease (PR):

1. The emergence of more virulent strains of PRV.
2. The change in swine production management from open-rearing to confinement operations.
3. With the eradication of hog cholera in the United States, the use of hyperimmune porcine serum, which contained some PRV antibodies, was discontinued.
4. Increased interest with awareness and recognition of the disease.
5. Better utilization of diagnostic services.
6. Improved reporting.

Two reviews detailing the early history and studies of Aujeszky's disease are recommended for further reading (Lourens, 1935; Galloway, 1938). More recently, Aujeszky's disease in pigs was reviewed by Baskerville et al. (1973). A chronological listing of references on the disease by Ryu (1975) covers the years 1903–1974.

B. Clinical Signs

1. Pigs

In the natural disease, the clinical signs vary according to the animal species and age.

Pigs of all ages and breeds are susceptible to infection with PRV. An infection may cause a mild to severe clinical illness, or an inapparent infection without clinical signs. The morbidity and mortality are highest in the very young pig, often reaching 100%. The morbidity and mortality decrease sharply as the age of the pig increases.

The disease has a very sudden onset. Death may occur within 48 hr in the newborn and in pigs from a few days old up to 4 or 5 weeks of age. Clinical signs consist of fever, anorexia, dullness, and muscular tremors in the young animal. As the disease progresses, the pigs become weak, ataxic, and uncoordinated. Paddling movements, convulsions, and prostration precede death. Respiratory signs are the characteristic clinical feature of some strains of virus. Vomition and diarrhea may occur, but are not consistent signs. Disoriented pigs, if not confined, will wander from the litter and die. They become a source of infection for predators.

The disease in feeder pigs is more sporadic. There are fewer sick animals at one time and less deaths than in the younger pigs. New cases in feeder operations may occur as late as 1 month after the addition of new animals. The clinical illness may linger from several days to a week after onset in the growing and feeder pigs; the protracted illness in pigs of this age often causes some confusion in making a diagnosis of pseudorabies. Temperatures of 41.5°C are common. Head and body tremors, circling, and paddling movements are characteristic clinical signs. Some animals may tilt their head slightly. These animals may go unnoticed. Animals may show a weakness in the hindquarters, which is followed by posterior paralysis. Death is preceded by convulsions and prostration.

The disease in sows and gilts is often manifested by fever, rhinitis, sneezing, and coughing which may be mistaken for influenza. A few animals may rub their noses, but pruritis (mad itch) is not a common feature in pigs. However, a marked generalized pruritis occurred in a group of experimentally infected gilts and in the contact-exposed gilts (Kluge and Maré, 1974).

Porcine abortions and fetal deaths occurred in Ireland (Gordon and Luke, 1955) and in Hungary (Csontos et al., 1962) before being recognized in the United States (Saunders et al., 1963). Since that time, resorption, fetal mummification, stillbirths, and abortions have occurred frequently in outbreaks. Very often, infected sows have fever, anorexia, and vomition at the time of farrowing or soon afterward. There is a marked decrease in lactation, or complete suppression of milk production. After recovery, infertility may persist in the herd. Occasionally, a sow or gilt will die.

The pathological findings of PR in pigs have been described in detail (Olander et al., 1966; Baskerville et al., 1973).

2. Cattle

Cattle of both sexes and of all ages and breeds are susceptible to infection.

Intense pruritus is the cardinal sign of pseudorabies infection in cattle; however, the disease may occur in cattle without evidence of pruritus (Sellers et al., 1949; Bitsch, 1975a; Beasley et al., 1980). Pruritus of the head is typically unilateral (Bitsch, 1975a). It is characterized by biting, licking, or rubbing the affected part so as to inflict an open wound. When present on the anterior portion of the body, the affected sites are frequently found on the nose, around the eyes, below the ear, and on the lower jaw. Posteriorly, the localized areas are usually seen on the hind leg, flank, udder, or perineum. Swelling and ulceration of the vulva have been observed. Rectal temperatures may reach 43°C. Infected cattle may not eat and often bellow and stamp their feet. The animal may chew continuously or intermittently, and salivate excessively. In lactating cows, there is a marked decrease in milk production. The animals may show aggressiveness, a staggering gait, and partial paralysis of the hindquarters. Animals usually die within 1 to 3 days of the appearance of pruritus.

In cases without pruritus, the animal may stand with head and neck extended, with excessive salivation and chewing motion (Fig. 1). These animals appear to be choking and will bloat and die very suddenly (Crandell, 1981).

Infections of cattle, with virus isolation from the fetus, have been reported in Brazil (Silva and Giovine, 1966) and Denmark (Bitsch, 1980). Silva and Giovine (1966) reported that a 9-month-old fetus removed from a cow after 8 days with clinical signs had PRV in the spleen, liver, and brain. The length of illness prior to death was long in this case as compared to the classic descriptions of the disease in cattle; however, PRV was recovered from the spinal cord and blood. The frequency of bovine abortions has increased in Denmark in recent years (Bitsch, 1980). A probable explanation of why bovine abortions have not been observed in the large PR outbreaks in cattle in America is that these outbreaks have occurred in feedlot animals that are not pregnant.

PR infections of cattle are considered to be fatal; however, several accounts of recovery are documented. Lourens (1935) reported the recovery of two animals which had been ill for approximately 15 days with clinical signs. One heifer aborted. More recently, Hagemoser et al. (1978) described the recovery of a 4-year-old beef cow in Iowa. Toma

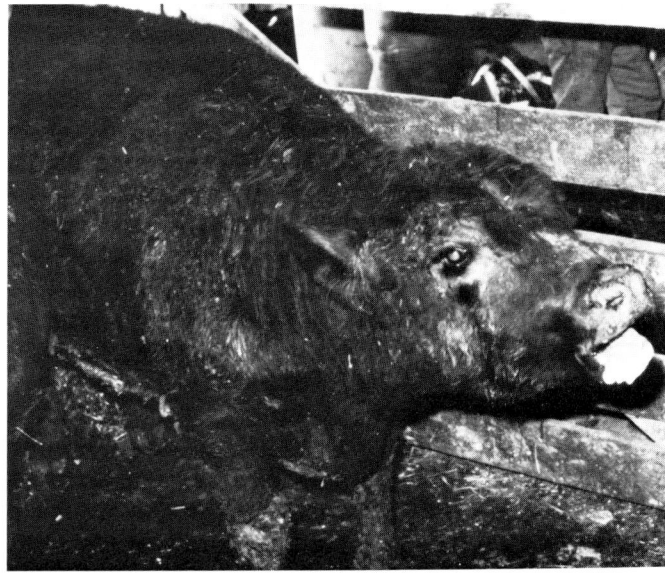

FIG. 1. Pseudorabies in a steer. Note open-mouth breathing with early signs of bloat including protrusion of the rumen over the left lumbar region.

and Gilet (1978) and Joubert et al. (1979) reported the recovery of cows in France. The affected animals showed a variety of clinical signs, and neutralization antibodies for PRV were demonstrated in the serum of some of the animals.

The pathological changes in natural and experimental bovine pseudorabies have been described (Dow and McFerran, 1962; Crandell et al., 1982).

3. Sheep and Goats

Sheep and goats are highly susceptible to infection with PRV by the respiratory route. The disease appears to be less common in goats. The virus is transmitted from pigs to sheep and goats by direct and indirect contact. Clinical disease in these small ruminants (Dow and McFerran, 1964; Baker et al., 1982) is characterized by intense pruritus, with open lesions from biting and rubbing the affected areas. Death occurs soon after the appearance of clinical signs. The pathology of the experimental disease in sheep has been reported (Dow and McFerran, 1964).

4. Dogs and Cats

There has been an increase in the number of dogs and cats infected with PRV during the past decade. Clinical signs occur within 24 to 72 hr after infection and may consist of hysteria, convulsions, lethargy, salivation, facial paralysis or tremors, ptosis, emesis, pruritus, and self-mutilation (Brown, 1939; Erdson *et al.*, 1953; Harris, 1968; Chastain *et al.*, 1973; Whitley and Nelson, 1980). A case characterized by depression, salivation, head pressing, and emesis without pruritus was described (Shell *et al.*, 1981). The disease in dogs is a rapid fatal illness with death occurring 24 to 48 hr after the onset of clinical signs (Boucher and Beran, 1977; Hugoson and Rockborn, 1972).

PRV infection in the cat is similar to that reported in dogs (Galloway, 1938).

5. *Horses*

Horses do not appear to be very susceptible to natural infection with PRV (Galloway, 1938). This author has never seen the disease in horses on farms where other livestock, dogs, and cats were infected with and dying of PRV. Kojnok (1962) has also reported that horses were unaffected on farms where cattle and sheep died of the disease. However, the natural disease has been reported in horses (Lourens, 1935; Galloway, 1938; Toneva, 1975). Iridocyclitis, blindness, ataxia, and posterior paresis are common signs reported in experimentally infected horses (Popescu, 1964; R. E. Mock, 1984, personal communication). Although pruritus does not occur, R. E. Mock (1984, personal communication) observed verrucous lesion of the skin on three of nine inoculated horses. All nine horses had seroconverted 14 days postinfection.

C. EPIZOOTIOLOGIC FEATURES

1. *Virus*

Antigenic Relatedness. Strains of PRV have been shown to be antigenically distinct from other herpesviruses and constitute one serotype. They do, however, share common antigens with some members of the herpesvirus family.

Sabin (1934) demonstrated slight antigenic relatedness between PRV and B virus by protection tests in guinea pigs and rhesus monkeys. This relationship was not confirmed by *in vitro* neutralization tests (Plummer, 1964). Some cross reactions were, however, shown by complement fixation (CF) among PRV, infectious bovine rhinotracheitis (IBR), and EHV 1. It had been shown earlier, by CF and gel diffusion, that IBR and EHV 1 shared common antigens (Carmichael and Barnes, 1961).

On the basis of immunodiffusion and immunoelectrophoresis, IBR and PRV viruses were shown to share two common antigens (Evans *et al.,* 1973). Crandell (1977) reported cross-neutralization between IBR and PRV by the tube neutralization test, using high potency serum. An antigenic similarity between these two viruses was later demonstrated in cattle by the delayed hypersensitivity skin reaction. Cattle with IBR antibodies elicited a delayed hypersensitivity reaction at the site of an intradermal inoculation with PRV (Aguilar-Setien *et al.,* 1979). These authors also reported the presence in cattle of neutralizing antibodies reacting against both IBR and PRV. Joubert *et al.* (1979) found the occurrence of antibodies against IBR and PRV in cattle serum to be a problem in the serodiagnosis of these 2 diseases.

PRV cross-reacted with Marek's disease virus using the fluorescent antibody test, but relatedness was not detected by gel diffusion, neutralization, or in cross-protection tests (Sharma *et al.,* 1972).

2. *Virus Strain Differences*

a. Biologic. Whenever live virus vaccines are used to control diseases, there is a need to differentiate the vaccine virus from the field virus isolates. In this regard, a number of biological characteristics of PRV have been studied in an effort to distinguish between virulent and vaccine strains of virus.

The cytopathology (CPE) induced in selected cell cultures indicates that the virulent strains are associated with syncytia formation, whereas attenuated strains are more apt to cause a rounding of the infected cell (Bodon and Greczi, 1966; Bodon *et al.,* 1968; Zuffa *et al.,* 1968; Golais and Sabo, 1976; Bitsch, 1980). The differences in the CPE in the study by Golais and Sabo (1976) appeared to be dependent upon the cell host. The type of CPE was not influenced in rabbit lung, BHK-21, and pig kidney cells infected with attenuated or virulent virus and incubated at 40°C (Golais *et al.,* 1977).

Attenuated strains of PRV produce small plaques, whereas virulent strains are reported to form larger plaques (Skoda *et al.,* 1964; Lomniczi, 1974; Platt and Maré, 1976; Tozzini, 1982a).

The susceptibility and response of rabbits to inoculation by vaccine and virulent strains of PRV have been investigated in search of markers. Skoda *et al.* (1964) and Platt *et al.* (1979) showed that rabbits receiving vaccine virus did not have pruritus, whereas those rabbits inoculated with virulent virus had pruritus. Rabbits inoculated with vaccine strains took longer to die than rabbits that received virulent virus (Bodon *et al.,* 1968; Platt *et al.,* 1979). The Shope strain was more virulent for rabbits and mink than the BUK-attenuated strain (Goto *et al.,* 1971).

In general, thermal resistance has been correlated with reduced virulence in PRV strains (Bodon et al., 1968; Bartha et al., 1969; Golais and Sabo, 1975; Lloyd and Baskerville, 1978; Platt et al., 1979); however, some vaccine strains (BUK) were shown to be heat sensitive and some virulent strains were considered to be heat resistant. Since various methods were employed in the studies, conclusions varied with regard to the usefulness of thermal inactivation for differentiating strains of PRV.

Similar data have been obtained by comparing the resistance to trypsin of vaccine strains with that of virulent strains (Bodon et al., 1968; Bartha et al., 1969; Lloyd and Baskerville, 1978; Platt et al., 1980).

Platt et al. (1980) demonstrated a significant difference in the mean times-to-death by inoculation with vaccine and virulent viruses. They showed that the mouse marker could be correlated with virulence for the pig by inoculating pigs with the vaccine and field strains. The pigs inoculated with the vaccines did not develop clinical signs, but seroconverted, whereas all of the pigs receiving the field strains developed a clinical illness.

PRV strains have been studied by electrophoresis methods to identify protein markers for virulence (Matis and Zuffa, 1969; Williams et al., 1982). The electrophoretic mobility of PRV and the isoelectric points were shown not to be associated with virulence of the virus for swine.

Lomniczi (1974) reported that avirulent strains were not neuropathogenic for chicks, whereas the virulent strains tested showed a distinct neurovirulence.

The K and BUK vaccine strains were differentiated from each other and from field strains by using the thermal inactivation and rabbit virulence marker in combination (Platt et al., 1980). Five strains of PRV isolated from fatal cases of bovine PR were determined to be attenuated by their effects on rabbits, in cell culture, and stability at 40°C (Sabo et al., 1979).

The general acceptance of these biological characteristics for differentiating strains is unlikely because of the observed variations within the virulent and vaccine strains, the techniques employed, and the lack of information with regard to their stability. Furthermore, the recently introduced technique of restriction endonuclease analysis is capable of determining nonidentity of PRV strains, and the current information indicates that these DNA fingerprints are a stable characteristic.

b. DNA Analysis. The genome of PRV is a linear, double-stranded DNA molecule of approximately 90×10^6 Da. The viral DNA consists of a short unique sequence, bracketed by an inverted repeat, and of a long unique sequence similar to EHV 1 DNA (Ben-Porat et al., 1979). Rixon and Ben-Porat (1979) mapped the genomic location of the restriction sites of PRV generated by the restriction endonucleases *Kpn*I and *Bam*HI.

Variations among strains of PRV have been demonstrated by a fingerprinting technique using the restriction endonuclease analysis of the DNA genomes. Studies on PRV have focused on the fingerprinting of modified, live, virus vaccines (Lawrence, 1982a; Gielkens and Berns, 1982; Paul et al., 1982) and field strains (Lawrence 1982b; Herrmann et al., 1984; Ludwig et al., 1982; Paul et al., 1982; Ben-Porat et al., 1984). Restriction enzyme analysis has been used in studies to identify the genes responsible for the virulence of PRV (Lomniczi et al., 1984; Kit et al., 1985), and in vaccine development (Kit et al., 1985).

It appears that this technique can clearly show strain differences, and thus it is an appropriate tool to use in the epidemiological investigation of PRV outbreaks. With this procedure, it is possible to determine whether one or more strains of PRV are circulating within a herd. The origin of a primary infection and the cause of secondary outbreaks can be traced, providing virus samples are available for comparison. A virus from recrudescence of latency can be differentiated from another strain introduced in the herd. The technique that has been used to compare the reactivated virus isolated from a latently infected pig to the virus believed to have caused the initial infection (Van Oirschot and Gielkens, 1984). The two viruses were indistinguishable and no changes were revealed in the PRV genome after latency. Whether a vaccine virus has the capacity to become latent, with subsequent shedding and transmission, can also be determined.

Ludwig et al. (1982) and Herrmann et al. (1984) described the restriction endonuclease DNA patterns of field strains as consisting of four main genome classes. They were clustered in distinct geographic areas of Northern Europe, Middle Europe, and Thailand. The isolates within each genome group were further subdivided according to geographic relatedness. It was postulated that the genome types emerged from the evolution of viruses in the distinct geographic region. A high degree of similarity in the DNA patterns of field strains of PRV was found, indicating stability of the genome under field conditions. Ben-Porat et al. (1984) analyzed the genomes of 12 PRV field isolates from different outbreaks and found their restriction patterns differed, thus allowing for differentiation from one another.

DNA fingerprints demonstrating strain variations in field strains of PRV prepared by Dr. W. Lawrence, University of Pennsylvania, are

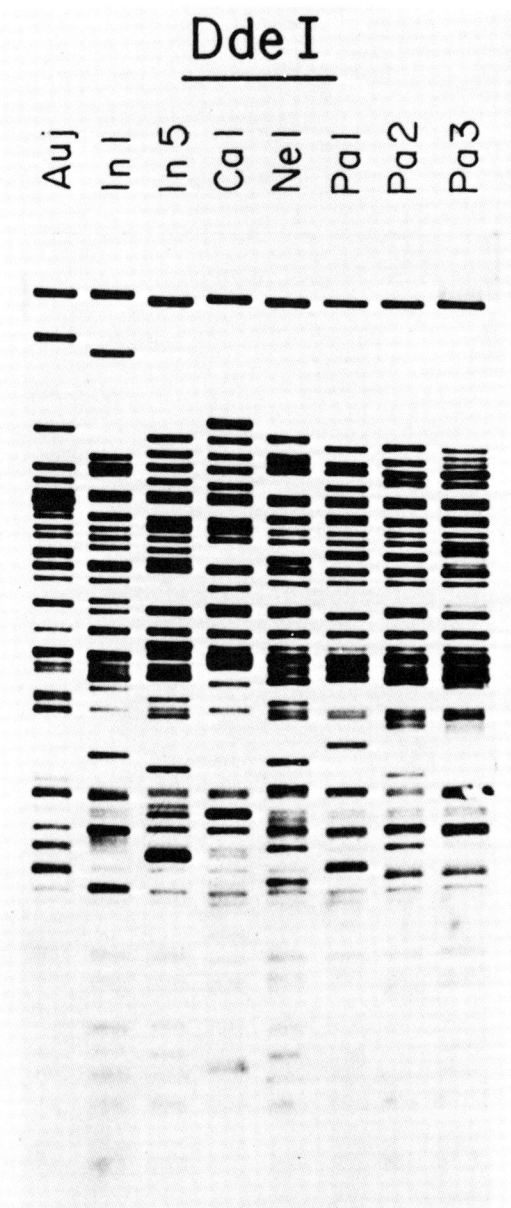

Fig. 2. Restriction patterns of field strains of PRV digested with *Dde*I. The virus strains are, from left to right: Aujeszky's, Indiana 1 and 5, California, Nebraska, Pennsylvania 1, 2, and 3. The viruses are from separate outbreaks of PR. (Courtesy of W. C. Lawrence and U.S. Animal Health Association.)

shown in Fig. 2. Briefly, virus labeled DNA was extracted from infected cells grown in media containing [^{3}H]thymidine. The DNA from each strain was digested with the indicated restriction enzyme (*Dde*I). The digestion products (fragments) were separated by agarose gel electrophoresis, and fluorograms of the dried gels were prepared (Lawrence, 1982b).

Each strain is distinguished by a different pattern of fragments. Since variations occur either in the number of cleavage sites or in the electrophoretic mobility of DNA fragments, a panel of restriction endonucleases are utilized to compare major and minor differences in the genomes of PRV strains.

Stability of fingerprints was demonstrated by the same procedure as above. Two strains of Aujeszky's original virus passed in different laboratories over a period of years in different hosts showed only minor variations in the size of two or three fragments, but no change in total number of fragments. Similarly, two strains of the Bucharest virus maintained under different conditions and at two laboratories revealed no major variations. The application of this technique to the epidemiologic study of PRV outbreak in sheep has shown its usefulness in identifying the source of infection (Van Alstine *et al.*, 1984).

In an investigation as to the source of PRV that killed 33 lambs, the genomes of the sheep isolates were compared to that of the Norden modified-live-virus (MLV) vaccine viral DNA. Paul *et al.* (1982) had reported earlier that the electrophoretic patterns of the Norden MLV and BUK strains had a unique *Bam*HI pattern and could be differentiated from field strains. The BUK strain is the parent strain of the Norden MLV vaccine. It was shown by Van Alstine *et al.* (1984) that the restriction endonuclease analysis of the DNAs of 2 sheep isolates were essentially identical and indistinguishable from that of the Norden MLV virus. On further investigation, it was learned that the 33 lambs had been injected with *Clostridium perfringens* C and D toxoid, tetanus antitoxin, and an antibiotic 7 days before the onset of illness. The syringe used to inject the lambs had been used to vaccinate pigs 3 days earlier with the Norden MLV vaccine. Although the syringe had been rinsed with water, it had not been disinfected. Horizontal transmission did not occur between the infected lambs and contacts.

3. Host Range

PRV has the broadest host range of the animal herpesviruses and the subject is well reviewed by Galloway (1938) and Baskerville *et al.* (1973).

Natural infections of pseudorabies have been observed in pigs, cattle, sheep, goats, horses, dogs, cats, rodents, mink, and wild animals. Although clinical illness occurs, the susceptibility, signs, and severity of infection vary among the species.

Human infections have been reported (Tuncman, 1938). However, current information indicates that pseudorabies is of no public health significance.

Replication of the virus with cytopathic changes occurs in cell cultures derived from a wide variety of animal species and has been reviewed (Baskerville et al., 1973).

a. *Laboratory Animals.* The rabbit is the most susceptible of the small laboratory animals to PRV (Galloway, 1938). The guinea pig, susceptible to infection by intranasal and parenteral routes, has been suggested as a model for studying the cellular and humoral responses to antigen stimulation (Ashworth et al., 1980). Suckling mice were most susceptible to intracerebral inoculation and least susceptible to infection by the oral route (Goto et al., 1971). Fraser and Ramachandran (1969) reported that unweaned mice were probably as suitable as rabbits for PRV isolation.

Although PRV has been propagated in embryonated hen eggs (Burnet et al., 1939) and in day-old chicks (Ramachandran and Fraser, 1971), the chick is not considered a very likely host for the natural disease. However, 10,000 3- and 4-day-old chicks died of PRV infection on a rearing farm in the Netherlands (Kouwenhoven et al., 1982). This uncommon outbreak in poultry is believed to have been caused by mistakenly injecting the newly hatched chicks with PRV alone, or together with the Marek vaccine virus.

b. *Wildlife.* In addition to the wild animal species listed by Galloway (1938) and Gustafson (1981) to be susceptible to PRV, the virus has also been isolated from a skunk (Crandell et al., 1976b) which died of a natural infection. PRV-neutralizing antibodies have been demonstrated in serum from feral swine in Florida (H. N. Becker and R. A. Crandell, 1979, unpublished data) and in Texas (R. A. Crandell and D. B. Lawhorn, 1984, unpublished data). Tozzini (1982b) demonstrated the susceptibility of wild swine in Italy to PRV infection by oral inoculation. This resulted in virus shedding and transmission to contact swine. These findings emphasize the importance of protecting domestic swine and other animals from comingling with feral swine. Although PRV has been recovered from a wide variety of wild animals, most attention has been directed toward the raccoon (*Procyon lotor*) and the wild Norway rat (*Rattus norvegicus*) because of their suspected role in the transmission of the virus in nature.

Results of recent experimental studies with PRV-infected wild and laboratory rats suggest that rats are not likely to be an important reservoir for PRV and that transmission of the virus to other animals would be limited to the consumption of an infected rat carcass (McFerran and Dow, 1970; Maes et al., 1979). These investigators found that large doses of virus were required to infect rats by the oral route and that oral infections were invariably fatal. Antibodies were not detected in serum from surviving rats, or from trapped rats on infected premises, nor was PRV recovered from their tissues. Transmission between rats was not observed in the laboratory or under natural field conditions.

Infected raccoons were found dead on PRV-infected swine premises in the midwestern states of the United States during the early 1970s, when the number of PRV outbreaks was on the increase (Crandell et al., 1976b).

Recently, three groups of researchers independently induced PRV infections in captive raccoons using different strains of virus, routes of administration, and dosages (Kirkpatrick et al., 1980; Wright and Thawley, 1980; Platt et al., 1983). Although the experimental approaches and methods differed, some common observations were demonstrated. Kirkpatrick et al. (1980) and Wright and Thawley (1980) agreed that a naturally infected raccoon would be a source of PRV for swine if the carcass were consumed. However, it is believed that the infected raccoon would probably not travel great distances after becoming infected. The authors differed in their respective conclusions concerning the role that the raccoon may play in perpetuating PRV in nature. Wright and Thawley (1980) concluded that the raccoon does not survive PRV infection and therefore is unlikely to serve as a reservoir host, whereas Platt et al. (1983) suggested that the raccoon has the potential of becoming a significant reservoir for PRV.

Raccoons were shown to be susceptible to infection with field and vaccine strains of PRV. In general, the responses in the animals were dose related. Fatalities increased and the mean number of days of illness decreased with a higher virus dose. Serum samples collected from raccoons in PRV-enzootic areas were found to be negative for neutralizing antibodies by Wright and Thawley (1980) and Kirkpatrick et al. (1980), whereas Platt et al. (1983) demonstrated a low titer in their study population. Although the possibility of a cross-reaction with a group antigen was considered, it was not ruled out. The latter group also demonstrated neutralizing antibody titers in the raccoons that survived the infection. Kirkpatrick et al. (1980) demonstrated interspecies transmission of PRV between raccoons and pigs, but attempts to demonstrate intraspecies transmission among raccoons were unsuccessful.

Platt et al. (1983) demonstrated virus shedding and anamnestic response in one raccoon when challenged 41 days after primary infection with the K strain of PRV. However, latency was not investigated in any of the raccoons surviving initial infection, or after challenge. It appears to this author that this is an important feature of the disease in raccoons that has to be considered with regard to their role as a reservoir host.

4. Pathogenesis

a. Pigs. The pathogenesis of PRV infection in swine has been reviewed by Baskerville *et al.* (1973) and studied recently by Wittman *et al.* (1980).

The respiratory tract is the natural route of infection. The primary site of virus replication is the nasopharyngeal region and the respiratory tract (McFerran and Dow, 1965; Sabo *et al.*, 1969; Wittmann *et al.*, 1980). The virus enters the olfactory nerves and travels along the glossopharyngeal nerve to the nucleus solitarius in the medulla, or to the pons and medulla by way of the trigeminal nerve (McFerran and Dow, 1965). The virus reaches the tonsils and local lymph nodes by way of the lymphatics. Transplacental infections also occur (Csontos *et al.*, 1962; Hsu *et al.*, 1980; Wohlgemuth *et al.*, 1978). The presence of viremia has been variable and may be strain related (Baskerville *et al.*, 1973; Donaldson *et al.*, 1983). The demonstration of PRV in white blood cells supports the suggestion of others that the virus may be transported by the blood to other organs.

The virus is excreted in nasal and oral secretions and vaginal discharge for varying periods after infection. Nursing pigs can acquire PHV from the milk of infected sows (Kojnok, 1957). PRV has been recovered from preputial swabs (Donaldson *et al.*, 1983), and the semen.

Recovery results in lasting immunity against clinical disease. Neutralizing antibodies are demonstrable in the serum between 7 and 10 days after infection and reach a maximum titer after 30 days. Animals with antibody titers can become reinfected and shed virus for a few days. Immune sows confer passive immunity to their offspring through colostrum (Kojnok and Surjan, 1963). The persistence of maternal antibodies is dependent upon the concentration acquired during the first few days of life.

Latent infection can be established in swine surviving the initial infection. Neurotropism has been demonstrated in naturally (Gutekunst *et al.*, 1980) and experimentally infected swine (Wittman *et al.*, 1983; Van Oirschot and Gielkens, 1984). Some clinically normal, recovered pigs will become latent carriers and shed PRV periodically

(Kojnok, 1965; Sabo and Grunert, 1971; Davies and Beran, 1980; Kemeny, 1981).

b. *Cattle.* An interesting aspect of the pathogenesis of bovine PRV is the recent recognition of extraneural virus in naturally and experimentally infected cattle. Since PRV has been demonstrated in the nasal mucosa (Bitsch, 1975a; Bitsch, 1975b), nasal secretions (Bitsch, 1975c; Crandell and Gebre-Mariam, 1980), and lung (Bitsch, 1975c; Beasley *et al.*, 1980) from naturally infected cattle, it has been suggested that this species may be a potential source of infection for other animals. This possibility is a concern in view of the current trend in the increase in number of cattle being infected in individual herds (Bitsch, 1975b; Joubert *et al.*, 1979; Beasley *et al.*, 1980). Therefore, the routes of infection and source of virus are important in understanding the epizootiology of this disease in cattle. Earlier studies by Dow and McFerran (1962) and McFerran and Dow (1964a) showed that cattle were susceptible to infection with PRV by intradermal, subcutaneous, intranasal, and oral inoculations and that PRV infections were strictly neurotropic in cattle. The location of lesions and virus distribution suggested virus dissemination via peripheral nerves to the related ganglia and, eventually, to the cord or brain. Similar virus neurotropism was also demonstrated in calves inoculated intravenously and intramuscularly (Dow and McFerran, 1966a). Significant lesions outside the central nervous system of calves inoculated intravenously were limited to the autonomic chains and the ganglionic neurons of the adrenal capsule and medulla. Virus was also isolated from the adrenal glands, pharynx, heart, kidney, and blood. Knowing where the virus is localized in the body is important in the selection of diagnostic specimens.

Bitsch (1975a,b) conducted an epidemiological study on bovine outbreaks in Denmark in an attempt to determine the natural routes of infection. He classified the bovine outbreaks according to the location of pruritus on the body, that is, as either anterior or posterior. It was concluded that the anterior pruritus cases were associated primarily with infections by the respiratory route, whereas the route of infection in the posterior (perineal) pruritus cases was obscure. However, some were found to be associated with vaginal infections. Human contamination was suggested as a possible source of some genital infections. This author has observed pigs nibbling or biting at the vulvas of cows that were lying down, and believes this to be a source of infection. Transmission of virus could easily occur from pig to cow, as the classic experiment by Shope (1935) in which he demonstrated the transmissibility of the virus from swine to rabbits. He successfully induced

PRV infection in rabbits by rubbing the nose of an infected pig against the freshly abraded abdominal skin of rabbits. Epidemiological data from a study by Beran et al. (1976) support the suggestion that the aerosol is a major source of virus and the respiratory tract is the major route of infection.

It is well established that, experimentally, the bovine is highly susceptible to infection to PRV by the nasal route and that clinical disease terminates inevitably in death (De Leeuw, 1982; Wittmann et al., 1982; Biront et al., 1982; Crandell et al., 1982). Differences in the distribution of virus in tissues and body fluids of experimentally inoculated cattle are reported. De Leeuw (1982) occasionally found virus in excretions (oral and pharyngeal fluids and nasal swabs) of 1.5-year-old cattle after they first showed clinical signs. However, virus was demonstrated in the nasal mucosa at slaughter. Wittmann et al. (1982) failed to isolate virus from the nasal secretions of infected 3- to 5-week-old calves, but isolated PRV from the nasal mucosa and thymus of a calf that died 3 days after inoculation. On the other hand, these authors demonstrated virus in nasal secretions in 1.5-year-old cattle as long as 6 days postinfection. Crandell et al. (1982) reported significant amounts of virus in nasal swabs from 4- to 5-month-old calves 1 to 4 days after intranasal inoculation. In addition, virus was also recovered from conjunctival swabs of two animals and tonsils of four animals at necropsy. Virus was not recovered from the olfactory lobes of all calves (Crandell et al., 1982), as reported by others (Dow and McFerran, 1962; Wittman et al., 1982), but was consistently isolated from the brain stem and trigeminal ganglia. Although pruritus is usually observed to be unilateral in naturally (Bitsch, 1975a) and in experimentally infected calves, the microscopic lesions and virus dissemination were found to be predominantly bilateral (Crandell et al., 1982). All studies clearly show that PRV is neurotropic in cattle and that the virus follows the nerve pathways to the brain and spinal cord. The role of the blood and lymphatics in the dissemination of virus throughout the body is a subject for further study.

There is no evidence to suggest virus spread between the bovine species. Transmission of virus did not occur experimentally between PRV-infected and contact calves (Masic, 1961; Crandell et al., 1982; De Leeuw, 1982); however, serological conversion of PRV did occur in a pig after contact with an experimentally infected calf (Crandell et al., 1982).

The length of contact time and shedding patterns of cattle are two factors which may explain the failure of horizontal transmission of PRV between cattle, in spite of the presence of moderate amounts of virus in the nasal passages. The exposure time to other animals would be shorter, since cattle die within a few days of becoming infected; in contrast to comingling with clinically normal, virus-shedding pigs. Pigs also have higher virus concentrations in their nasal secretions than cattle (Gutekunst and Pirtle, 1979; Wittmann et al., 1982). Virus shedding and contamination of the environment by the nasal secretions of cattle have not been studied. Currently, the pig remains the only known source of infection for cattle.

The pathogenesis of the PRV infections in pregnant cattle is unknown; the demonstration of PRV in the fetal tissues (Silva and Giovine, 1966; Bitsch, 1980) and in the blood (Silva and Giovine, 1966) of the cow suggests transplacental infection.

c. *Sheep.* Sheep are susceptible to infection by oral, intranasal, intraconjunctival, intradermal (by scarification) (McFerran and Dow, 1964b; Dow and McFerran, 1964), and subcutaneous (Dow and McFerran, 1966b) routes of inoculation by PRV. The distribution of lesions within the central nervous system is consistent with cephalad movement of the virus from the peripheral nerves to the related ganglia, and subsequently to the spinal cord or brain (Dow and McFerran, 1964). Although Dow and McFerran (1966b) demonstrated virus in the blood, pharynx, kidney, spleen, adrenal, and heart of some sheep that had been inoculated subcutaneously, the virus was recovered more consistently from the nervous tissue. In an earlier transmission study, McFerran and Dow (1964b) reported that sheep did not develop a viremia or excrete virus.

From an epidemiological review of reported cases of PR in sheep, it appears that the respiratory route is probably the most common route of infection for sheep, and that the pig is the source.

5. Latent and Persistent Infections

In the discussions to follow, latency is defined as that state following an initial infection when infectious virus is no longer isolated by routine cultural methods.

Latency is a characteristic of the herpesviruses and is the most troublesome feature of PRV infections in swine. Virus recovery from the nasal–oral–pharyngeal areas by conventional methods is limited to 10–25 days after infection (McFerran and Dow, 1964c; Sabo, 1969; Sabo and Blaskovic, 1970; Crandell et al., 1982; Maes et al., 1983). Several weeks after an initial infection in swine, the virus disappears from the nasopharyngeal region and enters into a quiescent stage referred to as the latent state. Recrudescence with virus excretion occurs after certain undefined stimuli or conditions. Spontaneous shedding of

PRV from latently infected pigs has occurred following stresses from extreme climatic conditions (Howarth, 1969), parturition (Davies and Beran, 1980), and shipping (Kemeny, 1981). The phenomenon of latency with reactivation of PRV has been recognized for years from epizootiological and clinical evidence.

The latency of PRV infections has been confirmed by various methods. Sabo and Rajcani (1976) demonstrated PRV in tonsil, cervical lymph node, nasal mucosa, and trigeminal (gasserian) ganglia by the tissue explant technique from hydrocortisone-treated pigs, which had been infected 160–181 days previously. In another study, Wittmann et al. (1982) demonstrated PRV latency in pigs by administering high doses of prednisolone 9.5 months after an initial infection. In an earlier study, Sabo (1969) was unsuccessful in demonstrating latency in pigs with a combination of hydrocortisone treatment, changing of the diet, and exposing them to heat and cold stresses. In another study, shocking PRV-infected pigs by the intravenous administration of egg albumin did not induce recrudescence (McFerran and Dow, 1964c). Smith (1979) was unsuccessful in causing recrudescence in vaccinated and naturally infected pigs by injecting some with 20 mg of dexamethasone and 5.0 mg of flumethasone and exposing others to ^{60}Co gamma rays to a total dose of 300 R. Virus isolation attempts were made in cell culture by inoculating nasal swabs and tissue suspensions. The use of low doses of corticosteroids and the inoculation of cell cultures with swabs and tissue suspensions may explain these earlier failures. Beran et al. (1980), combining the tissue explant and coculturing techniques, detected PRV in experimentally infected pigs 6 weeks to 13 months after infection. Virus was more consistently isolated from tonsil, trigeminal ganglia and pooled trigeminal ganglia, and olfactory and optic nerves than from other tissues. Virus was not isolated beyond 3 weeks after infection by conventional isolation techniques. However, since serial samples were not taken during the course of study, it is difficult to determine whether PRV persisted in these tissues for the extended periods of time as infectious virus, or if recrudescence had occurred. In addition, the cultural characteristics of their virus suggests latency. Under field conditions, PRV has been recovered from animals in a vaccinated, infected herd over a period of 11 months (Sabo and Grunert, 1971).

What is believed to be the first isolation of PRV from the trigeminal ganglia of a naturally latent, infected sow was accomplished by cocultivating minced fragments of the trigeminal ganglia in cell cultures of porcine kidney cells. A 2-year-old, PRV naturally infected, seropositive sow was injected with 200 mg of dexamethasone and, 5 days later, the tissues were removed for assay. The PRV genome was also demonstrated in the same trigeminal ganglia by the complementary RNA (cRNA)–DNA hybridization technique (Gutekunst et al., 1980).

The RNA–DNA hybridization technique had been used earlier to detect latency in the trigeminal ganglia of experimentally infected pigs (Gutekunst, 1979).

Another biochemical method used for the analysis of latent PRV infection is the Southern blot–DNA hybridization technique (Southern, 1975). With this technique, Lawrence (1983) successfully detected PRV genome sequences in trigeminal ganglia, medulla, and cervical cord from pigs infected 3–6 months earlier.

Rziha et al. (1984) employed the in situ hybridization, reassociation kinetic, and the Southern blot analyses to detect latent PRV DNA in tissues from experimentally infected swine. These investigators found, under their experimental conditions, that PRV latency was established by 7 weeks postinfection. The presence of viral DNA was demonstrated in single cells and it persisted predominantly in the neural tissues of the infected animals. The amount of PRV DNA in neural tissue was very small and it was suggested that the DNA occurs in a nonreplicable form. Blot hybridization of restriction fragments suggests the presence of PRV DNA in the white blood cells of latently infected pigs.

Latency has been reported in pigs vaccinated with a live virus vaccine (Mock et al., 1981; Van Oirschot, 1984), an inactivated vaccine (Wittmann et al., 1983; Wittmann et al., 1984), and in pigs born to vaccinated sows (Van Oirschot and Gielkens, 1984). Latency and the reactivation of virus occurred in spite of the presence of high titers of neutralizing antibodies. Virus shedding occurred in each group of pigs after administration of large doses of corticosteroids (prednisolone and dexamethasone).

The presence of virus was demonstrated by explant cultures (Van Oirshot and Gielkens, 1984) and cocultivation (Wittmann et al., 1983) of trigeminal ganglia, but not by the tissue suspension method (Mock et al., 1981; Wittmann et al., 1983). Van Oirshot and Gielkens (1984) suggested that the clinical signs they observed were probably a result of the effect of the corticosteroid treatment, since the signs were not correlated with virus shedding.

DNA analyses by restriction endonuclease of the reactivated virus revealed a fingerprint pattern indistinguishable from the initial isolate. The results also indicated that the virus remained genetically stable during latency (Van Oirschot and Gielkens, 1984). Gielkens

(1984) reported similar results, but, his recrudescent virus revealed an additional BamHI DNA fragment not present in the parent strain.

These findings clearly show that immunized pigs with neutralizing antibodies can be infected and become latent carriers of virulent virus. However, since higher doses of virus are required to infect immune pigs, it can be speculated that latency may occur less frequently in vaccinated animals.

Although PR immune animals may be reinfected, recent studies have shown that superinfection does not result in colonization of the ganglia of pigs previously infected with a virulent strain (Ben-Porat et al., 1984). Similar results were reported in rabbits using herpes simplex virus (HSV) type 1 (Centifanto-Fitzgerald et al., 1982). In this study the trigeminal ganglia of rabbits infected with HSV and superinfected with virulent strains were found to be colonized only by the initial infecting strain. It has been suggested by Centifanto-Fitzgerald et al. (1982) that an immune mechanism may play a role in the inhibition of the colonization of the superinfecting virus strain. However, it appears that the immune status of pigs vaccinated with PR MLV had no effect on the ability of a superinfecting virus to colonize or become latent (Mock et al., 1981). In addition, pigs with high concentrations of PRV maternal antibodies and those immunized with a PRV-inactivated virus will develop a latent infection after challenge with a virulent virus (Wittmann et al., 1983; Van Oirschot and Gielkens, 1984). The demonstration of the deletions in the genomes (Lomniczi et al., 1984) of two vaccine strains (Bartha and Norden) possibly related to virulence and latency could explain why the colonization by the Norden vaccine did not occur (Mock et al., 1981). Therefore, since this attenuated strain can no longer colonize, perhaps there is no genetic competition for a superinfecting virulent strain that would prevent colonization in an immune animal.

D. Diagnosis

In acute outbreaks, a clinical diagnosis should be confirmed as soon as possible by laboratory means. A definitive diagnosis is easily made by virus isolation, or by the fluorescent antibody tissue section technique (Meyling and Bitsch, 1967; Hill et al., 1977). The virus is readily isolated in cell cultures and identified by the serum neutralization test (SN) or by the fluorescent antibody test (FAT) (Stewart et al., 1967; Crandell and Gebre-Mariam, 1980). These diagnostic procedures (Carbrey, 1982) and the selection of tissues for diagnosis in cattle (Crandell, 1981) and in swine (Crandell, 1982) have recently been discussed.

Chronic infections without clinical illness are detected by serological methods.

A specific PRV antibody has been demonstrated by a number of serological procedures, which have been reviewed by Gustafson (1981) and Carbrey (1982). The serological tests that have been reported are SN, agar-gel immunodiffusion test (AGID) (Smith and Stewart, 1978), microimmunodiffusion test (MIDT) (Gutekunst et al., 1978b), the enzyme-linked immunosorbent assay (ELISA) (Snyder and Stewart, 1977), indirect solid-phase microradioimmunoassay (IRIA) (Kelling et al., 1978), modified direct complement-fixation (CF) (Eskildsen, 1975), countercurrent immunoelectrophoresis (CIET) (Papp-Vid and Dulac, 1979), and the indirect hemagglutination test (IHA) (Haffer et al., 1980).

The acceptability of each test is determined by its sensitivity, specificity, cost, and other factors such as serum toxicity and availability of cell cultures. Banks and Cartwright (1983) compared and evaluated the SN, CIET, MIDT, and ELISA tests for the detection of PRV antibodies in swine serum. They found the ELISA test to be the most suitable because of its sensitivity, speed, and cost.

Other investigators (Stewart et al., 1978; Gutekunst et al., 1978a; Johnson et al., 1983) have compared the sensitivity of MIDT with that of the standard SN test (Hill et al., 1977) with some differences in their results.

The Animal Plant Health Inspection Service (APHIS), the regulatory branch of the United States Department of Agriculture (USDA), has approved the recommended minimum standards for the SN (Hill et al., 1977) and the ELISA tests (Snyder and Erickson, 1981) to be used as official tests for the serodiagnosis of PRV.

The delayed hypersensitivity reaction (skin test) has been investigated as a field diagnostic test to identify swine herds infected with PRV (Haralambiev and Yotov, 1967; Skoda et al., 1968; Yotov, 1973; Smith and Mengeling, 1977; Scherba et al., 1978). Although the skin test was a promising test, results from a field trial indicate that it may not be sensitive enough, particularly in young animals, to detect herds with a low infection rate (Crandell et al., 1984). This lack of sensitivity, may, however, be overcome by the development of an improved antigen.

Another serodiagnostic test that has been proposed as a field diagnostic test is the radial immunodiffusion enzyme assay (RIDEA) (Joo et al., 1983). Although this test has not been approved as an official test, it is reported to be a simple, reliable, and rapid serological test for detecting and quantitating PRV antibody. As the name implies, the procedure is a combination of radial immunodiffusion and the ELISA test. Polystyrene plates are coated with PRV antigen and overlaid with agar. The test is performed by adding serum, or a drop of blood, to wells and allowing the antibody to diffuse and to bind with the antigen. The agar is removed and the antigen–antibody reaction is observed visually after adding enzyme-labeled, antiporcine antibody and substrate. The antibody is quantitated by measuring the diameter of the zone produced.

E. Prevention and Control

An understanding of the pathogenetic and epizootiologic features of the disease is necessary when considering prevention and control. Vaccination of swine was practiced for years in Eastern Europe without containing the spread of PRV infection. Use of vaccines reduced losses by cutting the duration of outbreaks and by preventing the occurrence of outbreaks in exposed herds (Csontos, 1977). However, vaccination of infected herds failed to eliminate the disease and to prevent pigs from becoming carriers (Sabo and Grunert, 1971; Csontos, 1977). Experimentally, it has been shown that pigs actively immunized with attenuated (Mock *et al.,* 1981; Van Oirschot, 1984) and inactivated PRV vaccines (Wittmann *et al.,* 1983) developed latency following superinfection with a virulent field strain of virus. It is this situation that creates concern when the present vaccines are employed indiscriminately as a control measure. In addition to being potential carriers, vaccinated animals cannot be distinguished from naturally infected animals by presently available serological methods.

Realizing the failure of vaccination to prevent the spread of PRV, Hungary initiated an eradication program to establish disease-free herds by vaccinating infected stock and selecting serologically negative offspring as replacement stock (Csontos, 1977).

Vaccines for pigs were introduced into the United States in 1977, with some controversy over their usefulness for controlling PR. Proponents of vaccines said they would save the industry, while those against mass vaccination programs claimed that the infections would continue to spread, making eventual control/eradication more difficult, if not impossible. Consequently, some states supported extensive vaccination, while others placed restrictions on its use. Data collected by national serological surveys of market hogs show that the infection in the United States has continued to increase slightly during the 1980s, but at a lower rate than in the 1970s.

Prevention of PRV infections is based on the control of swine movements—locally, nationally, and internationally. The importance of the carrier pig in the control of this disease cannot be overemphasized. McFerran *et al.* (1984) have reported that the majority of cases of PR occurs after the purchase of an apparently healthy animal. In an effort to control the spread of PRV, governments introduced legislation restricting the movements of infected swine, making the disease notifiable, and establishing control or eradication programs. In the United States, federal regulation (Part 85 Pseudorabies—Title 9 Code of Federal Regulations) became effective on May 17, 1979. This document primarily covers the restrictions on interstate movement of swine. The disease became notifiable in Great Britain (Goodhand, 1983) in 1979, and in Denmark (Anderson, 1982) and the Federal Republic of Germany (Pittler, 1982) in 1980. On March 14, 1983, a control and eradication policy was introduced in Great Britain (Goodhand, 1983). This control and eradication program involves the slaughtering of all herds in which PRV infection is confirmed (Goodhand, 1983). The program is a combined approach to disease eradication involving the government and the pig industry and is being accomplished without vaccination.

In the United States, several approaches to the elimination of PRV from swine herds are being used (Thawley *et al.*, 1982). The three basic procedures to achieve a neutralizing antibody-free (NAF) herd are (1) depopulation and repopulation, (2) test and removal, and (3) offspring segregation with various options. The extent of vaccination varies with the situation. Before a procedure is selected, an epidemiological evaluation of the herd must be conducted and all of the financial considerations for the producer must be considered.

Eradication of PRV has been achieved by similar programs of vaccinating and selecting serologically negative animals for replacement breeding stock in Ireland (McFerran *et al.*, 1984).

Currently, the federal government, in cooperation with some states, is conducting field studies to ascertain effective means for eradicating PRV.

Hyperimmune serum has been shown to be effective in reducing neonatal mortality in PRV-infected herds under field conditions, but its use has not been accepted as a control procedure (Kojnok and Greczi, 1957; Crandell *et al.*, 1977). However, the use of hyperimmune serum in combination with sow vaccination was recently reported for several farms in Taiwan, where PRV was enzootic (Hsu and Lee, 1984). The mean mortality in the pigs receiving immune serum was 5.6% and in the untreated controls the mortality was 47.7%. The mean reproductive failure rate in the vaccinated breeding sows was 1.9%, compared to 41.5% in the nonvaccinated animals.

Another approach to the management of PRV-infected herds is via embryo-transfer technology. This procedure has been used successfully to preserve genetic material from PRV-infected swine herds. James *et al.* (1983) reported that embryos collected from PRV-seropositive, recovered sows did not transmit PRV to recipients or their neonates. However, Bolin *et al.* (1982) presented evidence indicating that embryos exposed to PRV *in vitro* and those embryos collected from experimentally exposed donors transmitted the virus to recipient sows.

The virus can spread without the movement of swine; therefore, precautions should be taken in visiting neighbors, sale barns, and other facilities where pigs are handled. Trucks, trailers, and other vehicles should be cleaned after hauling swine, feed, and other supplies to reduce the risk of introducing the virus onto a premise. Recommended disinfectants are orthophenyl phenol compounds, 5% phenol sodium hypochorite calcium hypochlorite, 2% sodium hydroxide trisodium phosphate, quaternary ammonia, and chlorhexidine diacetate (Thawley *et al.*, 1982). Feeder pigs should not be introduced onto farms where farrowing operations exist. The disease can be prevented in cattle and sheep by not allowing them to comingle with, or to be in the proximity of infected pigs. Dogs and cats should not have access to buildings that house swine and should not be allowed to feed upon infected carcasses. Contaminated carcasses should be buried or burned. Efforts to control movement of wildlife are recommended.

F. Vaccines

The use of vaccines against porcine PRV infections has played an important role in reducing the economic losses due to this disease. The literature on the early vaccines has been reviewed (Baskerville *et al.*, 1973). Currently, both attenuated and inactivated virus vaccines are available for use in pigs, but neither prevents the latency of field strains. Recent studies with inactivated virus vaccines in cattle (Biront *et al.*, 1982) and dogs (Pensaert *et al.*, 1980) indicate that protection is not satisfactory.

Advances in molecular biology are being applied to the development of new kinds of PRV vaccines. Subunit vaccines prepared by extracting protective immunogens from the virus have been evaluated (Maes and Schutz, 1983; Platt, 1983). These vaccines prevented clinical signs in vaccinated pigs when challenged with virulent virus.

Reported advantages of these vaccines are that they do not contain live virus and, since some proteins are removed, the antibody raised against them has the potential of being differentiated from the antibody that results from natural infections. There is no available information to indicate whether the subunit vaccines will inhibit colonization after superinfection with a virulent virus.

A modified live PRV vaccine that is efficacious and more attenuated than present vaccines has been developed (Kit and Kit, 1984, personal communication). The vaccine is a deletion mutant of PRV constructed by genetic engineering techniques and has a negligible probability of reverting to virulence. The vaccine virus did not revert to thymidine kinase-positive plaques during cell culture passage. The vaccine virus carries a "corporate signature" so that it can be unequivocally differentiated from any field strain. Because of these properties, it may also be possible to develop a diagnostic serological test that would differentiate vaccinated pigs from naturally infected animals.

Important steps in the development of this vaccine were the deletion of a portion of the coding sequence of the PRV-encoded thymidine kinase gene and the selection of isolates which replicate at 39.1°C, as well as at 34.5°C. Similarly, previous studies have shown that the thymidine kinase-negative herpes simplex virus (Price and Khan, 1981) and herpesvirus tamarinus mutants (Kit et al., 1983) are highly attenuated for mice.

The vaccine did not produce clinical signs in calves and pigs. Studies have also shown that this vaccine virus will colonize in the ganglia of vaccinated pigs and that the prevention of latency after superinfection is dose dependent.

Lomniczi et al. (1984) mapped the genomes of the Norden and Bartha vaccine strains by restriction enzyme analysis. The studies revealed that these two attenuated vaccine strains have deletions of approximately 2.7×10^6 Da in the U_s sequence of their genome. It was further shown that the Norden vaccine strain contains a genome that is a class 3 herpesvirus DNA molecule. Herpesvirus simplex virus DNA is classified as a class 3 herpesvirus DNA, whereas PRV DNA is classified as a class 2 DNA molecule.

References

Aguilar-Setien, A., Pastoret, P. P., Burtonboy, G., Coignoul, F., Jetteur, P., Vandeputte, J., and Schoenaers, F. (1979). *Ann. Med. Vet.* **123**, 55–61.

Allen, G. P., O'Callaghan, D. J., and Randall, C. (1977). *J. Virol.* **24**, 761–767.

Allen, G. P., Yeargan, M. R., Turtinen, L. W., Bryans, J. T., and McCollum, W. H. (1983). *Am. J. Vet. Res.* **44**, 263–271.

Anderson, J. B. (1982). *In* "Aujeszky's Disease" (G. Wittmann and S. A. Hall, eds.), pp. 223–226. Nijoff, The Hague.

Anonymous. (1983). *Time* **121**, 60.

Ardans, A. A. (1982). *J. Am. Vet. Med. Assoc.* **181**, 1150–1153.
Ashworth, L. A. E., Baskerville, A., and Lloyd, G. (1980). *Arch. Virol.* **63**, 227–237.
Aujeszky, A. (1902). *Zentralbl. Bakteriol. Parasitenkd. Infektionskr. Hyg. Abt. 1 Orig.* **32**, 353–357.
Bagust, T. J. (1971). *Vet. Bull (London).* **41**, 79–92.
Baker, J. C., Esser, M. B., and Larson, V. L. (1982). *J. Am. Vet. Med. Assoc.* **181**, 607.
Banks, M., and Cartwright, S. (1983). *Vet. Rec.* **113**, 38–41.
Bartha, A., Belak, S., and Benyeda, J. (1969). *Acta Vet. Acad. Sci. Hung.* **19**, 97–99.
Baskerville, A., McFerran, J. B., and Dow, C. (1973). *Vet. Bull. (London).* **43**, 465–480.
Beasley, V. R., Crandell, R. A., Buck, W. B., Ely, R. W., and Thilsted, J. P., Jr. (1980). *Vet. Res. Commun.* **4**, 125–129.
Ben-Porat, T., Rixon, F. J., and Blankenship, M. L. (1979). *Virology* **95**, 285–294.
Ben-Porat, T., Deatly, A. M., Easterday, B. C., Galloway, D., Kaplan, A. S., and McGregor, S. (1984). *In* "Latent Herpes Virus Infections in Veterinary Medicine" (G. Wittmann, R. M. Gaskell, and H. J. Rziha, eds.), pp. 365–383.Nijhoff, The Hague.
Beran, G. W., Zierke, A. V., Hill, H. T., and Maré, C. J. (1976). *Proc. Int. Pig Vet. Soc. Congr.,* p. G.4.
Beran, G. W., Davies, E. B., Arambulo, P. V., Will, L. A., Hill, H. T., and Rock, D. L. (1980). *J. Am. Vet. Med. Assoc.* **176**, 998–1000.
Biront, P., Vandeputte, J., Pensaert, M. B., and Leunen, J. (1982). *Am. J. Vet. Res.* **43**, 760–763.
Bitsch, V. (1975a). *Acta Vet. Scand.* **16**, 420–433.
Bitsch, V. (1975b). *Acta Vet. Scand.* **16**, 434–448.
Bitsch, V. (1975c). *Acta Vet. Scand.* **16**, 449–455.
Bitsch, V. (1980). *Acta Vet. Scand.* **21**, 708–710.
Bodon, L., and Greczi, E. (1966). *Acta Microbiol. Acad. Sci. Hung.* **13**, 185–187.
Bodon, L., Mezaros, J., Papp-Vid, G., and Romvary, J. (1968). *Acta Vet. Acad. Sci. Hung.* **18**, 107–109.
Bolin, S. R., Runnels, L. J., Sawyer, C. A., and Gustafson, D. P. (1982). *Am. J. Vet. Res.* **43**, 278–280.
Borgen, H. C. (1972). *Arch. Gesamte Virusforsch.* **36**, 391–393.
Borgen, H. C., and Ludwig, H. (1974). *Intervirology* **4**, 189–198.
Boucher, J. D., and Beran, G. (1977). *Iowa State Univ. Vet.* **1**, 22–24.
Brown, J. H. (1939). *J. Am. Vet. Med. Assoc.* **95**, 230.
Bryans, J. T. (1969). *J. Am. Vet. Med. Assoc.* **155**, 294–300.
Bryans, J. T., and Prickett, M. E. (1970). *In* "Equine Infectious Diseases II" (J. T. Bryans and H. Gerber, eds.), pp. 34–40. Karger, Basel.
Buchman, T. G., Roizman, B., Adams, G., and Stover, B. H. (1978). *J. Infect. Dis.* **138**, 488–498.
Buchman, T. G., Roizman, B., and Nahmias, A. J. (1979). *J. Infect. Dis.* **140**, 295–304.
Buchman, T. G., Simpson, T., Nosal, C., and Roizman, B. (1980). *Ann. N.Y. Acad. Sci.* **354**, 279–290.
Bumgardner, M. K., Dutta, S. K., Campbell, D. L., and Myrup, A. C. (1982). *Am. J. Vet. Res.* **43**, 1308–1310.
Burek, J. D., Roos, R. P., and Narayan, O. (1975). *Lab. Invest.* **33**, 400–406.
Burgess, G. W., Stevenson, B. J., Buddle, J. R., and Lash, G. W. (1976). *N.Z. Vet. J.* **24**, 214–215.
Burnet, F. M., Lush, D., and Jackson, A. V. (1939). *Aust. J. Exp. Biol. Med. Sci.* **17**, 35–40.
Burrows, R., and Goodridge, D. (1973). *In* "Equine Infectious Diseases III" (J. T. Bryans and H. Gerber, eds.), pp. 306–321. Karger, Basel.

Burrows, R., and Goodridge, D. (1975). *J. Reprod. Fertil. Suppl.* **23,** 611–615.
Burrows, R., and Goodridge, D. (1984). In "Latent Herpes Virus Infections in Veterinary Medicine" (G. Wittmann, R. M. Gaskell, and H. J. Rziha, eds.), pp. 307–319. Nijhoff, The Hague.
Carbrey, E. A. (1982). *Off. Proc. Annu. Meet. - Livestock Cons. Inst.* pp. 132–139.
Carmichael, L. E., and Barnes, F. D. (1961). *Proc. Annu. Meet. U.S. Anim. Health Assoc.* **65**th, 384–388.
Centifanto-Fitzgerald, Y. M., Varnell, E. D., and Kaufman, H. E. (1982). *Infect. Immun.* **35,** 1125–1132.
Chastain, C. B., Andrews, J. J., and Rekemeyer, R. R. (1973). *J. Am. Vet. Med. Assoc.* **163,** 77.
Crandell, R. A. (1977). *Proc. Pseudorabies Fact-finding Conf.* pp. 23a–23d.
Crandell, R. A. (1981). In "Diseases of Cattle in the Tropics" (M. Ristic and I. McIntyre, eds.), pp. 91–106. Nijhoff, The Hague.
Crandell, R. A. (1982). *Vet. Clin. North Am.: Large Anim. Prac.* **4,** 321–331.
Crandell, R. A., and Angulo, A. B. (1985). *Vet. Med. Small Anim. Clin.* **1,** 73–75.
Crandell, R. A., and Gebre-Mariam, M. (1980). *Proc. Int. Symp. Vet. Lab. Diagn.* **2,** 392–395.
Crandell, R. A., Sells, D. M., and Gallina, A. M. (1976a). *Theriogenology* **6,** 1–19.
Crandell, R. A., Jelly, G. G., Hoefling, D. C., and Gallina, A. M. (1976b). *Proc. Am. Assoc. Vet. Lab. Diagn.* **19,** 13–20.
Crandell, R. A., Doby, P. B., Hill, R. O., Hoefling, D. C., Jelly, G. G., Norton, H. W., Spencer, P. L., Starkey, A. L., and Wu, C. H. (1977). *J. Am. Vet. Med. Assoc.* **171,** 59–63.
Crandell, R. A., Drysdale, S., and Stein, T. L. (1979). *Can. J. Comp. Med.* **43,** 94–97.
Crandell, R. A., Mesfin, G. M., and Mock, R. E. (1982). *Am. J. Vet. Res.* **43,** 326–328.
Crandell, R. A., Gustafson, D. P., White, R. C., and Adams, F. F. (1984). *J. Am. Vet. Med. Assoc.* **184,** 692–694.
Crowhurst, F. A., Dickinson, G., Burrows, R. (1981). *Vet. Rec.* **109,** 527–528.
Csontos, L. (1977). *Proc. Pseudorabies Fact-finding Conf.* p. 4.
Csontos, L., Hejj, L., and Szabo, I. (1962). *Acta Vet. Acad. Sci. Hung.* **12,** 17–23.
Davies, E. B., and Beran, G. W. (1980). *J. Am. Vet. Med. Assoc.* **176,** 1345–1347.
De Leeuw, P. W. (1982). In "Aujeszky's Disease" (G. Wittmann and S. A. Hall, eds.), pp. 127–128. Nijhoff, The Hague.
Dimock, W. W., and Edwards, P. R. (1932). *Kentucky Agr. Exp. Sta. Bull.* **333,** 291–339.
Dimock, W. W., and Edwards, P. R. (1933). *Suppl. Kentucky Agr. Exp. Sta. Bull.* **333,** 297–301.
Dimock, W. W., Edwards, P. R., and Bruner, D. W. (1947). *Cornell Vet.* **37,** 89–99.
Dinter, Z., and Klingeborn, B. (1976). *Vet. Rec.* **99,** 10–12.
Doll, E. R. (1961). *J. Am. Vet. Med. Assoc.* **139,** 1324–1330.
Doll, E. R., and Bryans, J. T. (1962a). *J. Am. Vet. Med. Assoc.* **141,** 351–354.
Doll, E. R., and Bryans, J. T. (1962b). *Am. J. Vet. Res.* **23,** 843–846.
Doll, E. R., and Bryans, J. T. (1963). *J. Am. Vet. Med. Assoc.* **142,** 31–37.
Doll, E. R., and Kintner, J. H. (1954). *Cornell Vet.* **44,** 355–367.
Doll, E. R., and Wallace, M. E. (1954). *Cornell Vet.* **44,** 453–461.
Doll, E. R., Richards, M. G., and Wallace, M. E. (1953). *Cornell Vet.* **43,** 551–558.
Doll, E. R., Bryans, J. T., McCollum, W. H., and Crowe, M. E. W. (1957). *Cornell Vet.* **47,** 3–41.
Donaldson, A. I., Wardley, R. C., Martin, S., and Ferris, N. P. (1983). *Vet. Rec.* **113,** 490–494.
Dow, C., and McFerran, J. B. (1962). *J. Comp. Pathol.* **72,** 337–347.

Dow, C., and McFerran, J. B. (1964). *Am. J. Vet. Res.* **25**, 461–468.
Dow, C., and McFerran, J. B. (1966a). *J. Comp. Pathol.* **76**, 379–385.
Dow, C., and McFerran, J. B. (1966b). *Br. Vet. J.* **122**, 464–470.
Dulac, G. C., and Binns, M. (1979). *Can. Vet. J.* **20**, 318–322.
Dutta, S. K., and Myrup, A. C. (1983). *Can. J. Comp. Med.* **47**, 64–69.
Dutta, S. K., Talbot, N. C., and Myrup, A. C. (1983). *Am. J. Vet. Res.* **44**, 1930–1934.
Erdson, M. E., Kissling, R. E., and Tierkel, E. S. (1953). *J. Am. Vet. Med. Assoc.* **123**, 34–37.
Eskildsen, M. (1975). *Bull. Off. Int. Epizoot.* **84**, 253–263.
Eugster, A. K., and Jones, L. P. (1977). *J. Tex. Vet. Med. Assoc.* **39**, 15–17.
Evans, D. L., Barnett, J. W., and Dmochowski, L. (1973). *Tex. Rep. Biol. Med.* **31**, 755–770.
Fraser, G., and Ramachandran, S. P. (1969). *J. Comp. Pathol.* **79**, 435–444.
Galloway, I. A. (1938). *Vet. Rec.* **50**, 745–762.
Gerber, J. D., Marron, A. E., Bass, E. P., and Beckenhauer, W. N. (1977). *Can. J. Comp. Med.* **41**, 471–478.
Gielkens, A. L. J. (1984). *In* "Latent Herpes Virus Infections in Veterinary Medicine" (G. Wittmann, R. M. Gaskell, and H. J. Rziha, eds.), pp. 385–386. Nijhoff, The Hague.
Gielkens, A. L. J., and Berns, A. J. M. (1982). *In* "Aujeszky's Disease" (G. Wittmann and S. A. Hall, eds.), pp. 3–13. Nijhoff, The Hague.
Gleeson, L. J., and Coggins, L. (1980). *Cornell Vet.* **70**, 391–400.
Golais, F., and Sabo, A. (1975). *Acta Virol. (Engl. Ed.)* **19**, 387–392.
Golais, F., and Sabo, A. (1976). *Acta Virol. (Engl. Ed.)* **20**, 70–72.
Golais, F., Sabo, A., and Svobodova, J. (1977). *Acta Virol. (Engl. Ed.)* **21**, 25–30.
Goodhand, R. H. (1983). *Proc. Annu. Meet. U.S. Anim. Health Assoc. 87th*, 454–458.
Gordon, W. A. M., and Luke, D. (1955). *Vet. Rec.* **66**, 591–597.
Goto, H., Burger, D., and Gorham, J. R. (1971). *Jpn. J. Vet. Sci.* **33**, 145–153.
Gustafson, D. P. (1981). *In* "Comparative Diagnosis of Viral Diseases, Vol. III: Vertebrate Animal and Related Viruses, Part A-DNA Viruses" (E. Kurstak and C. Kurstak, eds.), pp. 205–263. Academic Press, New York.
Gutekunst, D. E. (1979). *Am. J. Vet. Res.* **40**, 1568–1572.
Gutekunst, D. E., and Pirtle E. C. (1979). *Am. J. Vet. Res.* **40**, 1343–1346.
Gutekunst, D. E., Malmquist, W. A., and Becvar, C. S. (1978a). *Arch. Virol.* **56**, 33–45.
Gutekunst, D. E., Pirtle, E. C., and Mengeling, W. L. (1978b). *Am. J. Vet. Res.* **39**, 207–210.
Gutekunst, D. E., Pirtle, E. C., Miller, L. D., and Stewart, W. C. (1980). *Am. J. Vet. Res.* **41**, 1315–1316.
Haffer, K., Gustafson, D. P., and Kanitz, C. L. (1980). *J. Clin. Microbiol.* **11**, 217–219.
Hagemoser, W. A., Hill, H. T., and Moss, E. W. (1978). *J. Am. Vet. Med. Assoc.* **173**, 205–206.
Hanson, R. P. (1954). *J. Am. Vet. Med. Assoc.* **124**, 259–261.
Haralambiev, H., and Yotov, M. (1967). *C. R. Acad. Bulg. Sci.* **20**, 853–854.
Harris, A. L. (1968). *J. Am. Vet. Med. Assoc.* **152**, 54.
Hayward, G. S., Frenkel, N., and Roizman, B. (1975). *Proc. Natl. Acad. Sci. U.S.A.* **72**, 1768–1772.
Henry, B. E., Robinson, R. A., Dauenhauer, S. A., Atherton, S. S., Hayward, G. S., and O'Callaghan, D. J. (1981). *Virology* **115**, 97–114.
Herrmann, S., Heppner, B., and Ludwig, H. (1984). *In* "Latent Herpesvirus Infections in Veterinary Medicine" (G. Wittmann, R. M. Gaskell, and H. J. Rziha, eds.), pp. 387–401. Nijhoff, The Hague.

Hill, H. T., Crandell, R. A., Kanitz, C. L., McAdaragh, J. P., Seawright, G. L., Solorzano, R. F., and Stewart, W. C. (1977). *Proc. Am. Assoc. Vet. Lab. Diagn.* **20**, 375–390.
Horner, G. W. (1981). *N. Z. Vet. J.* **29**, 7–8.
Howarth, J. A. (1969). *J. Am. Vet. Med. Assoc.* **154**, 1583–1589.
Hsu, F. S., and Lee, R. C. T. (1984). *J. Am. Vet. Med. Assoc.* **184**, 1463–1466.
Hsu, F. S., Chu, R. M., Lee, R. C. T., and Chu, S. H. J. (1980). *J. Am. Vet. Med. Assoc.* **177**, 636–641.
Hugoson, G., and Rockborn, G. (1972). *Zentralbl. Veterinaermed., Reihe (B)* **19**, 641–645.
Jackson, T. A., and Kendrick, J. W. (1971). *J. Am. Vet. Med. Assoc.* **158**, 1351–1357.
Jackson, T. A., Osburn, B. I., Cordy, D. R., and Kendrick, J. W. (1977). *Am. J. Vet. Res.* **38**, 709–719.
James, J. E., James, D. M., Martin, P. A., Reed, D. E., and Davis, D. L. (1983). *J. Am. Vet. Med. Assoc.* **183**, 525–528.
Johnson, M. E., Thawley, D. G., Solorzano, R. F., and Wright, J. C. (1983). *Am. J. Vet. Res.* **44**, 28–30.
Jones, T. C., and Maurer, F. D. (1943). *Am. J. Vet. Res.* **4**, 15–31.
Jones, T. C., Gleiser, C. A., Maurer, F. D., Hale, M. W., and Roby, T. O. (1948). *Am. J. Vet. Res.* **9**, 243–253.
Joo, H. S., Lemon, A., and Molitor, T. (1983). *Proc. Annu. U.S. Anim. Health Assoc. 87th*, 451–453.
Joubert, L., Bijlenga, G., Keck, G., Ferry, R., Boch, F., Prave, M., and Chomel, B. (1979). *Rev. Med. Vet.* **130**, 979–1000.
Kaschula, V. R., Beaudette, F. R., and Byrne, R. J. (1957). *Cornell Vet.* **47**, 137–143.
Kelling, C. L., Staudinger, W. L., and Rhodes, M. B. (1978). *Am. J. Vet. Res.* **39**, 1955–1957.
Kemeny, L. J. (1981). *Am. J. Vet. Res.* **42**, 1987–1989.
Kirkpatrick, C. M., Kanitz, C. L., and McCrocklin, S. M. (1980). *J. Wildl. Dis.* **16**, 601–614.
Kit, S., Kit, M., and Pirtle, C. (1985). *Am. J. Vet. Res.* **46**, 1359–1367.
Kit, S., Qavi, H., Dubbs, D. R., and Otsuka, H. (1983). *J. Med. Virol.* **12**, 25–36.
Kluge, J. P., and Maré, C. J. (1974). *Am. J. Vet. Res.* **35**, 911–915.
Kojnok, J. (1957). *Acta Vet. Hung.* **7**, 273–276.
Kojnok, J. (1962). *Acta Vet. Hung.* **12**, 53–58.
Kojnok, J. (1965). *Acta Vet. Acad. Sci. Hung.* **15**, 283–295.
Kojnok, J., and Greczi, E. (1957). *Acta Vet. Hung.* **7**, 423–427.
Kojnok, J., and Surjan, J. (1963). *Acta Vet. Hung.* **13**, 111–118.
Kouwenhoven, B., Davelaar, F. G., Burger, A. G., and Walsum, J. van (1982). *Vet. Q.* **4**, 145–154.
Lawrence, W. C. (1982a). *Proc. Annu. Meet. U.S. Anim. Health Assoc., 86th*, 402–407.
Lawrence, W. C. (1982b). *Off. Proc. Annu. Meet. - Livestock Cons. Inst.* 139–145.
Lawrence, W. C. (1983). *Proc. Int. Symp. World Assoc. Vet. Lab. Diagn.* **1**, 131–133.
Lindemann, Von L., Petzoldt, K., and Merkt, H. (1967). *Berl. Muench. Tieraerztl. Worchenschr.* **80**, 425–427.
Little, P. B., (1974). *Vet. Rec.* **95**, 575.
Liu, I. K. M. (1983). *In* "Current Therapy in Equine Medicine" (N. Eward Robinson, ed.), pp. 4–5. Saunders, Philadelphia, Pennsylvania.
Liu, I. K. M., and Castleman, W. (1977). *J. Equine Med. Surg.* **12**, 397–401.
Lloyd, G., and Baskerville, A. (1978). *Vet. Microbiol.* **3**, 65–70.
Lomniczi, B. (1974). *Arch. Gesamte Virusforsch.* **44**, 205–214.
Lomniczi, B., Blankenship, M. L., and Ben-Porat, T. (1984). *J. Virol.* **49**, 970–979.

Lourens, L. F. D. E. (1935). *Bull. Off. Int. Eqizoot.* **10,** 199–240.
Ludwig, H., Heppner, B., and Herrmann, S. (1982). *In* "Aujeszky's Disease" (G. Wittmann and S. A. Hall, eds.), pp. 15–20. Nijhoff, The Hague.
McFerran, J. B., and Dow, C. (1964a). *J. Comp. Pathol.* **74,** 173–179.
McFerran, J. B., and Dow, C. (1964b). *Res. Vet. Sci.* **5,** 143–148.
McFerran, J. B., and Dow, C. (1964c). *Res. Vet. Sci.* **5,** 405–410.
McFerran, J. B., and Dow, C. (1965). *Am. J. Vet. Res.* **26,** 631–635.
McFerran, J. B., and Dow, C. (1970). *Br. Vet. J.* **126,** 173–179.
McFerran, J. B., McCracken, R. M., and Dow, C. (1984). *In* "Latent Herpes Virus Infections in Veterinary Medicine" (G. Wittmann, R. M. Gaskell, and H. J. Rziha, eds.), pp. 403–415. Nijhoff, The Hague.
Maes, R. K., and Schutz, J. C. (1983). *Am. J. Vet. Res.* **44,** 123–125.
Maes, R. K., Kanitz, C. L., and Gustafson, D. P. (1979). *Am. J. Vet. Res.* **40,** 393–396.
Maes, R. K., Kanitz, C. L., and Gustafson, D. P. (1983). *Am. J. Res.* **44,** 2083–2085.
Masic, M. (1961). *Acta Vet. (Belgrade)* **11,** 49–53.
Matis, J., and Zuffa, A. (1969). *Acta Virol. (Engl. Ed.)* **13,** 371–378.
Maurer, F. D., and Jones, T. C. (1943). *Am. J. Vet. Res.* **4,** 257–264.
Mayr, A., Bohm, H. C., Brill, J., and Woycrechowskas. (1965). *Arch. Gesamte Virusforsch.* **17,** 216–230.
Meyling, A., and Bitsch, V. (1967). *Acta Vet. Scand.* **8,** 360–368.
Mitchell, D. (1980). *In* "Current Therapy in Theriogenology" (D. A. Morrow, ed.), pp. 777–779. Saunders, Philadelphia, Pennsylvania.
Mock, R. E., Crandell, R. A., and Mesfin, G. M. (1981). *Can. J. Comp. Med.* **45,** 56–59.
Mumford, J. A., and Bates, J. (1984) *Vet. Rec.* **114,** 375–381.
O'Callaghan, D. J., Allen, G. P., and Randall, C. C. (1978). *In* "Equine Infectious Diseases IV" (J. T. Bryans and H. Gerber, eds.), pp. 1–32. Veterinary Publications, Princeton, New Jersey.
Olander, H. J., Saunders, J. R., Gustafson, D. P., and Jones, R. K. (1966). *Pathol. Vet.* **3,** 64–82.
Orr, C. M., Gaskell, C. J., and Gaskell, R. M. (1978). *Vet. Rec.* **103,** 200–202.
Papp-Vid, G., and Dulac, G. C. (1979). *Can. J. Comp. Med.* **43,** 119–124.
Patel, J. R., and Edington, N. (1983). *Vet. Microbiol.* **8,** 301–305.
Paul, P. S., Mengeling, W. L., and Pirtle, E. C. (1982). *Arch. Virol.* **73,** 193–198.
Pensaert, M. B., Commeyne, S., and Andries, K. (1980). *Am. J. Vet. Res.* **41,** 2016–2019.
Petzoldt, K. (1967). *Zentralbl. Bakteriol. Parasitenkd. Infektionskr. Hyg., Abt. 1 Ref.* **206,** 540.
Petzoldt, K. (1970). *Berl. Muench. Tieraerztl. Wochenschr.* **83,** 93–95.
Pittler, H. (1982). *In* "Aujeszky's Disease" (G. Wittmann and S. A. Hall, eds.), pp. 259–265. Nijhoff, The Hague.
Platt, K. B. (1983). *Off. Proc. Annu. Meet. - Livestock Cons. Inst.*, 145–147.
Platt, K. B., and Maré, C. J. (1976). *Proc. Int. Pig Vet. Soc. Congr.*, p. G.11.
Platt, K. B., Maré, C. J., and Hinz, P. N. (1979). *Arch. Virol.* **60,** 13–23.
Platt, K. B., Maré, C. J., and Hinz, P. N. (1980). *Arch. Virol.* **63,** 107–114.
Platt, K. B., Graham, D. L., and Faaborg, R. A. (1983). *J. Wildl. Dis.* **19,** 297–301.
Plummer, G. (1964). *Br. J. Exp. Pathol.* **45,** 135–141.
Plummer, G., and Waterson, A. P. (1963). *Virology* **19,** 412–416.
Plummer, G., Bowling, C. P., and Goodheart, C. R. (1969). *J. Virol.* **4,** 738–741.
Plummer, G., Goodheart, C. R., and Studdert, M. J. (1973). *Infect. Immun.* **8,** 621–627.
Popescu, Ar. (1964). *Lucr. Inst. Cercet. Vet. Bioprep. "Pasteur"* **3,** 21–30.
Price, R. W., and Khan, A. (1981). *Infect Immun.* **34,** 571–580.

Prickett, M. E. (1970). *In* "Equine Infectious Diseases II" (J. T. Bryans and H. Gerber, eds.), pp. 24–33. Karger, Basel.
Purdy, C. W., Ford, S. J., and Porter, R. C. (1978). *Am. J. Vet. Res.* **39**, 377–383.
Ramachandran, S. P., and Fraser, G. (1971). *J. Comp. Pathol.* **81**, 55–62.
Randall, C. C. (1955). *Proc. Soc. Exp. Biol. Med.* **90**, 176–178.
Rixon, F. J., and Ben-Porat, T. (1979). *Virology* **97**, 151–163.
Robinson, R. A., Henry, B. E., Duff, R. G., and O'Callaghan, J. O. (1980). *Virology* **101**, 335–362.
Robinson, R. A., Tucker, P. W., Dauenhauer, S. A., and O'Callaghan, D. J. (1981). *Proc. Natl. Acad. Sci. U.S.A.* **78**, 6684–6688.
Roizman, B., Carmichael, L. E., Deinhardt, F., de-The, G., Nahmias, A. J., Plowright, W., Rapp, F., Sheldrick, P., Takahashi, M., and Wolf, K. (1981). *Intervirology* **16**, 201–217.
Ryu, E. (1975). "Chronological Reference of Zoonosis: Aujeszky's Disease, Pseudorabies," pp. 1–52. Taipei, Taiwan, Republic of China.
Rziha, H. J., Mettenleiter, T., and Wittmann, G. (1984). *In* "Latent Herpes Virus Infections in Veterinary Medicine" (G. Wittmann, R. M. Gaskell, and H. J. Rziha, eds.), pp.429–444. Nijhoff, The Hague.
Sabin, A. B. (1934). *Br. J. Exp. Pathol.* **15**, 248–268.
Sabine, M., Robertson, G. R., and Whalley, J. M. (1981). *Aust. Vet. J.* **57**, 148–149.
Sabo, A. (1969). *Acta Virol. (Engl. Ed.)* **13**, 269–277.
Sabo, A., and Blaskovic, D. (1970). *Acta Virol. (Engl. Ed.)* **14**, 7–14.
Sabo, A., and Grunert, Z. (1971). *Acta Virol. (Engl. Ed.)* **15**, 87–94.
Sabo, A., and Rajcani J. (1976). *Acta Virol. (Engl. Ed.)* **20**, 208–214.
Sabo, A., Rajcani, J., and Blaskovic, D. (1969). *Acta Virol. (Engl. Ed.)* **13**, 407–414.
Sabo, A., Golais, F., and Grunert, Z. (1979). *Zentralbl. Veterinaermed.* **26**, 336–339.
Saunders, J. R., Gustafson, D. P., Olander, H. J. (1963). *Proc. Annu. Meet. U.S. Anim. Health Assoc. 67th*, 331–346.
Saxegaard, F. (1966). *Nord. Veterinaermed.* **18**, 504–512.
Scherba, G., Gustafson, D. P., Kanitz, C. L., and Sun, I. L. (1978). *J. Am. Vet. Med. Assoc.* **173**, 1490–1493.
Scott, J. C., Dutta, S. K., and Myrup, A. C. (1983). *Am. J. Vet. Res.* **44**, 1344–1348.
Sellers, A. F., Pomeroy, B. S., Sautter, J. H., Pint, L. H., and Schrafel, C. E. (1949). *J. Am. Vet. Med. Assoc.* **114**, 69–73.
Sharma, J. M., Burger, D., and Kenzy, S. G. (1972). *Infect. Immun.* **5**, 406–411.
Sheffy, B. E., and Rodman, S. (1973). *J. Am. Vet. Med. Assoc.* **163**, 850–851.
Shell, L. G., Ely, R. W., and Crandell, R. A. (1981). *J. Am. Vet. Med. Assoc.* **178**, 1159–1161.
Shope, R. E. (1931). *J. Exp. Med.* **54**, 233–248.
Shope, R. E. (1935). *J. Exp. Med.* **62**, 85–99.
Silva, R. A. da., and Giovine, N. (1966). *Pesqui. Agropecu. Bras.* **1**, 73–74.
Skoda, R., Brauner, I., Sadecky, E., and Mayer, V. (1964). *Acta Virol. (Engl. Ed.)* **8**, 1–9.
Skoda, R., Ivanicova, S. T., Jamrichova, O., and Sliepka, M. (1968). *Arch. Exp. Veterinaermed.* **22**, 925–926.
Smith, I. M., Girard, A., Corner, A. H., and Mitchell, D. (1972). *Can. J. Comp. Med.* **36**, 303–308.
Smith, P. C. (1977). *Proc. Annu. Meet. U.S. Anim. Health Assoc. 80th*, 149–157.
Smith, P. C. (1979). *Proc. Annu. Meet. U.S. Anim. Health Assoc. 83rd*, 432–443.
Smith, P. C., and Mengeling, W. L. (1977). *Can. J. Comp. Med.* **41**, 364–368.
Smith, P. C., and Stewart, W. C. (1978). *J. Clin. Microbiol.* **7**, 423–425.

Snyder, M. L., and Erickson, G. A. (1981). "Recommended Minimum Standards for Enzyme-linked Immunosorbent Assay (ELISA) in Pseudorabies Serodiagnosis," pp. 1–32. USDA, NVSL Publication.
Snyder, M. L., and Stewart, W. C. (1977). *Proc. Am. Assoc. Vet. Lab. Diagnost.* **20,** 17–32.
Southern, E. M. (1975). *J. Mol. Biol.* **98,** 503–517.
Stewart, W. C., Carbrey, E. A., and Kresse, J. I. (1967). *J. Am. Vet. Med. Assoc.* **151,** 747–751.
Stewart, W. C., Swanson, M. R., Snyder, M. L., and Kresse, J. I. (1978). *Proc. Am. Assoc. Vet. Lab. Diagn.* **21,** 43–51.
Studdert, M. J. (1974). *Cornell Vet.* **64,** 94–122.
Studdert, M. J. (1983). *Arch. Virol.* **77,** 249–258.
Studdert, M. J., and Blackney, M. H. (1979). *Aust. Vet. J.* **55,** 488–492.
Studdert, M. J., Simpson, T., and Roizman, B. (1981). *Science* **214,** 562–564.
Thawley, D. G., Gustafson, D. P., and Beran, G. W. (1982). *J. Am. Vet. Med. Assoc.* **181,** 1513–1518.
Thiry, E., Pastoret, P. P., Brochier, B., Kettmann, R., and Burney, A. (1983). *Ann. Med. Vet.* **127,** 29–36.
Thomson, G. R., Mumford, J. A., Campbell, J., Griffiths, L., and Clapham, P. (1976). *Equine Vet. J.* **8,** 58–65.
Thomson, G. W., McCready, R., Sanford, E., and Gagnon, A. (1979). *Can. Vet. J.* **20,** 22–25.
Toma, B., and Gilet, J. (1978). *Recl. Med. Vet.* **154,** 425–429.
Toneva, V. (1975). *Bull Off. Int. Epizoot.* **84,** 307–314.
Tozzini, F. (1982a). *In* "Aujeszky's Disease" (G. Wittmann and S. A. Hall, eds.), pp. 31–36. Nijhoff, The Hague.
Tozzini, F. (1982b). *In* "Aujeszky's Disease" (G. Wittmann and S. A. Hall, eds.), pp. 267–269. Nijhoff, The Hague.
Tuncman, Z. M. (1938). *Ann. Inst. Pasteur, Paris* **60,** 95–98.
Turner, A. J., Studdert, M. J., and Peterson, J. E. (1970). *Aust. Vet. J.* **46,** 90–98.
Turtinen, L. W., Allen, G. P., Darlington, R. W., and Bryans, J. T. (1981). *Am. J. Vet. Res.* **42,** 2099–2104.
Van Alstine, W. G., Anderson, T. D., Reed, D. E., and Wheeler, J. G. (1984). *J. Am. Vet. Med. Assoc.* **185,** 409–410.
Van Oirschot, J. T. (1984). *In* "Latent Herpes Virus Infections in Veterinary Medicine" (G. Wittmann, R. M. Gaskell, and H. J. Rziha, eds.), pp. 417–427. Nijhoff, The Hague.
Van Oirschot, J. T., and Gielkens, A. L. J. (1984). *Am. J. Vet. Res.* **45,** 567–571.
Veijalainen, P., Schulman, A., EK-Kommonen, C., and Neuvonen, E. (1982). *Nord Veterinaermed* **34,** 133–135.
Westerfield, C., and Dimock, W. W. (1946). *J. Am. Vet. Med. Assoc.* **109,** 101–111.
Whitley, R. D., and Nelson, S. L. (1980). *J. Am. Anim. Hosp. Assoc.* **16,** 69–72.
Williams, P. P., Pirtle, E. C., and Coria, M. F. (1982). *Can. J. Comp. Med.* **46,** 65–69.
Wittmann, G., Jakubik, J., and Ahl, R. (1980). *Arch. Virol.* **66,** 227–240.
Wittmann, G., Hahn, V., Weiland, F., and Bohrn, H. O. (1982). *In* "Aujeszky's Disease" (G. Wittmann and S. A. Hall, eds.), pp. 117–122. Nijhoff, The Hague.
Wittmann, G., Ohlinger, V., and Rziha, H. J. (1983). *Arch. Virol.* **75,** 29–41.
Wittmann, G., Ohlinger, V., and Rziha, H. J. (1984). *In* "Latent Herpes Virus Infections in Veterinary Medicine" (G. Wittmann, R. M. Gaskell, and H. J. Rziha, eds.), pp. 445–455. Nijhoff, The Hague.
Wohlgemuth, K., Leslie, P. F., Reed, D. E., and Smidt, D. K. (1978). *J. Am Vet. Med. Assoc.* **172,** 478–479.

Wright, J. C., and Thawley, D. G. (1980). *Am. J. Vet. Res.* **41,** 581–583.
Yotov, M. (1973). *Vet. Med. Nauki* **10,** 73–78.
Yurov, K. P., and Sologub, V. K. (1978). *In* "Equine Infectious Diseases IV" (J. T. Bryans and H. Gerber, eds.), pp. 43–48. Veterinary Publications, Princeton, New Jersey.
Zuffa, A., Matis, J., and Pleva, V. (1968). *Arch. Gesamte Virusforsch.* **24,** 396–405.

Index

A

Abortion
  equine herpesvirus 1 and, 283–284, 285, 289, 291, 293
  pseudorabies and, 297, 298
Acetohydroxamic acid, canine struvite urolithiasis and, 73–75, 79, 88
Acidification, therapy of canine struvite urolithiasis and, 82–86
Acquired immunodeficiency syndrome, cryptosporidiosis and, 160, 163–164
Adenovirus enteritis, in piglets, 185
Adhesins
  gastrointestinal microorganisms and, 208–209
  miscellaneous, 225–226
Aeromonas hydrophila, diarrhea in foals and, 192
Age, atrophic rhinitis in swine and, 260, 261
Alkalinity, of urine
  struvite uroliths and, 45
  urolith stoichiometry and, 35–36
Ammonia, in urine, 35–36, 75
Ammonium acid urate, 4, 9
  in canine uroliths, 16
  in feline uroliths, 15
Ampicillin, urolithiasis and, 79
Anaerobes, metabolic products of, 208
Animals, cryptosporidiosis in, 159–160
Antibiotics, atrophic rhinitis in swine and, 268
Antibodies, monoclonal, prevention ETEC diarrhea and, 147
Antigenic diversity, of rotaviruses, 108–109
Antigenic relatedness, of pseudorabies virus, 300–301
Antigenic variations, of rotaviruses, 114–115
  host response to, 115–116
Antigen(s)
  adhesive, of *E. coli,* 128
  of atypical rotaviruses, 117
Atrophic rhinitis in swine
  clinical and pathological features
    clinical signs, 244–245
    pathological changes, 245–246
  control of
    environment and management, 267
    eradication, 266–267
    medication, 267–268
    monitoring, 267
  diagnosis
    clinical, 262
    cultural, 263–265
    pathological, 262–263
    value of cultural and serological tests, 265–266
  epidemiology of, 259–262
  etiology
    environment and management, 248–249
    heredity, 246–247
    infection, 247–248
    nutrition, 247
  historical background, 240–241
  immunity and vaccination and, 268–269
    B. bronchiseptica, 269–271
    P. multocida, 271–274
  occurrence and importance, 242
    economic significance, 243
  pathogenesis
    Bordetella bronchoseptica, 249–254
    Pasteurella multocida, 254–259
Attachment
  and colonization
    by *B. bronchiseptica,* 249–251
    by *P. multocida,* 254–255
Aujeszky's disease, *see* Pseudorabies

INDEX

B

Bacteria, cell surface of
  capsule, 210–211
  fimbriae, 212–226
  lipopolysaccharide, 211–212
Bacterial infection, struvite uroliths and, 28–29, 31, 33
  experimental and clinical observations, 37–41
  overview, 34–35
  stoichiometry, 35–37
Bacteriocins, secretion of, 208
Bacteriophage, ETEC diarrhea and, 146–147
Biological behavior, of struvite uroliths
  in cats, 56
  in dogs, 54–56
  in humans, 57
  overview, 52
  recurrence, 52, 54
Biology, of equine herpesviruses, 286–287
Bone, changes, atrophic rhinitis in swine and, 245–246, 253, 257
Bordetella bronchiseptica atrophic rhinitis in swine and, 240–241, 242, 243, 244, 246, 247, 248, 254–255
  attachment and colonization, 249–251
  culture of, 263
  epidemiology and, 259–261
  immunity and vaccination and, 269–271
  lesions, 253–254
  production of toxins, 251–253
Breda/Berne virus, and other enteric viruses, calf diarrhea and, 178–179
Brush border, cryptosporidiosis and, 159–160
Brush border adhesion test, for *E. coli* antigens, 129–130
Brushite, 4

C

Calcium hydrogen phosphate, 4
  in canine uroliths, 16
Calcium hydrogen phosphate dihydrate, in feline uroliths, 15
Calcium oxalate dihydrate, 4
  in canine uroliths, 16
  in feline uroliths, 15
  shapes of crystals, 5
Calcium oxalate monohydrate, 4, 9
  in canine uroliths, 16
  in feline uroliths, 15
  shapes of crystals, 5
Calcium phosphate, 4, 9
  in canine uroliths, 16
  in feline uroliths, 15
Calf diarrhea
  epidemiology, 172–175
  infections specific to calves, 175–179
Calves
  E. coli infection in, 220, 223
  prevention of ETEC diarrhea in, 143–144
  rotavirus serotypes of, 111–112
  vaccination against rotavirus, 120–121
Campylobacter, calf diarrhea and, 176–178
Capsule, bacterial, 210–211
Carbohydrate, dietary, postweaning diarrhea and, 154
Carbonate apatite, 4
Carriers, atrophic rhinitis in swine and, 259
Cats
  biological behavior of uroliths in, 56
  clinical signs of pseudorabies in, 299–300
  medical management of struvite urolithiasis in
    clinical studies of sterile struvite, 89–93
    infected struvite, 93
    overview, 88
    prevention of recurrence, 93
  struvite uroliths in
    common characteristics of, 29, 30
    composition of matrix concretions, 33
  urethral plugs in
    characteristics of, 34
    gross appearance, 46
    males versus females, 48–49
    matrix composition, 48
    microscopic appearance, 46–47

mineral composition, 47–48
radiographic appearance, 46
uroliths
   composition of, 15, 49–50
   gross appearance, 49
   microscopic appearance, 49
   radiographic appearance, 49
Cattle, clinical signs of
   pseudorabies in, 298–299
   pathogenesis, 309–311
Cell cultures, propagation of *Cryptosporidium* in, 166
Cell surface
   bacterial
      capsule, 210–211
      fimbriae, 212–226
      lipopolysaccharide, 211–212
   of gastrointestinal epithelium, 226–228
Chemotherapeutic agents
   ineffective against crytosporidiosis, 167
   treatment of coccidiosis and, 184
Citrate, uroliths and, 22–23, 37
Clinical signs
   of atrophic rhinitis in swine, 244–245
   of equine rhinopneumonitis, 284–285
   of pseudorabies
      cattle, 298–299
      cats, 299–300
      dogs, 299–300
      goats, 298
      horses, 300
      pigs, 296–298
      sheep, 298
Clostridium perfringens type C, 176
   characteristics of disease, 168–169
   characteristics of organism, 169–170
   control of, 171–172
   diagnosis, 171
   in diarrhea in foals, 189–190
   mechanisms of diarrhea, 170–171
   prevalence in piglet enteritis, 179–180, 183
Coccidia, piglet enteritis and, 180, 181, 182, 183–184
Colostrum
   antibodies to *B. bronchiseptica* in, 269, 270
   ETEC antibodies in, 138, 144, 219, 221–222
   rotavirus antibodies in, 121–123, 182

Control
   of equine rhinopneumonitis, 294–295
   of necrotizing enteritis, 171–172
Coronavirus, prevalence in calf diarrhea, 172, 173, 174
Corticosteroids, latent pseudovirus infection and, 312–313
Corynebacterium, struvite uroliths and, 44
Cryptosporidiasis
   in animals, 159–160
   control of, 166–168
   diagnosis of *Cryptosporidium* infection, 164–165
   human, 160–164
   new advances in laboratory studies, 165–166
Cryptosporidium
   life cycle of, 159
   prevalence in calf diarrhea, 172, 173, 174
Crystallization-inhibition theory, of urolith formation, 22–23
Crystalloids, increased renal excretion of, 20
Crystalluria
   diagnosis of urolithiasis and, 59–61
   uroliths and, 2–3
Crystals, urinary, characteristics of, 59, 60
Crystal aggregation, urolith growth and, 25–26
Crystal growth, of uroliths, 24
Cultivation, *in vitro,* of rotavirus, 106–107
Cyclic adenosine monophosphate, diarrhea and, 132, 209
Cystine, 4
   in canine uroliths, 16

D

Dams, vaccination against rotavirus, 121–124
Deoxyribonucleic acid
   of equine herpesviruses, analysis of, 287–289

of pseudorabies virus, analysis of, 302–305
Diagnosis
  of *Cryptosporidium* infection, 164–165
  of equine rhinopneumonitis, 293–294
  of ETEC infection, 229–230
  of necrotizing enteritis, 171
  of pseudorabies virus infection, 314–316
  of struvite urolithiasis
    analysis of uroliths, 63–66
    crystalluria, 59–61
    overview, 57–58
    radiographic characteristics, 62–63
    urolith culture, 66–67
Diarrhea
  atypical rotaviruses and, 117
  cryptosporidiosis and, 161
    in immunologically compromised individuals, 163–164
  enterotoxigenic *E. coli* and
    development of vaccine, 137–145
    other methods of control, 145–148
  mechanisms of, *Clostridium perfringens* and, 170–171
Diet(s)
  calculolytic, canine struvite urolithiasis and, 77–81
  necrotizing enteritis and, 170
  struvite uroliths and
    infection stones, 42
    sterile stone, 42–45
Diseases, caused by *Clostridium perfringens* type C, 168–169
Diuresis, therapy of canine struvite urolithiasis and, 81–82
Dog
  biological behavior of uroliths in, 54–56
  clinical signs of pseudorabies in, 299–300
  medical management of struvite urolithiasis in
    acidification, 82, 86
    calculytic diets, 77–81
    control of urinary tract infections, 71
    diuresis, 81–82
    monitoring response to therapy, 86–87
    overview, 71

prevention of recurrence, 87–88
urease inhibitors, 73–77
struvite uroliths
  common characteristics of, 29, 30
  composition of matrix concretions, 33
uroliths, composition of, 16

E

Economic significance, of atrophic rhinitis in swine, 243
Embryonated eggs, propagation of *Cryptosporidium in*, 165
Energy level, dietary, postweaning diarrhea and, 155
Enterotoxin
  attachment of *E. coli* to mucosa and, 131
  E. coli pathogenic mechanisms and, 131
  heat-labile toxin, 132–133
  heat-stable toxin, 133–136
  fimbriae and, 218, 221, 224
  forms of, 209
Environment, atrophic rhinitis in swine and, 248–249, 267
Epidemiology
  of atrophic rhinitis in swine, 259–262
  of calf diarrhea, 172–175
  of piglet enteritis, 179–183
Epitaxial growth, of uroliths, 24–25
Epithelial cells, of gastrointestinal tract, surface of, 226–228
Epizootiologic features
  of equine rhinopneumonitis
    host range, 289–290
    latent and persistent infections, 292–293
    pathogenesis, 289–290
    virus strain differences, 286–289
  of pseudorabies
    host range, 305–308
    latent and persistent infections, 311–314
    pathogenesis, 308–311
    strain differences, 301–305
    virus, 300–301

Equine rhinopneumonitis
  clinical signs, 284–285
  diagnosis, 293–294
  epizootiologic features, 285–293
  introduction and history, 283–284
  prevention and control, 294–295
Eradication, of atrophic rhinitis in swine, 266–267
Escherichia coli
  enterotoxigenic, 125–126
    control of diarrhea, 137–148
    pathogenic mechanisms, 126–137
    postweaning diarrhea, 148–158
    prevalence in calf diarrhea, 172, 173, 174
    prevalence in piglet enteritis, 179–182
  Streptococcus durans infections in foals and, 188–189
Etiology, of atrophic rhinitis in swine
  environment and management, 248–249
  heredity, 246–247
  infection, 247–248
  nutrition, 247
Etiopathogenesis, of uroliths
  initiation and growth, 19–26
  overview, 18–19
  summary of formation, 27

F

Fat, dietary, postweaning diarrhea and, 155
Feces, detection of *Cryptosporidium* oocysts in, 164–165
Feeding methods, postweaning diarrhea and, 155–158
Fetus, equine herpesvirus infection in, 294
Fiber, dietary, postweaning diarrhea and, 154–155
Fimbriae, *see also* Pili
  bacterial cell surface and, 212
    CFA, 223–225
    F41, 223
    K88, 216–220
    K99, 220–222
    miscellaneous adhesins, 225–226
    type 1 or common, 213–216
    987P, 222–223
  in *B. bronchiseptica*, 250–251
  in clinical settings, 228–231
  E. coli mucosal attachment and, 126–127
Fluid, piglet weaner diet and, 156–157
Fluorofamide, as urease inhibitor, 77
Foals
  diarrhea in
    Clostridium perfringens type C, 189–190
    other enteropathogens, 191–192
    rotavirus, 186–188
    Streptococcus durans, 188–189
  rotavirus serotypes of, 112, 114

G

Ganglioside, *E. coli* heat-labile toxin and, 132
Gastrointestinal tract
  as ecosystem, 207–209
  epithelial cells, surface of, 226–228
Gene coding assignment, of rotaviruses, 107–108
Genetic diversity, of rotaviruses, 108–109
Genetic engineering, ETEC pilus vaccines and, 140–141
Genetics, struvite urolithiasis and, 45–46
Glycoproteins, adhesins and, 227
Glycosaminoglycans, matrix composition and, 33
Goats, clinical signs of pseudorabies in, 299
Group A rotaviruses, 109–110
  bovine, 111–112
  equine, 112–114
  host response to antigenic variation, 115–116
  minor antigenic variations, 114–115
  porcine, 110
Growth, of uroliths
  crystal aggregation and, 25–26
  crystal growth and, 24

INDEX

epitaxial growth, 24–25
growth versus time, 26–27
Guanite, 4

H

Heat-labile toxin, of *E. coli*
  characteristics of, 132
  detection of, 132–133
Heat-stable toxin, of *E. coli*
  characteristics of, 133–134
  detection of, 134–135
Hemagglutination, fimbriae and, 212, 214, 221, 223, 224
Heparin, uroliths and, 14–15
Heredity, atrophic rhinitis in swine and, 246–247
Herpesviridae, provisional designation and classification of, 282
Horses, clinical signs of pseudorabies in, 300
Host range
  of equine rhinopneumonitis virus, 289–290
  of pseudorabies virus, 305–308
Host response, to antigenic variations in rotaviruses, 115–116
Host specificity, of *Cryptosporidium*, 159–160
Human
  biological behavior of uroliths in, 57
  Campylobacter infections in, 177
  Clostridium perfringens infection in, 169
  cryptosporidiosis in
    immunologically compromised individuals, 163–164
    immunologically normal humans, 160–163
  enterotoxigenic strains of *E. coli* and, 137, 223–224
  rotavirus vaccines and, 124
  struvite uroliths
    common characteristics of, 29, 30
    composition of matrix concretions, 33
Hydrophilicity, of bacterial capsules, 210
Hydrophobicity
  CFA fimbriae and, 224
  K88 fimbriae and, 218
Hydroxyapatite, 4

I

Immunity
  epidemiology of *B. bronchiseptica* and, 260
  to pseudorabies virus, 308
Immunofluorescence, demonstration of ETEC and, 129
Indications, for medical management of urolithiasis, 67–68
Infections
  atrophic rhinitis in swine and, 247–248
  latent and persistent
    equine herpesvirus and, 292–293
    pseudorabies virus and, 308–309, 311–314
Inhibitors, of crystallization, in urine, 22–23
Initiation, of uroliths, 19–20
  crystallization-inhibition theory, 22–23
  matrix-nucleation theory, 21–22
  precipitation-crystallization theory, 20–21
  summary, 23–24
Isospora suis, piglet enteritis and, 183–184

K

Kidney, *P. multocida* toxin and, 258

L

Laboratory animals, pseudorabies virus and, 306
Laboratory studies, of *Cryptosporidium*, new advances in, 165–166
Lactic acid-producing bacteria, protection against ETEC and, 146

Lambs, *E. coli* infection in, 220
Laminations, of uroliths, 17–18
Lectins, bacterial capsules and, 211
Lesions
  B. bronchiseptica and, 253–254
  P. multocida and, 257–259
Leukocytes, equine herpesvirus and, 290–291, 292
Lipopolysaccharide, bacterial cell surface and, 211–212
Liver, *P. multocida* toxin and, 258

M

Mad itch, *see* Pseudorabies
Magnesium
  calculogenesis and, 23
  dietary, uroliths and, 43
Magnesium ammonium phosphate hexahydrate
  in canine uroliths, 16
  in feline uroliths, 15
  uroliths and, 3–4, 9
Magnesium hydrogen phosphate trihydrate, 4
  in canine uroliths, 16
Mannose
  epithelial cells and, 226–227
  hemagglutination and, 212, 214
Matrix composition
  of concretions, 14–15
  of feline urethral plugs, 48
  of uroliths, 10–14
  of struvite uroliths, 30–33
Matrix concretions
  of struvite uroliths
    in cats, 33–34
    in man and dogs, 33
  uroliths and
    occurrence of, 14
Matrix-nucleation theory, of urolith formation, 21–22
Matrix substance A, uroliths and, 21
Medical management, of struvite urolithiasis
  in canines, 71–88
  definition of urolith composition, 69
  in felines, 88–93

  increased urine volume, 69
  indications, 67–68
  objectives, 68–69
  overview, 67
Medication, atrophic rhinitis in swine and, 267–268
Methionine, therapy of sterile struvite and, 89
Mice, isolation of *P. multocida* and, 264
Mineral composition
  of feline urethral plugs, 47–48
  of struvite uroliths, 27–30
  of uroliths, 7–10
Monitoring, of atrophic rhinitis in swine, 267
Mucosa, attachment of *E. coli* to, 126–131
Mucus, attachment of *E. coli* and, 130

N

Necrotizing enteritis, *see Clostridium perfringens*
Neurotropism, of pseudorabies virus, 309, 310, 311, 312–313
Newberyite, 4
Nuclei, in uroliths, 15–18
Nutrition
  atrophic rhinitis in swine and, 247
  postweaning diarrhea and, 152
    carbohydrates, 154
    energy level, 155
    fat, 155
    feeding methods, 155–158
    fiber, 154–155
    protein, 153–154

O

Objectives, of medical management of urolithiasis, 68–69
Oncogenesis, equine herpesvirus and, 292
Opsonization, fimbriae and, 215

P

Pararotaviruses, significance of, 116–117
Pasteurella multocida
  atrophic rhinitis in swine and, 241, 242, 243, 244, 246, 247, 248, 252, 266–267
  attachment and colonization, 254–255
  culture of, 263–264
  epidemiology and, 259–262
  immunity and vaccination and, 271–274
  lesions, 257–259
  production of toxins, 255–257
  Pathogenesis
    of equine herpesvirus, 290–292
    of pseudorabies virus
      in cattle, 309–311
      in pigs, 308–309
      in sheep, 311
Pathogens, selective adsorption of, 209
Pathogenesis, type K88 fimbriae and, 218–219
Pathogenic mechanisms, of enterotoxogenic *E. coli*
  attachment to mucosa, 126–131
  enterotoxin production, 131–136
  serogroup and, 136–137
Pathological signs, of atrophic rhinitis in swine, 245–246
Peptides, synthetic, rotavirus vaccines and, 125
pH, urinary, urolith formation and, 20, 43
Phagocytosis, fimbriae and, 215
Phase variation, in *B. bronchiseptica*, 249–251, 252
Piglets
  E. coli infection in, 219, 222
  prevention of ETEC diarrhea in, 137–143
  rotavirus serotypes of, 110
Piglet enteritis
  epidemiology, 179–183
  infections specific to piglets, 183–185
Pig(s), clinical signs of
  pathogenesis, 308–309
  pseudorabies in 296–298
Pili, *see also* Fimbriae
  E. coli attachment to mucosa and, 127–128
  ETEC vaccines and, 140–143

Plasmids
  E. coli virulence and, 126–127, 138
  type K88 fimbriae and, 217, 219
  type K99 fimbriae and, 220
  type CFA fimbriae and, 224
Pneumonia
  atrophic rhinitis and, 259
  causes in swine, 244
Polysaccharide, capsular, *E. coli* colonization of small intestine and, 128
Porcine cytomegalovirus, *B. bronchiseptica* infection and, 253
Porcine epidemic diarrhea virus, epidemiology of, 185
Postweaning diarrhea
  influence of nutritional factors, 152–158
  prevention of, 147–148
  weaning and infection and, 149–152
Precipitation-crystallization theory, of urolith formation, 20–21
Prevention
  of equine rhinopneumonitis, 294–295
  of pseudorabies virus infection, 316–318
Protein
  dietary
    infection-induced struvite uroliths and, 42
    postweaning diarrhea and, 153
Proteus, struvite urolith formation and, 37, 38, 39
Pseudorabies
  clinical signs, 296–300
  diagnosis, 314–316
  epizootiologic features, 300–314
  introduction and history, 295–296
  prevention and control, 316–318
  reasons for epidemics, 296
  vaccines, 318–319
Pyrophosphates, calculogenesis and, 23

R

Rabbit, *E. coli* from, 225–226
Racoons, pseudorabies virus and, 307–308
Radiography, diagnosis of urolithiasis and, 62–63

Raffinose, type K88 fimbriae and, 217
Rats, pseudorabies virus and, 306–307
Reassortment, cultivation of rotaviruses and, 106–107
Receptors
  on epithelial cell surface, fimbriae and, 226–228
  on gastrointestinal epithelial cells, 208
  for K88 *E. coli,* 130, 131
Recombinant DNA, immunoassays of ETEC and, 129
Recurrence, of uroliths, 52, 54
  prevention of, 87–88, 93
Reoviridae, rotavirus and, 105
Resistance, to ETEC, selection for, 145–146
Restriction endonuclease
  equine herpesvirus DNA and, 287–288
  pseudorabies virus DNA and, 303–305
Rotavirus
  characteristics of, 105–106
  development of vaccine, 119–125
  gene coding assignment, 107–108
  genetic and antigenic diversity, 108–109
  group A rotaviruses, 109–116
  other rotavirus groups, 116–119
  postweaning diarrhea and, 150–152
  prevalence
    in calf diarrhea, 172, 173, 174
    in diarrhea in foals, 186–188
    in piglet enteritis, 180–182
  in vitro cultivation, 106–107
Rotavirus strains, recognized as distinct serotypes among human and animal strains, 113
Ruminants, struvite uroliths in, diet and, 44

S

Salmonella
  adhesins of, 225
  and other enteric bacteria
    calf diarrhea and, 176
    in foals, 191
Serogroup, enterotoxigenicity of *E. coli* and, 136–137
Serological tests
  for *B. bronchiseptica,* 264–265

for *P. multocida,* 265
for pseudorabies virus, 314–316
Serology
  of atypical rotaviruses, 118–119
  equine herpesvirus and, 293–294
Serotyping, lipopolysaccharide and, 211
Sheep, clinical signs of
  pseudorabies in, 299
  pathogenesis, 311
Silicon dioxide, 4
  in canine uroliths, 16
  shapes of uroliths, 5
Sneezing, atrophic rhinitis in swine and, 244
Snout deformation, atrophic rhinitis in swine and, 244, 245
Sodium acid urate monohydrate, 4
  in canine uroliths, 16
Staphylococcus, struvite urolith formation and, 37, 38, 39, 40, 55, 75
Stilbestrol, urolith formation and, 44
Stoichiometry, of struvite uroliths, bacterial urinary tract infections and, 35–37
Strain differences, in pseudorabies virus
  biologic, 301–302
  DNA analysis, 302–305
Streptococcus durans, diarrhea in foals and, 188–189
Streptococcus faecium, ETEC diarrhea and, 146, 188, 231
Struvite, composition of, 3
Struvite urolithiasis
  alkaline urine and, 45
  bacterial urinary tract infections, 34–41
  biological behavior of, 52–57
  composition of matrix concretions, 33–34
  diagnosis, 57–67
  diet, 42–45
  feline urethral plugs versus feline struvite uroliths, 46–51
  genetics, 45–46
  matrix composition, 30–33
  medical management of, 67–93
  medical versus surgical management of, 93–94
  mineral composition, 27–30
  ureaplasma urinary tract infection, 41–42
Struvite uroliths

infected, treatment in cats, 93
sterile, clinical studies in cats, 89–93
Surgery
versus medical management, 93–94
removal of uroliths and, 54, 67–68
Symptoms, of cryptosporidiosis, in normal humans, 161

T

Tamm-Horsfall mucoprotein, urolith matrix and, 13, 22
Tetracyclines, atrophic rhinitis in swine and, 268
Therapy, of canine struvite urolithiasis, monitoring response to, 86–87
Thyroid hormone, receptors for adhesins and, 228
Time, growth of uroliths and, 26
Toxin
Campylobacter and, 177–178
lipopolysaccharide and, 211, 212
Pasteurella multocida and, 248, 255–257
production by *B. bronchiseptica,* 251–253
released by *Clostridium perfringens,* 169–170
demonstration of, 171
Trace elements, in uroliths, 9
β-Tricalcium phosphate, 4
Trypsin, *in vitro* cultivation of rotaviruses and, 106
Turbinate atrophy, atrophic rhinitis in swine and, 244, 245, 253, 257, 262–263
Type CFA fimbriae, characteristic of, 224
Type F41 fimbriae, characteristic of, 223
Type K88 fimbriae, characteristic of, 217
genes for, 217
Type K99 fimbriae, characteristics of, 220
Type 1 (common) fimbriae, characteristics of, 213–214
Type 987P fimbriae, characteristics of, 222

U

Ureaplasma, urinary tract infections, struvite uroliths and, 41–42
Urease inhibitors, canine struvite urolithiasis and, 73–77
urolith formation and, 35–36, 38–39
Urethral plugs, in felines, characteristics of, 34
Uric acid, 4, 9
in canine uroliths, 16
in feline uroliths, 15
Uric acid dihydrate, 4
Urinary tract infections, complicated
classification of identifiable causes of, 53–54
eradication or control of, 71
Urine
flora, struvite uroliths and, 40
increasing volume, treatment of urolithiasis and, 69
Urolithiasis, terminology and, 3
Uroliths
analysis of, 63–66
chemical and physical characteristics of
matrix composition, 10–15
mineral composition, 7–10
nuclei and laminations, 15–18
overview, 6–7
crystalluria and, 2–3
culture of, 66–67
definition of composition, 69, 70
etiopathogenesis of
initiation and growth, 19–26
overview, 18–19
summary of formation, 27
matrix composition, 10–14
names of, 3–6
shapes of, 5–6
terminology and
names of uroliths, 3–6
urolithiasis, 3
uroliths and crystalluria, 2–3

V

Vaccines
for control of ETEC diarrhea, 137–138, 230

factors affecting vaccine efficiency, 144–145
genetically engineered pilus vaccines, 140–143
prevention of diarrhea in calves, 143–144
purified bacterial components and, 138–140
whole cell vaccines, 138–139
pseudorabies and, 316, 317, 318–319
against rotavirus, 119–120
calves and, 120–121
dams and, 121–124
future vaccines, 124–125
humans and, 124
Vectors, of *B. bronchiseptica,* 260
Viremia
equine herpesvirus and, 290–291
pseudorabies virus and, 308
Virus
of equine rhinopneumonitis, strain differences in, 286–289
of pseudorabies, antigenic relatedness, 300–301

W

Water balance, urolith formation and, 20
Weaning, recommended feeding methods, 158
Weddellite, 4
Whewellite, 4
Whitlockite, 4
Whole cells, *E. coli* vaccines and, 138–139
Wildlife, pseudorabies virus and, 306–308

X

Xanthine, 4